DECENTERING EPISTEMOLOGIES AND CHALLENGING PRIVILEGE

CAREWORK IN A CHANGING WORLD
Amy Armenia, Mignon Duffy, and Kim Price-Glynn, Series Editors

The rise of scholarly attention to care has accompanied greater public concern about aging, health care, child care, and labor in a global world. Research on care is happening across disciplines—in sociology, economics, political science, philosophy, public health, social work, and others—with numerous research networks and conferences developing to showcase this work. Care scholarship brings into focus some of the most pressing social problems facing families today. To study care is also to study the future of work, as issues of carework are intertwined with the forces of globalization, technological development, and the changing dynamics of the labor force. Care scholarship is also at the cutting edge of intersectional analyses of inequality, as carework is often at the very core of understanding gender, race, migration, age, disability, class, and international inequalities.

Sophie Bourgault, Maggie FitzGerald, and Fiona Robinson, eds., *Decentering Epistemologies and Challenging Privilege: Critical Care Ethics Perspectives*

Mignon Duffy, Amy Armenia, and Kim Price-Glynn, eds., *From Crisis to Catastrophe: Care, COVID, and Pathways to Change*

Fumilayo Showers, *Migrants Who Care: West Africans Working and Building Lives in U.S. Health Care*

DECENTERING EPISTEMOLOGIES AND CHALLENGING PRIVILEGE

Critical Care Ethics Perspectives

EDITED BY
SOPHIE BOURGAULT, MAGGIE FITZGERALD,
AND FIONA ROBINSON

RUTGERS UNIVERSITY PRESS
New Brunswick, Camden, and Newark, New Jersey
London and Oxford

Rutgers University Press is a department of Rutgers, The State University of New Jersey, one of the leading public research universities in the nation. By publishing worldwide, it furthers the University's mission of dedication to excellence in teaching, scholarship, research, and clinical care.

Library of Congress Cataloging-in-Publication Data

Names: Bourgault, Sophie, editor. | FitzGerald, Maggie, 1990– editor. | Robinson, Fiona, editor.
Title: Decentering epistemologies and challenging privilege : critical care ethics perspectives / edited by Sophie Bourgault, Maggie FitzGerald and Fiona Robinson.
Description: New Brunswick : Rutgers University Press, [2024] | Series: Carework in a changing world | Includes bibliographical references and index.
Identifiers: LCCN 2023049488 | ISBN 9781978835030 (hardcover) | ISBN 9781978835023 (paperback) | ISBN 9781978835047 (epub) | ISBN 9781978835061 (pdf)
Subjects: LCSH: Caring. | Privilege (Social psychology) | Feminist ethics. | Knowledge, Theory of.
Classification: LCC BJ1475 D43 2024 | DDC 177/.7—dc23/eng/20240528
LC record available at https://lccn.loc.gov/2023049488

A British Cataloging-in-Publication record for this book is available from the British Library.

This collection copyright © 2024 by Rutgers, The State University of New Jersey
Individual chapters copyright © 2024 in the names of their authors
All rights reserved

No part of this book may be reproduced or utilized in any form or by any means, electronic or mechanical, or by any information storage and retrieval system, without written permission from the publisher. Please contact Rutgers University Press, 106 Somerset Street, New Brunswick, NJ 08901. The only exception to this prohibition is "fair use" as defined by U.S. copyright law.

References to internet websites (URLs) were accurate at the time of writing. Neither the author nor Rutgers University Press is responsible for URLs that may have expired or changed since the manuscript was prepared.

∞ The paper used in this publication meets the requirements of the American National Standard for Information Sciences—Permanence of Paper for Printed Library Materials, ANSI Z39.48-1992.

rutgersuniversitypress.org

CONTENTS

	Introduction SOPHIE BOURGAULT, MAGGIE FITZGERALD, AND FIONA ROBINSON	1
1	Indigenous Voices and Relationships: Insights from Care Ethics and Accounts of Hermeneutical Injustice CHRISTINE KOGGEL	15
2	Epistemic Injustice, Face-to-Face Encounters, and Caring Institutions SOPHIE BOURGAULT	31
3	Privilege and the Denial of Vulnerability: When Care Ethics Meets Epistemologies of Ignorance MARIE GARRAU	47
4	Learning through Care: Decentering an Epistemology of Domination to Theorize Caring Men at the "Center" RIIKKA PRATTES	62
5	Decenterings Elsewhere and the Epistemic Dimensions of Care VRINDA DALMIYA	78
6	The Commitment to Care: An Unwavering Epistemic Decentering MAGGIE FITZGERALD	94
7	Indigenous and Feminist Ecological Reflections on Feminist Care Ethics: Encounters of Care, Absence, Punctures, and Offerings ANDREA DOUCET, EVA JEWELL, AND VANESSA WATTS	109
8	Crafting a New Corpo-Reality in Care Ethics: Contributions from Feminist New Materialisms and Posthumanist Ethics ÉMILIE DIONNE	128
9	Diffracting Care and Posthuman Ethics: Responsibility, Response-ability, and Privileged Irresponsibility VIVIENNE BOZALEK	145

10   "Do You Really Want to Know about This?":
     Critical Feminist Ethics of Care as a Project of Unsettling   159
     MASAYA LLAVANERAS BLANCO

11   The Operation(s) of Abolitionist Care: Healing, Care Ethics,
     and the Movement for Black Lives   176
     CHRISTOPHER PAUL HARRIS

12   When Facts Only Go So Far: Decentering What It Means
     to Know and Understand as a Care-Ethical Researcher
     in a Polarized, Post-Truth Era   194
     ALISTAIR NIEMEIJER AND MEREL VISSE

     Acknowledgments   209
     Notes on Contributors   211
     Index   215

DECENTERING EPISTEMOLOGIES
AND CHALLENGING PRIVILEGE

INTRODUCTION
SOPHIE BOURGAULT, MAGGIE FITZGERALD, AND FIONA ROBINSON

In 1980, Sara Ruddick's essay "Maternal Thinking" made an important claim when it underscored the fact that mothering entailed not only "labour" and "feeling" but also extensive and valuable "thought" and "knowledge" (Ruddick 1980). Two years later, Carol Gilligan's *In a Different Voice* introduced the world of Anglo-American moral philosophy to the language of "care"—a "non-hierarchical vision of human connection" (Gilligan 1982, 62). Susan Hekman has described Gilligan's contribution as a "radical decentering" of traditional moral theory, where the "disembodied knower" is replaced by the "relational self" (Hekman 1995, 30). Since these works were published, feminists have been creating "ever more nuanced critiques of reason and clearer accounts of alternative ideas of rationality" (Ruddick 1995, x). Several of them have indeed argued that women's experiences were not reflected in the dominant, masculinist approaches to ethics. An ethics of care challenged these approaches by positing ethics as relational, contextual, embodied, and realized through practices rather than abstract principles of right action.

Although the tremendous influence of Gilligan and other early care ethicists is undeniable, it is also evident that care ethics was not received with equal enthusiasm by all feminists. Notably, Gilligan's approach was perceived as essentialist—either "biologically" (Kerber 1986) or in its erasure of "other perspectives" such as race, class, and sexual orientation (Fraser and Nicholson 1990). Indeed, both Gilligan and Ruddick felt compelled to respond, in the prefaces to the second editions of their books, to critiques of their "universalizing tendencies" (Ruddick 1995, xvii). In 1995, Uma Narayan pointed to the use of "colonialist care discourses" to provide a moral justification for imperialism (Narayan 1995). More recent challenges have centered on care ethics' "Western-centrism" (Raghuram 2016), its heteronormativity (Malatino 2020), and the insufficient attention it pays to race and intersectionality (Hankivsky 2014). Once again, scholars of care are responding to these challenges and reflecting on the need to decenter care. For example, Joan Tronto (2020) explicitly calls upon care ethics scholars to reflect on how to make care ethics "travel" without becoming justifications for colonial and imperial domination (Tronto 2020).

This volume also takes up this challenge, paying particular attention to Tronto's important concept of "privileged irresponsibility," whereby willful ignorance serves to "prevent the relatively privileged from noticing the needs of others" (Tronto 1993, 121). As many of the contributors to this volume demonstrate, the notion of privileged responsibility leads us, inevitably, to considering questions of epistemology. Specifically, it requires us to think about epistemic privilege and what we might call "epistemic irresponsibility"—the power of those whose privilege means that they do not need to "care to know" (Bernasconi 2012; Medina 2013; Dalmiya 2016; Casalini 2020). Thus, "privileged irresponsibility" provides a helpful starting point from which to begin thinking critically about the intersections between care and epistemology, by foregrounding the relations between various forms of power and hierarchy, knowledge and the ethics and practices of care.

Vrinda Dalmiya's 2002 essay "Why Should a Knower Care?" already explored the care perspective as a basis for an alternative epistemology—one that confronts directly the harms that come from epistemologies of privileged irresponsibility. In fact, her entire body of work, which examines the intersections of care ethics, comparative philosophy, and epistemology, provides a model for much-needed scholarship in these areas (see esp. *Caring to Know*; Dalmiya 2016). This volume builds on this important work and on the growing interest in the intersections between care ethics and alternative ways of knowing, especially in relation to various hierarchies of power/knowledge and privilege that inhere to the context of modernity.

It could be argued that questions of epistemology—and its decentering—have always been at the heart of care ethics (especially in Gilligan's work), although not always explicitly addressed. For instance, feminist standpoint epistemology has always existed in close relationship with care ethics. Hartsock's (1983) account of a feminist standpoint as a superior vision produced by the political conditions and distinctive work of women is based specifically on caring labor—work that is overwhelmingly done by women and is "characteristically performed in exploitative and oppressive circumstances" (Ruddick 1995, 130). Of course, feminist standpoint epistemology has been the target of much criticism—specifically, the idea that there can be a single women's point of view, regardless of other identity aspects of culture, ethnicity, race, sexuality, or class. These criticisms have led to lively debates regarding the meaning of "woman," especially as understood by "largely white-dominated academic feminism" (Hirschmann 1998, 74). Despite these criticisms, the basic premise of feminist standpoint—that it is located in and produced by the culturally constructed social relations of household production and reproduction in late capitalism—is an important resource for understanding *what* and *how* we know from the perspective of care ethics. But if feminist standpoint theory is to be an "ally," care ethicists must continue paying close attention to relations of power and privilege not only within the gendered division of labor but in a range of social contexts.

Care ethics' emphasis on relationality and attentiveness to others within specific and varied contexts also suggests a rejection of abstract reasoning and an embrace of emotion and affect in the way we "know"; this undoubtedly resonates with earlier feminist work on the role of emotions, including love, in epistemology (Jaggar 1989; Collins 2003). Indeed, Collins (2003, 64) describes an "ethic of caring"—characterized by expressiveness, emotions, and empathy—as central to her Afrocentric feminist epistemology. It is, she explains, an "epistemology of connection, in which truth emerges through care." While writing in a somewhat different register, hooks (2000, 55) similarly highlights how self-love and love for others allow us to know, to "live consciously," and to think "critically about ourselves and the world we live in." Here, love, which can perhaps be thought of as a type of care, is again a critical epistemic tool that may allow us to work toward emancipatory practices geared to making the world more livable. Importantly, these ways of knowing are not abstract and transcendent but material and embodied—an idea that has been taken up by care ethics scholars (see esp. Hamington 2004; Vaittinen 2015).

More recently, care ethics has begun to engage with posthumanism and the new materialisms. María Puig de la Bellacasa's work, for example, connects a feminist materialism and critical thinking on care with debates on more-than-human ontologies and ecological practices (Puig de la Bellacasa 2012, 2017). Starting from a position of situated knowledges (Haraway 1988), posthumanist epistemology accounts for one's locations in terms of both space (geopolitical or ecological) and time (Braidotti 2019, 34). Here, again, there is an emphasis on immanence, but, crucially, all matter is understood as deeply relational—as "one"—thus decentering the human subject. These insights have been central, since time immemorial, to many Indigenous onto-epistemologies that are based on relationality—including relations with the nonhuman world, especially the land itself. A decentered care ethics must pay attention to these ways of knowing and their implications for the way we live in and with this earth, now and in the future.

The contributions in this volume build on these scholarships and offer diverse approaches, tools, and methods for decentering epistemology—most specifically in relation to the ethics of care. But while our volume grapples with such decentering from a variety of perspectives and considers distinct ethicopolitical issues, there are nevertheless a few core themes and claims that run throughout the collection. First, several chapters in this volume underscore the urgency and complexity of articulating critiques of epistemic privilege and epistemic irresponsibility. For instance, Marie Garrau explores the many mechanisms (social, psychological, etc.) by which the privileged are able to sustain a denial of their mutual vulnerability. Focusing on embodied practices, Riikka Prattes discusses how many of the men in her study were able to avoid mundane practices of care like cleaning; in this way, their privilege meant that they failed to know, and most significantly care for, the spaces in which they lived. Likewise, Vivienne Bozalek and Vrinda Dalmiya begin their chapters with the concept of privileged irresponsibility and consider a variety of tools—including diffractive methodologies (Bozalek) and epistemic humility (Dalmiya)—that might counter the harms attached to the privilege of not having to care or of not knowing *how* to care.

Second, many contributors to this volume demonstrate a commitment to analyzing knowing as something necessarily embodied and material. How do emotions like grief shape our care knowing or, perhaps more accurately, allow us to embrace and better navigate the ambiguity of epistemic claims (Dalmiya)? How does the complex interplay between our corporeal senses and our imaginations both help and, perhaps paradoxically, hinder our attempts to connect with others and address their care needs and concerns (FitzGerald)? How does our relational and embodied being facilitate thicker forms of noticing and witnessing, and how can such attentiveness facilitate richer forms of responsibility and care (Dionne)? In exploring these questions, our volume seeks to attune us to the body and its epistemological resources and thus foregrounds how our own knowledge claims always come from some body, somewhere.

Relatedly, several of our contributors make a powerful case for caring about the epistemic importance of place, of landscapes, and of the nonhuman world. For example, Prattes challenges us to think about how practices like cleaning connect us to space and cultivate an orientation toward caring for our homes—an orientation that can be expanded to include caring for our environments in a broader sense. Bozalek urges us to consider how privileged irresponsibility allows many of us to neglect our "damaged planet" and limits our horizons for thinking about possible future configurations of our entanglements with the earth. And Doucet, Jewell, and Watts use Indigenous epistemologies to foreground how different places—and different relations to different places—constitute different knowledges. Taken together, these contributions emphasize that our bodies are always connected to the geographies and material world in which we find ourselves and that it is through a weaving together of these places and ourselves that care knowing emerges and is tested. More simply, as Masaya Llavaneras Blanco writes in her chapter, "The concept of care is necessarily situated: it exists in place."

It is also from such a situated, embodied, and embedded epistemology that the sociopolitical *consequences* of rendering certain voices and agents invisible/inaudible are best revealed, as several of our contributors suggest. Epistemologies premised on narrow notions of reason often delegitimize other knowledge claims and ways of knowing/telling, which can lead to alienation, exclusion, low self-esteem, and poor mental health.[1] Making these injustices discernible and creating more space for marginalized voices are thus pressing ethical tasks, as many authors in this volume underscore (e.g., Koggel; Llavaneras Blanco; Bourgault; Dionne; Doucet, Jewell, and Watts). Moreover, by making such exclusions perceptible, other large-scale harms that are directly implicated in these epistemic injustices can also be brought to the fore. For example, Bozalek's piece in this volume illustrates how epistemic irresponsibility is intimately tied to environmental destruction, while Niemeijer and Visse show how epistemic injustices can often undermine civic trust and increase polarization.

Now, while contributors to this volume unanimously embrace the view that care scholarship ought to attend to less audible voices or underappreciated knowledges, the question of *how* to proceed to address these epistemic exclusions elicits more varied answers. Indeed, our authors offer distinctive rejoinders to the following set of questions: How exactly can one attend to marginalized voices in a nonpaternalistic and respectful manner, and who is best equipped to do so? How can our acknowledgment of "absences" in our epistemologies, legal structures, healthcare systems, or universities be meaningful rather than superficial, and how can they be nonexploitative or "nonextractivist" (to use the term discussed by Prattes in this volume)? Moreover, how can scholars attend to groups and communities struggling with epistemic marginalization, violence, or health inequities tied to colonialism without falling prey to what Unangax̂ scholar Eve Tuck (2009) calls "damage-based research"—that is, research that overly emphasizes deficits, pain, and failures and that underplays desire, hope, and self-determination? (On this last issue, Watts, Hooks, and McLaughlin [2020] have provided powerful evidence for the urgency of addressing this within Canadian sociological research.) While none of our contributors believe they offer exhaustive or definitive answers to these admittedly complex questions, they all share the hope that their reflections might elicit long overdue conversations in years to come.

Some of these conversations will likely entail examining how one might come to *unlearn* old cognitive patterns and epistemic practices that reinforce cultural imperialism and patriarchal frameworks. And certainly "unlearning" is another theme that is discussed through much of our volume—discussions that give pride of place to epistemic humility and to attentive listening (e.g., in this volume, Dalmiya, Bourgault, Koggel, Dionne). Many of our contributors underscore that privilege and power can sometimes lead to unreflexivity/laziness, arrogance, and narrow vision and, as such, that privilege can sometimes be "one's *loss*," to use Spivak's terms (1990, 10).[2] As contributors like FitzGerald and Garrau indicate, for instance, the task of "unlearning" (a word that partially captures what decentering is about) entails a long and difficult process, difficult in part because the process requires a willingness to engage in self-criticism, but also because it ought to lead—if this unlearning is to be meaningful—to a commitment to significant social transformation, structural changes, and time investments. As the chapters by Harris and by Doucet, Jewell, and Watts underscore, it will not suffice to sit with the status quo, to merely tweak our existing sociopolitical institutions, or to adjust our course syllabi to make a bit of room for previously marginalized knowledges; much more is required.[3]

This takes us to another claim that traverses several chapters in our book: namely, the desirability of embracing what could be called an ethics or a politics of refusal—whether it be a refusal of patriarchal norms (Prattes), of Western epistemologies of mastery (Dionne, Bozalek), of colonial epistemic frameworks (Doucet, Jewell, and Watts), or of racial capitalism and of the carceral state (Harris). Many contributors also underscore the intimate ties between refusal and desire as well as those between refusal and healing/repair.[4] For the authors who tackle (directly or implicitly) the issue of refusal in this volume, refusals ought to be seen as generative, joyful, and *affiliative*—and as closely linked to hopeful "expansive" futures (see particularly Doucet, Jewell, and Watts).

In some chapters of our book, readers will be presented not only with theoretical reflections on what decentering ethics and research could mean but also with concrete, vivid attempts to carry out such decentered ways of doing and communicating research. For instance, Vrinda Dalmiya explicitly describes her own chapter as *performing* a kind of "epistemic disobedience" vis-à-vis mainstream Western philosophy. Moreover, fellow contributors Alistair Niemeijer and Merel Visse propose a chapter that is anchored in experiential knowledge and that conceives of the humble task of the care ethical researcher as facilitating the interplay of plural and sometimes conflicting narratives. Last but not least, the piece by Doucet, Jewell, and Watts offers a polyphonic and highly collaborative series of reflections on Indigenous and feminist ecological thought. The three authors' voices remain distinct in a chapter that beautifully weaves in autoethnographic narratives with a careful analysis of texts.

A final theme that emerges is that which concerns the important role played by self-care in struggles for social justice. While the term "self" in self-care can be read, narrowly, as referring to one's own body and psyche, it can also be read more broadly as referring to the members of one's community or militant organization, which is partially the type of care famously celebrated as "warfare" by Audre Lorde (1988) and Sara Ahmed (2014).[5] While care is widely known to require a decentering of the self and a commitment to "other-regardingness," feminist scholars (including Gilligan) have consistently alerted us to the dangers of self-erasure (see FitzGerald's essay in this volume on the importance of recentering the self). The significance of self-care is also briefly underscored in Llavaneras Blanco's chapter, which brings readers' attention to the care practices taken up by Haitian migrant workers to care for one another while taking care of *others*. While at first glance these "ordinary" practices may seem banal and at a distance from things commonly understood as "political," what the chapters of Llavaneras Blanco and Harris indicate is that these practices in fact play a crucial role in solidarity and resistance, joy and healing.

What readers may gather from this brief and nonexhaustive list of the themes and issues that run through our book is that this collection of essays ultimately foregrounds the ambivalence of care. Care can be steeped in violence, domination, resentment, and anger but also in peace, solidarity, love, and empathy. In light of this, it should come as no surprise to readers that our discussions of the intersections between care and *epistemology* should also be characterized by tensions and complexity. The chapters of our volume have been written from distinct sociohistorical, cultural, and national contexts—and are informed by the methodological sensibilities and concerns of different academic disciplines (philosophy, sociology, education, political science), thus contributing to their richness and diversity. But despite the polyphonic nature of *Decentering Epistemologies and Challenging Privilege*, contributors speak in one voice in their commitment to the arduous work of decentering their own epistemological claims and practices. In so doing, they demonstrate how "knowing can be seen as a patient and relentless labor of weaving together the individual self and other to create social units that are either strengthened or weakened by (supportive or disabling) social, cultural, political, and institutional contexts." Such a "weaving epistemology . . . recognizes that knowledge is simultaneously individual and collective, independent and relational, aware of power symmetries yet not determined by them" (Confortini and Ruane 2013, 79, 88). In this volume, we join with our contributors in considering care ethics as an ongoing commitment to relationality, to decentering, and to challenging—via attentive listening, learning, unlearning, and refusals—various forms of epistemic power and privilege that silence marginalized voices.

OVERVIEW OF THE VOLUME

This volume considers various facets of epistemic oppression and of epistemic irresponsibility through the lens of care ethics. Most of our contributors here respond to Joan Tronto's twofold invitation in *Caring Democracy: Markets, Equality, and Justice* (2013) to consider more closely the ties between privileged irresponsibility and gender and racial inequalities in the distribution of care as well as the ties between privileged irresponsibility and the willful marginalization of certain bodies of knowledge. Several of our contributors also seek to decenter Western ethics and epistemologies through critical encounters with a variety of different moral voices and epistemological frameworks, proposing perspectives that might help care ethics better tackle questions pertaining to race, Indigeneity, class, gender, the environment, and nonhuman beings/agents.

In chapter 1, Christine Koggel uses accounts of hermeneutical injustice and a "feminist relational political orientation" to build upon, but also go beyond, the relational moral orientation of care. In particular, Koggel argues that we need to examine how oppressed and marginalized groups often can and do make sense of their experiences but are forced to supplant or suppress these experiences and their knowledge in favor of understanding and adopting the collective interpretative resources of the oppressor. In this way, she builds on both relational care ethics and Miranda Fricker's 2007 account of hermeneutical injustice in order to shed light on Indigenous-settler relations in Canada. Focusing on the Truth and Reconciliation Commission final report, Koggel emphasizes the need to first uncover the ontological, epistemological, and political assumptions underlying modernity's ties to colonialism to reveal more robust and attentive ways of seeing, hearing, understanding, and knowing.

Like Koggel, Sophie Bourgault (chapter 2) seeks to show the relevance of Fricker's work for care ethics but also its limitations. More specifically, Bourgault assesses the two main means proposed by Fricker to diminish epistemic injustices in public institutions: one that entails the *unveiling* of particulars (attending to context and to the specifics of each individual case) and another that involves the *veiling* of particulars (e.g., the concealing of names, of bodily features, etc.). In addition to showing how care ethics can offer healthy correctives to Fricker's work, the chapter underscores the basic tension attached to any effort to create more caring/inclusive institutions (a key goal pursued by countless feminist care scholars). More generally, Bourgault insists on the significance of temporal conditions and face-to-face contact in public service delivery as well as the need for scholars to analyze epistemic wrongs within the context of an economy of credibility and attention.

The following chapter also attends to the complexity of diminishing epistemic injustices in our communities. More specifically, Marie Garrau proposes to rearticulate contemporary feminist debates over the question of vulnerability in terms of epistemic ignorance and privilege. Building on the research of Joan Tronto, Pascale Molinier, Carol Gilligan and Naomi Snider, and José Medina (in particular, the latter's *Epistemology of Resistance*), Garrau argues that relations of domination and various constructions of privilege are the most crucial obstacles to the wide acknowledgment of our vulnerability and hence to the creation of a more caring society. The chapter offers a detailed discussion of the various ideological, psychological, material, and epistemic forces that help sustain the ignorance or outright denial of vulnerability (of oneself and of others). In her concluding section, Garrau also briefly considers how we might proceed in order to tap into the greater epistemic lucidity of the dominated and into the power of epistemic friction (Medina).

Riikka Prattes pursues these reflections on how to challenge epistemic ignorance in the next chapter (chapter 4) via an understanding of knowledge as place- and practice-based. Drawing upon feminist and Indigenous scholarship that foregrounds the embodied and located nature of all knowledge claims, Prattes illustrates how such epistemologies differ from the dominant Western epistemology, which is premised on objective, decontextualized, and abstracted knowledge claims. Next, she draws on her fieldwork studying men and the ways they clean (or not) their homes to indicate that when privileged men undertake this work—when they are brought closer to the "center" of care practices—they can often learn/embody a care epistemology that attentively considers what is needed to make and maintain their home environment, their place. Prattes's chapter also discusses the dangers of epistemic extractivism, that is, of problematically co-opting other epistemes (e.g., Indigenous ones) by importing them into different contexts. In foregrounding this risk, Prattes demonstrates a way to learn from other epistemologies while consciously working to avoid extractivist practices.

In the following chapter, Vrinda Dalmiya invites care ethicists to travel in time and in space by orchestrating a rich conversation between a non-Western classical text (the *Mahabharata*) and feminist care ethics. More specifically, the focus of her chapter is the ties between embodiment, vulnerability, and ethical relationships. Dalmiya offers readers an act of "epistemic disobedience"—a methodological decentering of both Western political philosophy and care ethics (thanks to her turn to classical Indian thought) as well as a more substantive decentering of standard accounts of vulnerability (by foregrounding *epistemic* vulnerability). Providing rich insights about grief along the way, this chapter proposes that at the core of care ethical agency is a willingness to relinquish mastery and control. Moreover, Dalmiya argues that it is this humble willingness to be hospitable to ambivalence and failure that is absolutely crucial for undoing privileged irresponsibility and for building greater sociopolitical solidarity.

Maggie FitzGerald, in chapter 6, shows that because care ethics conceives of "how we know" as an ongoing and iterative process of decentering the self to know the other, it necessarily and continually results in a decentering of "what we know," including what we know care itself to be. In this way, FitzGerald argues that care ethics, and the epistemology inherent in a commitment to care, demands that all care knowers undertake the difficult work of interrogating critically their knowledges, including understandings of both care practices and values, in an ongoing way. This epistemic work, FitzGerald foregrounds, is tough work; while we have several epistemic resources that help us in this task—most notably our bodies, imagination, and humility—these resources must also be decentered at times as we attempt to know the other without losing our own voices. As FitzGerald concludes, we cannot, however, turn away from this tough work: it is only through epistemic decenterings that knowledge and deed can be tested, evaluated, and revised, helping us move toward more caring worlds.

In chapter 7, Andrea Doucet, Eva Jewell, and Vanessa Watts observe that while Indigenous and feminist ecological interventions have often attended to parallel concerns (particularly in their shared critiques of the modern, capitalistic, patriarchal, and colonial epistemologies that dominate knowledge ecologies), little work exists on the nexus of these approaches and care ethics. The dialogue between Doucet, Jewell, and Watts in this chapter begins to address this gap by weaving together two important stories. On one hand, these authors demonstrate the need to make space for abandoned and invisible worlds of care and for acknowledging the absence of Indigenous concepts and onto-epistemologies in care ethics literature. On the other hand, they also outline shared principles that tie the ethics of care, feminist ecological approaches, and Indigenous (specifically Anishinaabe and Haudenosaunee) imaginaries together and demonstrate how these imaginaries inform their research on Indigenous family lives. In so doing, these scholars demonstrate the potential of the relational autonomy between them as they cowrote this piece and between feminist care ethics and various articulations of Indigenous care concepts.

Émilie Dionne's chapter (chapter 8) again seeks to expand the ethics of care in ways that confront the harms of epistemic ignorance, but this time via a dialogue with posthumanist theories like feminist new materialism, critical science and technology studies, and material ecocriticism. Dionne proposes new ethical and epistemological sensibilities and corporeal dispositions that might enable care ethics to hear and bear witness to others, particularly "others" that are invisibilized in dominant discourses. Further, Dionne foregrounds the productive nature of these new epistemological sensibilities: moving toward thicker forms of noticing and witnessing could allow us to better relate and be accountable for that which we are noticing. Dionne's contribution thus offers original insights into Gilligan's old challenge: how to make different moral voices be heard *and* understood in and on their own terms and how to be responsive to these voices and the relations they enact.

In chapter 9, Vivienne Bozalek reads care ethics through posthuman ethics in order to consider what might be done to bring about better prospects for those who coinhabit our "damaged planet." Specifically, Bozalek uses a "diffractive methodology" (Haraway 1992; Barad 2007) that engages affirmatively with difference in order to "think-with" Tronto's (1993) notion of privileged irresponsibility. By mobilizing concepts such as "hauntology" (Barad 2010), "grievable lives" (Butler 2004), "shadow places" (Plumwood 2008), "non-innocence" (Haraway 2008, 2016), "entangled empathy" (Gruen 2015), and "transcorporeal culpability" (Alaimo 2016), Bozalek demonstrates how the relational ontology of both care ethics and posthuman ethics reveals the entanglements and "intra-actions" between human and nonhuman entities. In this way, Bozalek enriches care ethics' relational ontology and Tronto's privileged irresponsibility in part by emphasizing the need to "render each other capable" of responding to our own entanglement with the planet and to its past, present, and future.

Masaya Llavaneras Blanco's contribution (chapter 10) draws upon extensive fieldwork to discuss the effects of racialization, class, and migratory status on the ways care needs are understood and attended to by Haitian migrant domestic workers in the Dominican Republic. Llavaneras Blanco unearths "non-innocent genealogies" of care (Murphy 2015) by centering care practices carried out by subaltern women, practices that have often been marginalized by interlocutors in positions of privilege. In so doing, her feminist, critical, and global approach to care illuminates the ways in which care ethics has the potential to foreground class- and race-based forms of inequality and thereby serve as a political ethic that is attuned to power relations and to the ways in which these relations shape care, care needs, and care work across diverse forms of life. The chapter also briefly underscores the importance of certain caring practices (e.g., hair braiding) offered by Haitian migrant workers to one another and exclusively to their "own" group.

Christopher Paul Harris (in chapter 11) continues the discussion initiated by Llavaneras Blanco regarding the care done *within* community or militant groups. Drawing in part on his experience as a member of the Black Youth Project 100 (New York City chapter), but also on key sources in Black feminist thought (e.g., those by Lorde, Collins, Sharpe, Woodly), Harris offers illuminating reflections on the care practices and ethics operating within the Movement for Black Lives. According to Harris, this ethics ought to be seen chiefly as a praxis of interdependence that seeks to challenge anti-Blackness and the legitimacy of the liberal, heteropatriarchal, carceral, and capitalist state. The chapter also tackles the very complex questions of how to "undo" worlds and institutions and of what repair requires. Here the insights of Black feminist thought and praxis are drawn upon not only to stress the desirability of having adequate spaces for healing and joy within militant groups but also to indicate the significance of accountability and of *attending* to difference. Harris's chapter considers not only the most joyful moments of solidarity within the Movement for Black Lives but also the conflicts, organizational problems, disappointments and difficulties that traverse it.

Finally, in the closing chapter, Alistair Niemeijer and Merel Visse consider the potential strategies for "knowing with care" in the context of the increasingly polarized, post-truth era, when factual claims and expert knowledge are looked at with distrust. Starting from the care ethical commitment to plurality and revisability in moral knowledge, Niemeijer and Visse argue that this commitment can be rendered precarious in these polarized and epistemically unstable times. Using a methodology of "generative critique" and using a wide range of examples (including some from the COVID-19 pandemic), the authors propose "precarious knowing"—a "polyvocal, collaborative approach"—as a timely approach to truth-seeking and socially engaged care ethical research.

Interestingly, the rise of the post-truth era has put questions of epistemology on the table for many who have rarely had to consider the struggle to have their own ways of knowing recognized, heard, or believed. That struggle has been and continues to be commonplace, however, for individuals and groups outside of the "center." From the start, care ethics has been about listening to those "different" voices and about recognizing relational practices as moral knowledge. But as the chapters in this volume demonstrate, care ethics must be mindful of the need to follow its own professed epistemological commitments to humility and revisability; it must work constantly to decenter itself—to recognize its own silences, omissions, and assumptions about what constitutes "caring knowledge." By inquiring more deeply into notions such as "privileged (epistemic) irresponsibility," this volume seeks to reveal the specific sites/places and structures—including those of gender, race, and coloniality—wherein this work must take place. While the solutions are not always evident, we hope that the chapters in this book will stimulate many lively conversations about the necessary "unlearning" required to recenter marginalized voices in the context of care ethics' ongoing commitment to nonhierarchical modes of relationality and connection.

NOTES

1. For insightful discussions of these consequences (and many additional ones), see Kidd, Medina, and Pohlhaus (2019).
2. See also Spivak (1990, 30).
3. As fellow contributor Harris (2021, 908) emphasized elsewhere, "The problem is not a matter of ignorance but design, and no amount of 'counter-hegemonic discourses' or 'caring to

know' will disrupt extant anti-Black institutions without undoing them altogether. Recourse to already existing concepts and practices will reproduce already existing grammars of captivity and subjection. It will not point us towards something else."

4. On the latter and its ties to refusal, readers may wish to consult the work of Leanne Betasamosake Simpson (2017), Audra Simpson (2014), and Eve Tuck and K. Wayne Yang (2014).

5. On the importance of care within social movements, see most notably Deva Woodly's *Reckoning: Black Lives Matter and the Democratic Necessity of Social Movements* (2021).

REFERENCES

Ahmed, Sara. 2014. "Self-Care as Warfare." *Feminist Killjoys*, August 25, 2014. https://feministkilljoys.com/2014/08/25/selfcare-as-warfare/.

Alaimo, Stacy. 2016. *Exposed: Environmental Politics and Pleasures in Posthuman Times*. Minneapolis: University of Minnesota Press.

Barad, Karen. 2007. *Meeting the Universe Halfway: Quantum Physics and the Entanglement of Matter and Meaning*. Durham, NC: Duke University Press.

———. 2010. "Quantum Entanglements and Hauntological Relations of Inheritance: Dis/continuities, Spacetime Enfoldings, and Justice-to-Come." *Derrida Today* 3: 240–268.

Bernasconi, Robert. 2012. "On Needing Not to Know and Forgetting What One Never Knew: The Epistemology of Ignorance in Fanon's Critique of Sartre." In *Race and Epistemologies of Ignorance*, edited by Shannon Sullivan and Nancy Tuana, 231–239. Albany: State University of New York Press.

Bourgault, Sophie. 2022. "Jacques Rancière and Care Ethics: Four Lessons in (Feminist) Emancipation." *Philosophies* 7 (3): 62. https://doi.org/10.3390/philosophies7030062.

Braidotti, Rosa. 2019. "A Theoretical Framework for the Critical Posthumanities." *Theory, Culture & Society* 36 (6): 31–61.

Butler, Judith. 2004. *Precarious Life: The Powers of Mourning and Violence*. London and New York: Verso.

Casalini, Brunella. 2020. "Care and Injustice." *International Journal of Care and Caring* 4 (1): 59–73.

Collins, Patricia Hill. 2003. "Toward an Afrocentric Feminist Epistemology." In *Turning points in Qualitative Research: Tying Knots in a Handkerchief*, edited by Yvonna S. Lincoln and Norman K. Denzin, 47–72. Lanham, MD: Rowman & Littlefield.

Confortini, Catia C., and Abigail E. Ruane. 2013. "Sara Ruddick's *Maternal Thinking* as Weaving Epistemology for *Justpeace*." *Journal of International Political Theory* 10 (1): 70–93.

Dalmiya, Vrinda. 2002. "Why Should a Knower Care?" *Hypatia* 17 (1): 34–52.

———. 2016. *Caring to Know*. Oxford: Oxford University Press.

Fraser, Nancy, and Linda Nicholson. 1990. "Social Criticism without Philosophy." In *Feminism/Postmodernism*, edited by Linda Nicholson, 19–38. New York: Routledge.

Fricker, Miranda. 2007. *Epistemic Injustice: Power and the Ethics of Knowing*. New York: Oxford University Press.

Gilligan, Carol. 1982. *In a Different Voice*. Cambridge, MA: Harvard University Press.

Gruen, Lauren. 2015. *Entangled Empathy: An Alternative Ethic for Our Relationships with Animals*. New York: Lantern Books.

Hamington, Maurice. 2004. *Embodied Care*. Urbana: University of Illinois Press.

Hankivsky, Olena. 2014. "Rethinking Care Ethics: On the Promise and Potential of an Intersectional Analysis." *American Political Science Review* 108 (2): 252–264.

Haraway, Donna. 1992. "The Promises of Monsters: A Regenerative Politics for Inappropriate/d Others. In *Cultural Studies*, edited by Lawrence Grossberg, Cary Nelson, and Paula Treichler, 295–337. New York: Routledge.

———. 1988. "Situated Knowledges: The Science Question in Feminism and the Privilege of Partial Perspective." *Feminist Studies* 14 (3): 575–599.

———. 2008. *When Species Meet*. Minneapolis: University of Minnesota Press.

———. 2016. *Staying with the Trouble: Making Kin in the Chthulucene*. Durham, NC: Duke University Press.

Harris, Christopher Paul. 2021. "(Caring for) the World That Must Be Undone." *Contemporary Political Theory* 20:890–925.

Hartsock, Nancy. 1983 "The Feminist Standpoint: Developing the Ground for a Specifically Feminist Historical Materialism." In *Discovering Reality: Feminist Perspectives on Epistemology, Metaphysics, Methodology, and Philosophy of Science*, edited by Sandra Harding and Merrill B. Hintikka, 283–310. Boston: Kluwer Academic Publishers.

Hekman, Susan. 1995. *Moral Voices, Moral Selves*. University Park: Pennsylvania State University Press.

Hirschmann, Nancy. 1998. "Feminist Standpoint as Postmodern Strategy." *Women & Politics* 18 (3): 73–92.

hooks, bell. 2000. *All about Love: New Visions*. New York: HarperCollins.

Jaggar, Alison M. 1989. "Love and Knowledge: Emotion in Feminist Epistemology." *Inquiry* 32 (2): 151–176.

Kerber, Linda. 1986. "Some Cautionary Words for Historians." *Signs: Journal of Women in Culture and Society* 11 (2): 304–310.

Kidd, Ian James, José Medina, and Gaile Pohlhaus Jr., eds. 2019. *The Routledge Handbook of Epistemic Injustice*. New York: Routledge.

Lorde, Audre. 1988. *A Burst of Light*. Ithaca, NY: Firebrand Books.

Malatino, Hil. 2020. *Trans Care*. Minneapolis: University of Minnesota Press.

Medina, José. 2013. *The Epistemology of Resistance: Gender and Racial Oppression, Epistemic Injustice, and Resistance Imaginations*. Oxford: Oxford University Press.

Murphy, Michelle. 2015. "Unsettling Care: Troubling Transnational Itineraries of Care in Feminist Health Practices." *Social Studies of Science* 45 (5): 717–737.

Narayan, Uma. 1995. "Colonialism and Its Others: Consideration on Rights and Care Discourses." *Hypatia* 10 (2): 133–140.

Plumwood, Val. 2008. "Shadow Places and the Politics of Dwelling." *Australian Humanities Review* 44 (1): 139–150.

Puig de La Bellacasa, María. 2012. "Nothing Comes without Its World': Thinking with Care." *The Sociological Review* 60 (2): 197–216.

———.2017. *Matters of Care: Speculative Ethics in More Than Human Worlds*. Minneapolis: University of Minnesota Press.

Raghuram, Parvati. 2016. "Locating Care Ethics beyond the Global North." *ACME: An International Journal for Critical Geographies* 15 (3): 511–533.

Ruddick, Sara. 1980. "Maternal Thinking." *Feminist Studies* 6 (2): 342–367.

———. 1995. *Maternal Thinking*. 2nd ed. Boston: Beacon.

Simpson, Audra. 2014. *Mohawk Interruptus: Political Life across the Borders of Settler States*. Durham, NC: Duke University Press.

Simpson, Leanne Betasamosake. 2017. *As We Have Always Done: Indigenous Freedom through Radical Resistance*. Minneapolis: University of Minnesota Press.

Spivak, Gayatri Chakravorty. 1990. *The Post-colonial Critic: Interviews, Strategies, Dialogues*. Edited by Sarah Harasym. New York: Routledge.

Tronto, Joan C. 1993. *Moral Boundaries: A Political Argument for an Ethic of Care*. New York: Routledge.

———. 2013. *Caring Democracy: Markets, Equality, and Justice*. New York: New York University Press.

———. 2020. "Caring Democracy: How Should Concepts Travel?" In *Care Ethics, Democratic Citizenship and the State*, edited by Petr Urban and Lizzie Ward, 181–198. Amsterdam: Springer.

Tuck, Eve. 2009. "Suspending Damage: A Letter to Communities." *Harvard Educational Review* 79 (3): 409–427.

Tuck, Eve, and K. Wayne Yang. 2014. "R-Words: Refusing Research." In *Humanizing Research: Decolonizing Qualitative Inquiry with Youth and Communities*, edited by Django Paris and Maisha T. Winn, 223–248. Thousand Oaks, CA: Sage.

Vaittinen, Tiina. 2015. "The Power of the Vulnerable Body." *International Feminist Journal of Politics* 17 (1): 100–118.

Watts, Vanessa, Gregory Hooks, and Neil McLaughlin. 2020. "A Troubling Presence: Indigeneity in English-Language Canadian Sociology." *Canadian Review of Sociology / Revue canadienne de sociologie* 57:7–33.

Woodly, Deva. 2021. *Reckoning: Black Lives Matter and the Democratic Necessity of Social Movements*. Oxford: Oxford University Press.

1 · INDIGENOUS VOICES AND RELATIONSHIPS

Insights from Care Ethics and Accounts of Hermeneutical Injustice

CHRISTINE KOGGEL

A decade after the publication of *In a Different Voice*, Carol Gilligan reflects on how her work has been misunderstood and sets out to clarify what she tried to do in the book first published in 1982. I continue to find the following passage from the "Letter to Readers, 1993" illuminating: "My questions are about our perceptions of reality and truth; how we know, how we hear, how we see, how we speak. My questions are about voice and relationship." She adds, "To have a voice is to be human. To have something to say is to be a person. But speaking depends on listening and being heard; it is an intensely relational act" (1993, xiii, xvi). Three broad areas are identifiable in these quotations: ontological issues of being and doing that shape *what* we know, what we see, what we hear, and what we say; epistemological issues of *how* we know, how we see, how we speak, and how we hear; and political issues of power that shape *who* is taken to know and *who* is heard and not heard.

In this chapter, I begin in the second and third sections with recent accounts of care ethics to explore the significance and implications of these ontological, epistemological, and political aspects of what we know, how we know, and who is taken to know. Joan Tronto, Fiona Robinson, and Maggie FitzGerald all highlight facts and features of relationships that can account for perceptions of reality and truth and of the power to speak and be heard. And each of these accounts places the voice of care into the political realm and as relevant to public institutions and policy making. In the fourth section I use insights from FitzGerald's account of a care as a critical political theory to connect the ontological and epistemological. FitzGerald applies her account to what can be learned about the value of care for government policy at the national level, but I want to go broader. In the fifth section I begin to draw out broader political implications in and through the concept of hermeneutical injustice first introduced by Miranda Fricker and yet to be fully examined in the care ethics literature. Hermeneutical injustice captures the idea of gaps in the collective interpretative resources of those who are dominant and powerful and those who are marginalized and oppressed. I build on Fricker's account by applying hermeneutical injustice to broad areas of gaps in collective interpretative resources in colonial histories that have shaped relationships between non-Indigenous and Indigenous peoples. In the final sections I turn to an account of this history and its shaping of relationships in Canada's settler-colonial context by discussing parts of Canada's Truth and Reconciliation Commission (TRC) final report. I show how questions about what is known, how it is known, and who knows have been and continue to be central to the shaping of Canada's settler-colonial history as one in which Indigenous ways of being and knowing have been dismissed, denigrated, and ignored.

TRONTO ON CARE ETHICS AND INSTITUTIONS

I often return to Tronto's *Moral Boundaries: A Political Argument for an Ethic of Care* (1993) for the kind of complex account of care ethics that is needed to shift the focus from personal, dyadic relationships to networks of relationships in public and political spheres. Tronto's account of care is meant to be broad and general, as captured in the description that she and Berenice Fisher provided in their early work on care: "We suggest that caring be viewed as a species activity that includes everything that we do to maintain, continue, and repair our 'world' so that we can live in it as well as possible. That world includes our bodies, our selves, and our environment, all of which we seek to interweave in a complex, life-sustaining web" (Fisher and Tronto 1990, 40; Tronto 1993, 103). As the subtitle of *Moral Boundaries* indicates, the boundaries delineated in mainstream liberal theory between the moral and political that place care practices in the private moral domain are challenged in Tronto's formative work in making the case for a political argument for an ethic of care.

In her more recent "Creating Caring Institutions: Politics, Plurality, and Purpose," Tronto (2010, 162) takes us right to where the focus needs to be in applying an account of good care to policy making in public and political institutions: "To imagine a world organized to care well requires that we focus on three things: *politics*: recognition and debate/dialogue of relations of power within and outside the organization of competitive and dominative power and agreement of common purpose; *particularity and plurality*: attention to human activities as particular and admitting of other possible ways of doing them and to diverse humans having diverse preferences about how needs might be met; and *purposiveness*: awareness and discussion of the ends and purposes of care." The four Ps come together for Tronto in addressing relationships of power (gendered, racialized, and hierarchical aspects of caregiving and care receiving), in attending to needs and preferences in all their diversity and context specificity, and in settling conflicts in and through democratic processes that "are highly deliberate and explicit about how to best meet the needs of the people who they serve" (2010, 169).

When I use Tronto's article in my courses, it always prompts questions about whether her account of caring institutions can be applied to political institutions more generally. Tronto is well aware that the caring institutions she envisions are necessarily nested in broader social, economic, and political relationships that shape the deliberations that can take place and that often set policy agendas that thwart possibilities for actualizing the kinds of caring institutions that Tronto has in mind. For example, long-term care facilities, even the best ones, are hamstrung by too few caregivers and limited budgets—conditions that can be said to have been exacerbated and made all the more visible in times of COVID-19. In a subsection of "Creating Caring Institutions" called "Seven Warning Signs That Institutions Are Not Caring Well," warning sign 6 has Tronto (2010, 165–166) identify some of the policy and institutional problems that affect the ability of an institution to provide good care: "(6) Care givers see organizational requirements as hindrances to, rather than support for, care. Many care-giving institutions split hands-on care giving from higher 'management' functions. Managers are generally better compensated than direct care workers, and their work is less subject to control. Frequently, institutions cut budgets by cutting direct care workers, not managers. Care givers frequently complain that they have inadequate resources for their tasks at hand. When care givers find themselves saying that they care despite the pressures and requirements of the organization, the institution has a diminished capacity to provide good care." However, Tronto's focus is on what deliberative practices *within* caring institutions can achieve by discussing and working out the context specific details of the four Ps identified earlier: the *politics* of recognizing and debating relations of power within and outside the institution; the *particularity and plurality* of attending to "human activities as particular and admitting of other possible ways of doing them and to diverse humans having diverse preferences about how needs might be met" (2010, 162); and the *purposiveness* of deliberation about the ends and purposes of care within the institution. Yet what is possible by way of deliberation and decision making within an institution is shaped and affected by deliberation and decision making in broader social and political contexts. The issues will also need to be about how to influence and change the broader social and political contexts. Sophie Bourgault's "Epistemic Injustice, Face-to-Face Encounters, and Caring Institutions" elucidates the "dark sides of care" (2020, 91) when those with the authority to make decisions about the nature and quality of care are outside the institutions of care on which Tronto focuses. In these cases, those in power do not listen, hear, or "care" to understand or respond to needs as articulated by care receivers or caregivers within institutions. In other words, the four Ps within an institution are necessarily embedded in and shaped by the politics of social and political power outside the institution.

A brief sketch of how contemporary discussions about each of the four Ps have been affected by COVID-19 inside and outside institutions of care can heighten awareness of the significance of the broader political context of state, national, and global policies. Early data about the elderly contracting COVID-19 and dying at rates higher than those in the general population made visible what has been happening in many long-term care facilities for some time and merely magnified through COVID-19. Bourgault points out that attempts at "making institutions more caring and more inclusive" (2020, 93) come up against the lack of power of those in these institutions to challenge the very policies of cuts to staff and pay or to have their concerns about regulations that dictate time for completing tasks and for interacting with care receivers be heard. In this context (and with respect to COVID-19), Tronto's call for deliberative practices regarding the four Ps cannot really be effectively enacted: the politics of cuts to health care that create shortages of care workers, who are then hampered in being able to do the work of taking care of basic bodily needs (thus the elderly left in beds and wheelchairs); particularity and plurality being suspended in the face of low pay for care workers that forced many of them to take up work in a number of facilities at a time (thus increasing exposure to COVID-19 for themselves and the elderly); and power and purpose being in the hands of mandates by managers of for-profit facilities and of regulations by government officials (thus investigations into conditions that have been ongoing and exacerbated through COVID-19). While the deliberations that Tronto calls for within an institution are important, a basic and crucial question is whether and how an account of care ethics can provide insight into how to challenge and change the broader policy issues that are in place outside of institutions that, in the end, shape what these institutions can do to provide good care. The question, as FitzGerald (2020, 248) puts it, is this: How can we broaden the scope of care ethics policy to policy areas not generally viewed as care related or care relevant?

BROADENING THE SCOPE OF CARE ETHICS: FITZGERALD AND ROBINSON

In "Reimagining Government with the Ethics of Care," FitzGerald (2020) identifies two strands in care ethics, one that focuses on *practices and activities of care* and one that explores the transformative power of care ethics as a *critical political theory*. She follows Robinson in defending the latter in that it "allows for a radical critique of institutions and governing norms, and inherently destabilizes the dominant understandings of the purpose, structure, and role of government and public policy" (FitzGerald 2020, 248). Before discussing what FitzGerald does by way of building a positive account of what the second strand can do, I briefly discuss Robinson's account of the two strands and the objections she raises to the first. In "Resisting Hierarchies through Relationality in the Ethics of Care," Robinson (2020, 12) describes the pitfalls of the first strand:

I argue that these criticisms—that care ethics privileges gender and is "Western-centric"—are not wrong *per se*, but licensed by a particular view of care ethics that seeks to provide the normative and conceptual basis from which to develop more effective care policy and even "caring societies" (Glenn, 2000). Specifically, I argue that these criticisms are most likely to arise in one of two contexts: first, when care ethics is viewed as an advocacy framework that is "applied" to the work of caring, or to policy and practice related to care; and, second, when care ethics is treated as more or less interchangeable with care work.

The first thing I want to note is that while many care ethicists do focus on the practices and activities of care as such, Tronto's account, as sketched above, goes beyond this and is, thus, not susceptible, in my view, to the criticisms that her account privileges gender or is Western-centric. While it can be said that Tronto discusses what good care looks like, it is in the context of a constant examination and questioning of and within the institutions and structures that provide care. But does the second strand provide more than can be found in Tronto? To counter the limitations of the first strand that has care ethics focus on practices and activities of care and to answer the objections raised against this account, Robinson (2020) offers a reading of care ethics that has it be a *critical political theory*: "Against these charges, and following the recent work of Carol Gilligan, I offer a reading of the ethics of care as a critical feminist political theory. Understood in this way, I argue that care ethics has the conceptual and critical resources to counter these most recent challenges related to difference. The significance of this extends beyond these particular critiques; indeed, the broader contribution of this article is to offer an account of care ethics that responds to difference by resisting oppositional hierarchies in *favour of relationality*" (12, emphasis added). Much of my own research uses the lens of relationality and, more specifically, of feminist relational theory to draw out the effects of relationships of power (Koggel 2012, 2014, 2018; Koggel, Harbin, and Llewellyn 2022). While relationality and the significance of relationships of power are certainly present in Tronto's work, I think that making relationships the explicit lens through which to debate issues of power, plurality, particularity, and purpose can help highlight the potential of care ethics as a critical feminist political theory. After all, relationships of power that exist in institutions are themselves nested in broader political contexts and structures of power. I take this to be key to Robinson's (2020, 12) account of care as a critical feminist political theory that resists "oppositional hierarchies."

Building on Robinson, FitzGerald (2020, 249) says of the care as practices and activities strand that "this approach to care ethics in some ways misses a key aspect of the transformative potential of the ethics of care, particularly when care ethics is instead understood as a critical political theory." I want to draw out the transformative potential of care ethics as a critical political theory by examining FitzGerald's critique and then returning to a discussion of the triad of ontological (how we know), epistemological (what we know), and political (who is taken to know) that underlies the Robinson and FitzGerald accounts.

FITZGERALD ON THE INTERCONNECTEDNESS OF THE EPISTEMOLOGICAL AND ONTOLOGICAL

For FitzGerald (and care ethicists more generally), the epistemological is taken to be what is known and what can be spoken when the *relational moral orientation of care* as responsibility for meeting the needs of others is the starting point. This relational moral orientation of care uncovers ways of being and ways of knowing shaped by the embodied and engaged practices and activities in which care is located. Most importantly for FitzGerald (and for Tronto and Robinson as well) is the need to situate practices and activities of care in social, economic, and political contexts. FitzGerald's basic argument is that care ethics needs to focus less on *practices and activities of care* and more on the transformative power of care ethics as a critical political theory that "allows for a radical critique of institutions and governing norms, and inherently destabilizes the dominant understandings of the purpose, structure, and role of government and public policy" (2020, 248). As articulated by FitzGerald, care ethics that is a critical political theory brings the ontological and epistemological together in revealing assumptions in mainstream liberal theory that "legitimizes moralities based on autonomous individuals, and which privileges those who use such moralities, abstract principles, and binary categories to guide their reasoning and actions" (2020, 253). The ontology of liberal individualism is tied to the epistemology of what is "known" about how to reason about the world and morality.

FitzGerald argues that what needs to be foregrounded is the epistemological roots found in Gilligan that can highlight the broader ontological and epistemic issues of care as a relational moral orientation that challenges the reliance on rationalist, universalist, individualist, and abstract principles found in mainstream liberal moral *and* political theory. The epistemology that emerges from a relational moral orientation of care reveals what we know about relationships, responsibilities, and the world and worlds in which we are situated and embedded. This has us return to Gilligan's statement of her project as answering questions about "our perceptions of reality and truth; how we know, how we hear, how we see, how we speak" (1993, xiii) and the corresponding warning that these processes depend on "listening and being heard" (xvi). A relational moral orientation of care, one that shows the inseparability of the ontological fact of relationships and the epistemologies/perceptions/knowledges that are shaped in and through them, opens up spaces for interrogating the political and the corresponding relations of power "that shape and operate through our governing norms, values, and moral thinking" (FitzGerald 2020, 253).

FitzGerald (2020, 249) builds on Robinson's idea of the transformative power of care ethics as a critical political theory: "The ethics of care, as critical political theory, requires much more than a prescriptive analysis of how policies fail to facilitate care; rather, a critical political ethics of care foregrounds the transformative potential of care ethics as it necessitates a rethinking of the governing norms (Koggel 2012, 74) and values which underpin current policy structures and government organisations more broadly." FitzGerald references my work, but it will be useful for understanding the connection of this work with the literature on epistemic injustice in the next section if I make my own position (as referenced in FitzGerald) more explicit. I take one of the central features and strengths of a feminist relational approach to be its ability to uncover and challenge dominant norms. When the focus is on relationships, who is oppressed and thereby silenced and marginalized shapes and entrenches the norms, structures, and institutions that reflect the world of the oppressors. This factor shapes, as the Gilligan quotations that open this chapter highlight, who gets to speak and be heard, who is taken to know, and what they are not taken to know.

We therefore return to Gilligan's point that how we know, how we hear, how we see, and how we speak are relational processes that depend on "listening and being heard" (1993, xvi). These relational processes open spaces for interrogating relations of power and oppression "that shape and operate through our governing norms, values, and moral thinking" (FitzGerald 2020, 253). In "Reimagining Government with the Ethics of Care," FitzGerald points to the "type of political institution or organisation that could result from such a rethinking and reformulation of the values that govern our lives" (261). Going beyond Tronto's account of what constitutes good care in institutional settings, FitzGerald discusses the ways in which a department of care at the national level can uncover and critique male-biased epistemologies, ontologies, and policies that value autonomy and individualism over dependency, that ignore facts of our interdependency, and that denigrate care as a relational moral orientation: "Instead of focusing on how care ethics can help illuminate better practices of care in the context of politics—that which already exists—the ethics of care, as a broader political theory and critique of existing hierarchies which value certain moral epistemologies over others, has the potential to transform governing norms, the institutions shaped by these norms and values, and most radically, the current configuration of 'the political' itself" (FitzGerald 2020, 261). The worldview and ways of being in the world shaped by a relational moral orientation of care are privileged vantage points from which to notice and pay attention to the lived realities of our daily lives as relational and needy beings who are always interdependent and whose levels of dependence and independence change throughout a lifetime. I applaud FitzGerald's thought experiment on what a department of care can offer: "It would bring to the fore the ways in which these responsibilities have been historically distributed and are distributed today, and to commit to the on-going evaluation of how we can better distribute these responsibilities to enhance all caring relations" (257). As she points out, her account of care as a government department can challenge and inform other departments such as finance that are currently "viewed as the most significant measures of collective well-being" (260).

Yet there are features of the epistemological/ontological/political in addition to those explored thus far with respect to a relational *political* orientation that I take to be distinct from a relational *moral* orientation of care. Two points can clarify what I set out to show in the remaining sections: (1) additional features emerge when the focus is on the moral/political *and* the epistemological as intertwined and emerging from an ontological conception of the relational self; and (2) there is more at stake in uncovering an ontology and epistemology that is male-biased with respect to concepts such as autonomy, individualism, independence, and abstract principles so valued in mainstream liberal theory. This involves interrogating relations of power beyond those of caring relations and of using insights from feminist relational theory's starting point of describing and analyzing broad networks of relationships at all levels—from personal to public to national to global.

I argue that a feminist relational approach can reveal how relationships of power and oppression are shaped by governing norms and structures in ways that shape what one knows, how needs are articulated and prioritized, and how bodies and ways of knowing are perceived (Koggel 2008, 2012, 2022). The epistemological/ontological framework emerging from care as a critical feminist political theory intersects with my work on a feminist relational approach in explaining how and why some voices are privileged as morally significant and valuable while others are dismissed, denigrated, or devalued—all as created and shaped in and through relationships of power. While care as a critical feminist political theory zeroes in on how political/hierarchical/power structures can lead to a loss/absence/devaluing of care and caring relations, a *relational political orientation* differs in attending to the broad range of political/hierarchical/power structures as ones that shape and maintain relationships of power and oppression more generally. Looking ahead, the broader focus can capture how the triad of ontology, epistemology, and politics shapes how, what, and who knows in ways that dismiss and denigrate voices, relationships, and people themselves beyond those of caring relations. I argue that the concept of epistemic injustice can help elucidate the epistemic and moral/political failures to hear, listen to, or understand voices outside of those in power.

When placed in histories of settler-colonial contexts, ways of knowing and being are shaped by broad lifeworld activities of interacting with others through practices, laws, institutions, and language-making activities that shape what one knows, what one claims to know, and what those in power take to be ignorance rather than knowledge. Norms, laws, institutions, practices, languages, and activities are shaped and reshaped in and through relationships of power and oppression of all kinds and at all levels from the personal to the public and national to the global. In the ever-growing literature on epistemic injustice these ways of knowing are referred to as hermeneutical or collective interpretative resources.

HERMENEUTICAL INJUSTICE: MOVING BEYOND FRICKER'S ACCOUNT

In coining the concept of "epistemic injustice," Fricker distinguishes two kinds: testimonial injustice and hermeneutical injustice. The former describes the "wrong done to someone specifically in her capacity as a knower" (2007, 20). Testimonial injustice captures cases where one's credibility is negatively affected by bias on the part of the hearer based on the social identity of the speaker. On Fricker's account, the social identity of the speaker affects whose testimony is likely to be credible and whose is likely to be discredited. The concept of social identity means that on Fricker's account, testimonial injustice is placed in contexts of power and oppression. Yet Fricker's account of testimonial injustice tends to have power and oppression in the background in her descriptions of individuals responding negatively to the testimony of other individuals. That testimonial injustice needs to foreground accounts of power and oppression will become evident when I apply the discussion of epistemic injustice to settler-colonial relations in Canada.

Hermeneutical injustice, according to Fricker, is *structural* in form and "occurs at a prior stage when a gap in *collective interpretative resources* puts someone at an unfair disadvantage when it comes to making sense of their social experience" (2007, 1, emphasis added). Much more attention has been paid to the two categories of testimonial and hermeneutical and to questions about what each captures or fails to capture than I can cover here. Elsewhere, for example, I have argued that the delineation of testimonial and hermeneutical injustice may not be so clear and that Fricker's account of testimonial injustice is too individualist (Koggel 2018). In this chapter, my focus is on hermeneutical injustice and the criticism of Fricker's too narrow account of the gap in collective interpretative resources.

Though her definition of hermeneutical injustice references collective interpretative resources, for Fricker it tends to be the group or persons experiencing the gap who cannot make sense of their social experience (thus her example of women not making sense of sexual harassment until the concept was formulated and described). I suggest that there is more to hermeneutical injustice than the creation of concepts that can then fill the gap. I agree with critics who have argued that there are different kinds and levels of hermeneutical injustice other than that given by Fricker (Medina 2012; Pohlhaus 2012). But I also think that Fricker's example of women needing to have the concept "sexual harassment" before they could understand their *experiences* of sexual harassment is flawed. A discussion of what is missing and flawed will reveal that the core of the *injustice* in hermeneutical injustice is that collective interpretative resources reflect the norms, structures, and institutions of the dominant and powerful who are positioned to not see, hear, or know the collective interpretative resources of those who are marginalized and without power. To the dominant and powerful, the collective interpretative resources of the marginalized and oppressed are invisible, not taken to be resources, ignored, dismissed, or denigrated.

In her discussion of Carmita Wood, Fricker interprets her as unable to understand what was happening to her when she was targeted by her supervisor, who would make inappropriate gestures toward her and touch her without consent. Yet Wood can be seen as resisting these advances in actions that had her avoid him, in experiencing stress-related symptoms of neck and back pain, in quitting her job, and in applying for unemployment insurance and having her claim be rejected. According to Fricker's account, when a claim investigator questioned her about why she quit her job, Wood was unable to understand her experiences of "sexual harassment" and said that it was for personal reasons (Fricker 2007, 150). Another way to interpret what was going on is to acknowledge that although Wood may not have had the concept of sexual harassment, she did understand that her supervisor had power over her, that she could be fired if she didn't comply, that she was being targeted and was unable to stop the advances except by quitting her job, that she felt alone and isolated in her thoughts about what she experienced, and that what was happening to her was wrong and unjust. In other words, there were many women like Wood who would have shared these experiences of being "sexually harassed" and who would have had their own collective interpretative resources for understanding the physical, mental, and emotional toll, and all before the concept "sexual harassment" was created to name the experiences in the mid-1970s.

Revealing the injustice in hermeneutical *injustice* is about examining the "gaps" in ways of being and knowing in relationships between those with power and privilege and those whose voices are dismissed, ignored, or denigrated. But this account of hermeneutical injustice already takes us beyond Fricker's account, in which she specifies the gap in terms of those who are oppressed or marginalized not being able to make sense of their experiences (as her example of women who could not make sense of experiences of sexual harassment happening to them until the concept was formulated and put into law). I argue that while women may not have had the concept, they knew about needing to be silent to keep their jobs and about the injustice of the dominant understanding of the behavior as acceptable.

Critics such as Gaile Pohlhaus Jr. (2012) and José Medina (2012) broaden the scope of Fricker's account of hermeneutical injustice by arguing that while the social experiences of marginally situated knowers may be obscured from the dominant collective interpretative resources, they are not necessarily obscure to marginally situated knowers or to marginally situated communities. By developing new interpretive resources or retrieving collective interpretative resources that have been denigrated or dismissed by the dominant and powerful, marginalized knowers can achieve robust understandings of their experiences even while their experiences remain misunderstood and/or obscured from the hermeneutically dominant and powerful (Pohlhaus 2012, 719; Medina 2012, 207).

We need to examine how oppressed and marginalized groups often can and do make sense of their experiences but are forced to supplant or suppress these experiences and their knowledge in favor of understanding and adopting the collective interpretative resources of the oppressor (as assimilation policies make clear). I take these cases to be better able to explain how the collective interpretative resources of the oppressed (as shaped in and through their own histories, practices, institutions, traditions) are ignored or dismissed and sometimes even become objects for erasure by oppressors. The literature on willful hermeneutical ignorance is important for highlighting that those with power are positioned to willfully ignore the collective interpretative resources of the marginalized and oppressed (Pohlhaus 2012). My application of hermeneutical injustice in relationships between settler-colonial and Indigenous peoples shows a layer of complexity of who knows and what they know that highlights the importance of distinguishing between oppressor and oppressed and between dominant and marginalized collective interpretative resources. This broader perspective on a *relational* moral *and political* orientation that emerges from and is embedded in and shaped by histories and processes of colonization raises questions that are not so easily answered either by care ethics conceived as a critical political theory or in the mainstream literature on epistemic injustice.

In the case of Carmita Wood, creating the concept of sexual harassment and implementing it in law meant that oppressors were forced to at least recognize that their behavior could and would have consequences. In the case of sexual harassment, the dominant collective interpretative resources were challenged and changed as a result, and, it can be said, sexual harassment gained standing and acceptance in the dominant discourse / collective interpretative resources. This could happen within the framework of existing laws that now clarified the category of sexual harassment and delineated punishments that could result for those guilty of sexual harassment. While this continues to be an ongoing project of challenging male biases in law and policy, it was law and policy that changed through women's efforts to fight and challenge what was allowed or assumed in the workplace. And even if resisted by some, these policies also changed what were taken to be appropriate relationships in the workplace.

Canada's settler-colonial history reveals a different story of possibilities for challenge and change because Indigenous collective interpretative resources were and continue to be ignored, dismissed, and denigrated. These collective interpretative resources were not deemed to be resources and were openly targeted for erasure through the residential school systems (Koggel 2018). Canada's history of the colonization of Indigenous peoples, from the moment of arrival of European settlers, has shaped and continues to shape relationships of power and domination between settler-colonial and Indigenous peoples. These relationships are built on government policies of the forced assimilation of Indigenous peoples— through, for example, the residential school system—and they reflect the dismissal and denigration of the collective interpretative resources, the ways of being and knowing, of Indigenous peoples. Indigenous scholars such as Glen Coulthard (2014) and Audra Simpson (2014) describe Indigenous ways of being and knowing as themselves relational moral orientations that situate Indigenous peoples on the land, in communities, and in interaction with each other and nonhuman animals in ways that have shaped and continue to shape the laws, institutions, practices, languages, and traditions that constitute their collective interpretative resources. These are precisely the kinds of collective interpretative resources that Western enlightenment and modernity do not take to be knowledge-based claims at all. Before turning to a discussion of the relevance of hermeneutical injustice to Canada's TRC in the section that follows, consider three examples of recent work that applies these insights on the role of modernity and of colonialism with respect to the denigration or dismissal of non-Western and Indigenous collective interpretative resources. Katharina Hunfeld examines the relevance and dominance of Western linear accounts of time in global justice and development literature and "calls for alternative ways of narrating, conceptualising, and experiencing temporality in a way that resists the preproduction of the persistent coloniality in Western linear assumptions about time" (Hunfeld 2022, 101). Bourgault also discusses the relevance of time but in the context of communicative interactions that assume an "economy of credibility," one that works against listeners taking time to seek additional information or to gather information through face-to-face encounters (2020, 93). FitzGerald's *Care and the Pluriverse: Rethinking Global Ethics* takes a broad approach to collective interpretative resources to highlight features of Indigenous worldviews of "more-than-human beings" (2022, 195) that contrast with and can better inform the taken-for-granted ontologies and epistemologies of modernity. In all cases, modernity reflects collective interpretative resources that assume and exploit relationships of power over oppressed peoples, nonhuman entities, and nature.

HERMENEUTICAL INJUSTICE IN CANADA'S SETTLER-COLONIAL CONTEXT

While there is perhaps greater awareness of the facts that shape the context within which Canada's TRC emerged from the Indian Residential Schools Settlement Agreement (IRSSA), less explored are the hermeneutical gaps in the collective interpretative resources of Indigenous and settler-Canadian understandings of Canada's history. A strong message emerging from the final report of the TRC is that for reconciliation to be possible at all, non-Indigenous Canadians need to be reeducated about Canada's history—to unlearn what is taught in the official accounts of its history and to learn about the histories of laws, practices, and traditions as told by Indigenous peoples. Dominantly situated settlers recorded and continue to control narratives about the "history of Canada." This "history" shapes the collective interpretative resources that are taken to be legitimate, and these, in turn, shape the relationships between Indigenous and non-Indigenous peoples. Importantly, acknowledging who gets to tell the stories and how the stories are told shapes Canada's *collective history* as one that is reflected in the collective interpretative resources *of settler-colonial peoples*.

The Indian Act of 1876 contained clauses that allowed the federal government to establish Indian residential schools. The result was that over one hundred federally supported schools were set up in most provinces across Canada and functioned for well over a century. Most schools operated as joint ventures with Catholic entities and with Anglican, Presbyterian, or United churches. Indian residential schools separated over 130,000 Indigenous children from their families and communities and had the explicit objective of removing and isolating children from the influence of homes, families, traditions, laws, languages, and cultures with the goal of assimilating them into the dominant culture. Remarkably, the last of the residential schools closed only in 1996.

On May 10, 2006, the government of Canada announced approval of the IRSSA drawn up with legal representatives of former students of residential schools, legal representatives of the churches involved in running those schools, the Assembly of First Nations, and other Indigenous organizations. The IRSSA was approved by the courts and came into effect on September 19, 2007. The settlement set out five main components: a common experience payment (CEP) for all eligible former students of residential schools, an independent assessment process (IAP) for claims of sexual or serious physical abuse, measures to support healing, commemorative activities, and the establishment of a TRC.

On June 11, 2008, then–Prime Minister Stephen Harper, along with leaders of the other federal political parties, formally apologized in the House of Commons for the harms caused by the residential school systems. The TRC part of the settlement began its work in 2008, with hearings across Canada that included public testimonies from residential school survivors and many others who participated in their national events and community hearings. More than six years of research culminated in the TRC's closing ceremonies held in Ottawa in June 2015 and a final six-volume report that outlines the history and legacy of residential schools and puts forward ninety-four "calls to action" identifying concrete steps to be taken on the path toward reconciliation. Many of the calls to action put forth in the TRC final report involve ways and means for learning about and giving credence to Indigenous collective interpretative resources that have survived despite Canada's history of repeated attempts to erase them through practices and policies that dispossessed them of land, ignored treaties, forced children into residential schools, and so on. In bringing these aspects of the dismissal of Indigenous knowledge to the fore, the TRC itself can be said to have adopted a broad mandate of recording hermeneutical rather than testimonial injustice. Perhaps more accurately, there is no longer any significant distinction to be drawn between testimonial and hermeneutical injustice when testimony is always and only interpreted in terms of the norms, structures, and institutions of the dominant and powerful.

The epistemological/ontological/political framework also reveals that Indigenous collective interpretative resources were and continue to be shaped by their histories, laws, institutions, activities, and practices in and through their interactions and embeddedness on land and in Indigenous communities. In the face of attempted erasures through residential schools, their collective interpretative resources have had to be remembered, retrieved, and recorded by the many people in communities of Indigenous peoples across Canada, in the work of Canada's TRC, and post-TRC in the research centers set up to retrieve and record lost languages, laws, traditions, and practices.

Returning to FitzGerald's (2020) defense of a department of care, we can now grasp that, in a settler-colonial context, such a department may miss the point insofar as it may still fail to recognize and acknowledge Indigenous collective interpretative resources of, for example, the meaning of care as it connects with Indigenous worldviews of the interconnectedness of humans with land and nonhuman animals.[1] The point is that a relational moral orientation of care may capture epistemological and ontological male biases in government structures and policies but fail to capture a relational moral and political orientation shaped by Indigenous languages, laws, institutions, policies, and traditions. What is seen, heard, and known are *dominant* collective interpretative resources reflecting the laws, institutions, structures, languages, and policies imposed in and through settler and colonial processes of taking land, negotiating (and often ignoring) treaties, negating or ignoring Indigenous-based constitutions and laws, and installing and protecting capitalist modes of production and resource extraction. Through the lens of Indigenous voices not heard and not recognized as legitimate perspectives, the concepts used by colonizers and the policies that emerge from them can be said to be tainted by a long history of relationships and processes of colonization that are ongoing.

Whether the dominant and powerful advocate for Indigenous peoples by using the language of rights, justice, care, recognition, reconciliation, self-determination, or sovereignty, how these concepts are understood is from the top-down perspective and collective interpretative resources of settler-colonial accounts of what these concepts mean. Coulthard (2014) has argued forcefully that recognition, for example, is framed in terms of policies of multiculturalism that allow the state to "recognize" what counts as Indigenous "culture"—thereby ignoring the importance of recognizing already existing and long-standing Indigenous laws, legal orders, treaties, and institutions. The point is also made with respect to the concept of sovereignty. As Courtney Jung (2018, 257) notes, "It is precisely Canadian sovereignty that is the root cause of Indigenous land dispossession and loss of sovereignty." Moreover, liberal theorists who defend the importance of the rule of law assume a constitution and a set of laws to which all are subjected (Koggel 2018).

These dominant collective interpretative resources operate at all levels: of perverted notions of care actualized in the institutional structures of the residential school system and the sixties scoop; of assumptions about the impartiality and neutrality of the rule of law that actually and only reflects the Canadian Constitution and Canada's laws more generally; of understandings of land and property; of mandates and policies as set out by the government and its departments (including the departments of Crown-Indigenous Relations and Northern Affairs Canada); of corporate interests in developing pipelines and extracting resources for profit; of finance and fiscal policies that prioritize resource extraction and industry over providing clean drinking water, health care, and so on. And so, we return to my central argument that builds on but also goes beyond an account of care as a critical political theory.

CONCLUSION

I have argued that a discussion of forms and levels of hermeneutical injustices, when applied to the settler-colonial context of Canada, can provide a deeper analysis of the epistemological/ontological/political triad than have the accounts of a *relational moral orientation of care* examined in this chapter. I've referred to the broader lens and perspective as a feminist relational political orientation that situates hermeneutical injustices in histories and contexts of oppression that reveal how gaps in understanding emerge from those in power being positioned to ignore, dismiss, and denigrate all that lies outside the collective interpretative resources they control, maintain, and assume. I have suggested that a critical feminist political theory of care may need to reach further into realms and perspectives beyond those revealed by a relational moral orientation of care. If the descriptions and analyses of networks of relationships are insufficiently broad, what may get missed are the ways in which accounts of practices and activities of care may themselves be shaped by colonial processes, histories of oppression, and historic injustices. This may be but one reason that Indigenous peoples have resisted a language of care that assumed they needed to be removed from their families and communities to be properly cared for. I have used the lens of feminist relational theory to reveal hermeneutical injustices at the broad level of worldviews, what FitzGerald (2022) refers to as a "pluriverse," to highlight the interconnectedness of the ontological, epistemological, and political. By uncovering the ontological, epistemological, and political assumptions underlying modernity's ties to colonialism, new and better ways of seeing, hearing, understanding, and knowing are thereby revealed.

NOTE

1. It should be noted that FitzGerald addresses some of these points in her book *Care and the Pluriverse: Rethinking Global Ethics* (2022).

REFERENCES

Bourgault, Sophie. 2020. "Epistemic Injustice, Face-to-Face Encounters, and Caring Institutions." *International Journal of Care and Caring* 4 (1): 91–107. Reprinted in this volume, chapter 2.

Coulthard, Glen Sean. 2014. *Red Skin, White Masks: Rejecting the Colonial Processes of Recognition*. Minneapolis: University of Minnesota Press.
Fisher, Berenice and Joan C. Tronto. 1990. "Toward a Feminist Theory of Caring." In *Circles of Care: Work and Identity in Women's Lives*, edited by Emily K. Abel and Margaret K. Nelson, 36–54. Albany: State University of New York Press.
FitzGerald, Maggie. 2020. "Reimagining Government with the Ethics of Care: A Department of Care" *Ethics and Social Welfare* 14 (3): 248–265.
———. 2022. *Care and the Pluriverse: Rethinking Global Ethics*. Bristol: Bristol University Press.
Fricker, Miranda. 2007. *Epistemic Injustice: Power and the Ethics of Knowing*. New York: Oxford University Press.
Gilligan, Carol. 1993. *In a Different Voice: Psychological Theory and Women's Development*. 2nd ed. Cambridge, MA: Harvard University Press.
Hunfeld, Katharina. 2022. "The Coloniality of Time in the Global Justice Debate: Decentring Western Linear Temporality." *Journal of Global Ethics* 18 (1): 100–117. https://doi.org/10.1080/17449626.2022.2052151.
Jung, Courtney. 2018. "Reconciliation: Six Reasons to Worry." *Journal of Global Ethics* 14 (2): 252–265.
Koggel, Christine. 2008. "Agency and Empowerment: Embodied Realities in a Globalized World." In *Agency and Embodiment*, edited by Letitia Meynell, Sue Campbell, and Susan Sherwin, 313–336. University Park: Pennsylvania State University Press.
———. 2012. "A Relational Approach to Equality: New Developments and Applications." In *Being Relational: Reflections on Relational Theory and Health Law and Policy*, edited by Jocelyn Downie and Jennifer Llewellyn, 63–88. Vancouver: University of British Columbia Press.
———. 2014. "Relational Remembering and Oppression." *Hypatia* 29 (2): 493–508.
———. 2018. "Epistemic Injustice in a Settler Nation: Canada's History of Erasing, Silencing, Marginalizing." *Journal of Global Ethics* 14 (2): 240–251.
Koggel, Christine, Ami Harbin, and Jennifer Llewellyn. 2022. "Feminist Relational Theory." *Journal of Global Ethics* 18 (1): 1–14. https://doi.org/10.1080/17449626.2022.2073702.
Medina, José. 2012. "Hermeneutical Injustice and Polyphonic Contextualism: Social Silences and Shared Hermeneutical Responsibilities." *Social Epistemology* 26 (2): 201–220.
Pohlhaus, Gaile, Jr. 2012. "Relational Knowing and Epistemic Injustice: Toward a Theory of Willful Hermeneutical Ignorance." *Hypatia* 27 (4): 715–735.
Robinson, Fiona. 2020. "Resisting Hierarchies through Relationality in the Ethics of Care." *International Journal of Care and Caring* 4 (1): 11–23.
Simpson, Audra. 2014. *Mohawk Interruptus: Political Life across the Borders of Settler States*. Durham, NC: Duke University Press.
Tronto, Joan C. 1993. *Moral Boundaries: A Political Argument for an Ethic of Care*. New York: Routledge.
———. 2010. "Creating Caring Institutions: Politics, Plurality, and Purpose." *Ethics and Social Welfare* 4 (2): 158–171.

2 · EPISTEMIC INJUSTICE, FACE-TO-FACE ENCOUNTERS, AND CARING INSTITUTIONS

SOPHIE BOURGAULT

Canada's Chief Public Health Officer released a damning report in 2019 concerning the significant effects of stigma and prejudice on the provision of health care across the country. This report showed that some health inequities are closely linked to the way nurses and doctors interact with, and listen to, their patients (Government of Canada 2019b). As several of the interviews conducted highlighted, many racialized, LGBTQ+, and Indigenous Canadians hold the view that their testimonies are not taken seriously or genuinely listened to within healthcare settings (Government of Canada 2019b, 35). But of course, there was nothing new about the 2019 report; similar research has documented for decades some of the serious consequences of these failures in listening. Indeed, countless studies have shown the impact of prejudice or implicit bias on the communication between health professionals and racialized patients—for instance, less time spent with the latter than with white patients, less credibility given to their testimonies or to their reporting of pain, and less participation of these patients in decision making (e.g., Dovidio et al. 2008; Penner et al. 2012; Goodman et al. 2017).

The communicative dysfunctions documented here are in part what philosopher Miranda Fricker has termed "epistemic injustices"—forms of harm that entail speakers' testimonies being unduly ignored or downgraded. These are discursive dysfunctions that take place regularly in our hospitals, but also in our courts, schools, workplaces, and social service counters (Dotson 2012; Kidd, Medina, and Pohlhaus 2017). Epistemic injustices can be tied to both what is said (the *content* of claims) and *how* it is said (the style of delivery—e.g., a speaker's accent, gaze, body posture). As Fricker (2007, 1) argues in her very influential *Epistemic Injustice*, these injustices generally take two forms: "Testimonial injustice occurs when prejudice causes a hearer to give a deflated level of credibility to a speaker's word: hermeneutical injustice occurs at a prior stage, when a gap in collective interpretive resources puts someone at an unfair disadvantage when it comes to making sense of their social experiences." One of the goals of this ever-growing literature on epistemic injustice is to show that when someone is not adequately heard because of their skin color, class, sexual orientation, or gender, what this person suffers is a serious harm, an *injustice*; one is marginalized and undermined in one's capacity as "knower"—as a participant and giver of information in an epistemic community. As scholars in the field argue, this epistemic marginalization is *fueled by* other types of injustices and marginalization (socioeconomic, political, cultural, etc.), and it ends up reinforcing them.

Fricker's book describes at length the harms caused by epistemic injustices (e.g., nonrecognition, humiliation, unemployment, loss of confidence); it also proposes a virtue that could help mitigate some of these dysfunctions: namely, epistemic justice or what Fricker often refers to as "virtuous hearing." Having spent years thinking chiefly about what epistemic justice entails for individuals, she has increasingly turned her attention to what it would mean for an *institution* to possess this virtue and to showing how critical the latter is for making our political lives more inclusive and democratic (Fricker 2012, 2013, 2016).

This chapter's main objective is to discuss two of Fricker's numerous proposals concerning how to increase epistemic justice. The chapter argues that these two proposals pull us in different directions: the first entails the *unveiling of particulars*, whereas the other involves the *veiling* of particulars (e.g., the concealing of names, bodily features, accents). The first route calls upon us to eliminate epistemic injustices by cultivating a capacity to understand the other—that is, a hermeneutic generosity on the part of the civil servant / employee that requires attention to *particularity*. The second involves structuring decision making such that public employees are in fact prevented from allowing unconscious biases to impair their impartiality. If the latter route rests on a lack of trust in judgment, I argue that the former is anchored in a more optimistic view of human beings' ability to exercise judgment, to exercise practical reason decently, under adequate temporal conditions.

The chapter's second objective is to assess Fricker's proposals from the perspective of care ethics, which has of late been concerned with a similar project to that of Fricker's: namely, to render institutions more inclusive, responsive, and democratic (e.g., Robinson 2011; Tronto 2013; Barnes et al. 2015). Many have emphasized the urgent need to decrease constraints on democratic participation and decrease domination; others have argued for better dialogical skills in that project—particularly *attentive listening*. As such, Fricker's reflections on what "virtuous hearing/listening" entails for ethicopolitical practice (particularly in large bureaucratic organizations) is of utmost relevance for care ethics.

To marry a discussion of bureaucratic institutions with care ethics might seem an odd thing to do: after all, numerous care ethicists have criticized bureaucracies for their impersonality, hierarchy, and standardization. Many have lamented the fact that caregivers and workers within large bureaucratic organizations often experience painful contradictions between institutional rules/procedures and their desire to provide *personalized* care (e.g., Tronto 2010; Glenn 2000; cf. Stensöta 2010; Engster 2020). What this chapter shows is that there is indeed an essential tension, a basic ambivalence, at the heart of public service delivery when it comes to issues like epistemic justice and that any attempt at *improving* public service ethics—at making institutions more caring and more inclusive—will come face-to-face with a dissonance between principles. As such, the fact that Fricker's proposals push us in opposite directions is not a sign that she is confused; it is, rather, revelatory of the trade-offs entailed in the push to deliver public services in a manner that is not compromised by epistemic injustices. This chapter also indicates that care ethics has pertinent correctives to offer to the likes of Fricker—particularly regarding the significance of time and embodied contact as well as the need to consider epistemic wrongs within the context of an economy of credibility and with an eye to larger, more radical *structural* changes.

UNVEILING PARTICULARS: DISCRETION, LISTENING, AND JUDGMENT

In *Street-Level Bureaucracy*, Michael Lipsky (1990) underscored the significant amount of discretion possessed by street-level bureaucrats—that is, public employees who have regular face-to-face encounters with citizens (e.g., police officers, social welfare administrators). His study showed that these public servants have substantial freedom when they apply and interpret policies—discretion is inscribed in the very nature of their work. But what Lipsky (1990) also underscored is that several factors affect the quality of this discretionary work—e.g., limited financial resources, unclear policy goals, insufficient time and energy. Because of these pressures, frontline workers must often resort to mental "short-cuts" and stereotypes to perform their tasks: "At best, street-level bureaucrats invent benign modes of mass processing that more or less permit them to deal with the public fairly, appropriately and thoughtfully. At worst, they give in to favoritism, stereotyping, convenience" (1990, xiv). While not all consequences of bureaucrats' resorts to stereotypes are dire, they can reinforce existing socioeconomic inequalities (e.g., Hastings 2009).

That class, gender, or racial prejudice can sometimes corrupt face-to-face encounters between public institutions' employees and citizens, that they can corrupt the exercise of discretion (making it arbitrary or highly partial), is also central to the literature on epistemic injustice and oppression. It is claimed that when prejudices compromise the way doctors, police officers, and judges listen to an individual and exercise judgment, this individual is harmed in her capacity as an epistemic subject. In *Epistemic Injustice*, Fricker (2007) analyzes at length these intricate connections between prejudices and injustice (and their various upshots). What I wish to focus on here is chiefly what she has to say about how to diminish the pull of prejudice.

As noted above, the main corrective Fricker proposes is the virtue of "epistemic justice." This "virtuous hearing" is a type of attention and listening that entails at least two things on behalf of listeners:[1] first, a critical awareness of the impact our power and identities have on how we speak and assess one another in communicative exchanges; second, an *upward compensation in our judgment* when there is a possibility that negative prejudices (or limited collective interpretative resources) might cause us to regard a speaker as untrustworthy, unintelligible, or unreliable. The goal of this upward compensation is to bring one's assessment of the person's credibility to what it *might have been* had the person not been associated with a negative group stereotype. It is very important to note here that the only credibility adjustments that Fricker is concerned with are upward ones (i.e., those needed to address credibility *deficits*). She is not concerned with the issue of correcting for the *excess* in credibility given, say, to a doctor or professor. Fricker (2007, 20–21) believes that credibility excesses are not deeply problematic and do not constitute a harm (an issue we will return to).

Now, Fricker admits that in ambiguous situations it might be too demanding to expect individuals to make these credibility adjustments when they fear the impact of prejudice on their work; if so, they should withhold judgment. But if the listener has *sufficient time* and resources, he ought to seek additional information (e.g., consult other people with similar experience or sociodemographic background). What specific form the epistemic virtue will take in practice varies from context to context; much remains unspecified. But consider one passage where Fricker (2007, 171–172, emphasis added) describes succinctly what "virtuous hearing" might entail:

> In practical contexts *where there is enough time* and the matter is sufficiently important, the virtuous hearer may effectively be able to help generate a more inclusive hermeneutical micro-climate through the appropriate kind of dialogue ... such dialogue involves a more pro-active and more socially aware kind of listening.... This sort of listening involves listening as much to what is *not* said as to what is said. Such virtuous behavior by a hearer will be more or less difficult to achieve depending on the circumstances, and in particular, *depending on how much or how little is shared with the speaker in terms of relevant social experience.*

Two elements are worth underscoring in this passage: first, the effect that shared or similar socioeconomic experiences can have on discursive exchanges. The uptake for us here (one Fricker does not spell out) is that one remedy for communicative failures in socioinstitutional life might be to decrease disparities in wealth and sociocultural goods. Second, note Fricker's all-too-brief mention of time's importance for epistemic justice and decent institutional practice—a claim she does not develop either. This is surprising given the great significance of temporal resources for institutional practice: as we observed above (with Lipsky 1990), it is largely because of time constraints that street-level bureaucrats often resort to stereotypes. Kidd and Carel (2017) have also shown how critical time pressures are as a key source of communication failure and of epistemic injustices within healthcare settings.

Care ethics might enrich these discussions by inviting scholars of social epistemology to look even more closely at the significance of time. Care theorists have forcefully shown that temporal factors are critical for providing care that is competent and responsive to particular needs (e.g., Damamme and Paperman 2009; Tronto 2003). They have also underscored the extent to which decent face-to-face encounters, which often require a slow rather than fast pace, are threatened by the gospel of neoliberalism and calls for austerity. Some have also insisted that it is up to (time-privileged) tenured scholars and policy makers to push back against neoliberal discourse, including against the latter's unquestioned view that more time is something we simply cannot afford (Bourgault 2016). Note that for Tronto (2013) it is not solely for a specific situation like hospital care that we need more time. More generally, *it is our political communities as a whole* that require more significant time investments; it is time *spent together* that is one of the backbones of solidarity and trust, which matter for decreasing sociopolitical marginalization. If care itself is about relationships (as care ethics has always emphasized), "relationships require, more than anything else, two things: sufficient time and proximity" (Tronto 2013, 166).

Care theorists and scholars working on epistemic injustice ought to join forces to think critically about the impact of neoliberal management practices and social acceleration, for these weigh heavily on institutional responsiveness and our ability to offer particularized and nonprejudicial public services—whether health, justice, or education (e.g., Hartman and Darab 2012). In these joint efforts, it is crucial in my view to keep in mind a fairly simple (yet often overlooked) fact: namely, that time and attentiveness are radically *finite* resources. When we listen attentively to a particular individual (whether a subordinated or a highly privileged person), these are temporal and cognitive resources that do *not* go to someone else.

Differently put: the attentive hearing, recognition, or credibility we accord individuals is something finite and comparative—two claims Fricker rejects (2007, 20–21). Contra Fricker, I think that we should not only concern ourselves with credibility *deficits* that marginalized people experience but also consider the unduly high levels of credibility and attention offered to the privileged or powerful (i.e., credibility *excesses*). Deficits and excesses cannot be disentangled, as José Medina (2011, 21) has rightly underscored. Put most simply, my point here is that we ought to consider epistemic injustices within the context of a more global economy of attention and credibility.

Let us now look a bit more closely at what is entailed in Fricker's "virtuous hearing." Particularly relevant here is an essay by Fricker (2012) about silence and institutional prejudice, where she discusses the case of a young Black man whose encounter with the police and judiciary was compromised by discrimination. Dwayne Brooks,

Fricker writes, was "not properly heard; he was silenced... the police at the scene were not ready to hear him without prejudice" (2012, 301–302). But if Brooks was silenced (and here silence is characterized as an ill), Fricker observes that *there is not one but several kinds of silence*. Reminiscent of what several care scholars have argued (Robinson 2011; Tronto 2013; Bourgault 2016), Fricker insists that there is one positive type of silence that is critical for decent institutions and justice: namely, that entailed in listening, in a caring, *attentive silence*. Drawing briefly on philosophers Simone Weil and Iris Murdoch (who have both been important for care theorists), Fricker (2012, 287) describes epistemic justice in terms of *silent listening*—describing it as a "kind of silence [that] belongs with a moral attitude of attention to others—an openness to who they are and what they have to say."

Quite significantly, this "who they are" entails an attunement and respect for the *particular* individual one is faced with—whether in a police station or a hospital's triage room. For Fricker (2012, 296), "This capacity for attention—the ability to see through prejudice to real human individuals is indispensable in ethical life." Epistemic justice in her view entails attending to distinct, embodied beings whose social situatedness (class, neighborhood, gender, racial background) shapes sociopolitical encounters. One ought not to pretend to be capable of a kind of difference blindness—rather, the public employee should understand the specific social situations of those they are serving, and that knowledge should inform the judgments they make.

This call for attentive listening is certainly appealing enough. But it is far from clear how one could foster this in institutions (beyond ensuring that public employees have sufficient time, which is, again, critical), nor is it obvious how we might go about "operationalizing" the credibility adjustments called for by Fricker. Some might suggest that general rules/guidelines ought to be established to orient a doctor or a civil servant in their credibility adjustments (if they suspect that sexism, racism, or ageism might affect their judgments). But Fricker (2007, 91) disagrees: there can be no "across-the-board" policy regarding credibility adjustments given the multilayered nature of social identity. We simply cannot come up with detailed enough rules that would capture the complexity of the world and power differentials.

To recapitulate, what we saw in this section is that virtuous hearing is for Fricker a matter of making adjustments based on *more information* about the *particular* person we are dealing with, and that there are no rules for the exercise of this virtue. What undergirds Fricker's main route to cultivating epistemic justice (i.e., unveiling/attending to particulars, and *correcting* for particulars) is a fairly *high degree of trust in human judgment*—a trust in our hermeneutic skills and ability to reach a context-sensitive, situated judgment without codes/rules.

However, despite the fact that she does not wish to propose guidelines for credibility adjustments, Fricker does emphasize (albeit too briefly) one concrete measure that might help foster spontaneous credibility adjustments: plain old human contact or familiarity. With regular exposure to sociodemographic diversity, many markers that feed prejudicial stereotypes might vanish in her view:

"An initially socially loaded accent gets normalised with habituation; a socially alien conversational style becomes familiar; the colour of someone's skin becomes irrelevant; their sex no longer impinges; their age is forgotten" (Fricker 2007, 96). Here, what Fricker (2007, 96) has in mind is particularly the familiarity gained "over the course of a conversation, or perhaps a more sustained acquaintance."

The social science related to the effects of direct, face-to-face interaction on prejudice is complex and multilayered. Much depends on the type of interaction and the particular geographic, economic, and historical circumstances. I certainly do not wish to suggest that contact *always* decreases prejudices or that absence of contact *necessarily* feeds racism (the nuanced findings of Canadian political scientists Antoine Bilodeau and Luc Turgeon [2014] are worth taking seriously). Nonetheless, there is still some evidence that Fricker is correct; many have shown the significance of contact and familiarity for challenging ambient prejudices (e.g., Vezzali and Stathi 2016). And certainly Fricker's insistence on the importance of closeness and embodied contact is echoed loudly in care ethics scholarship, such as that of Hamington (2004), Tronto (2013), and Brugère (2011, 121; my translation): the latter insists on the urgency of "public services finding anew the route of proximity with users". But as we will see, to call for frequent, embodied contact and for familiarity is precisely what runs counter to the other route proposed by Fricker and political scientists interested in diminishing prejudicial discretion—a route to which we now turn.

VEILING PARTICULARS: OF SCREENS, ANONYMIZATION, AND ALGORITHMS

In the vast multidisciplinary literature on epistemic injustice and oppression, several scholars have shown that certain bodily markers (skin color, weight, gender) can be closely associated with negative group stereotypes that affect the way testimonies are received. As such, if bodily presence and physiological features are one significant source of discriminatory practice in institutions, one might be tempted to suggest that the veiling or hiding of some of these physiological markers (e.g., ethnicity or gender) could be one way to prevent corrupt judgment on the part of doctors, civil servants, and teachers. One might also consider the veiling of names or of age as one way to prevent unfavorable institutional treatment based on gender, age, capacity, or ethnic traits.

This is precisely one of the paths Fricker (2016) explores in recent work on epistemic injustice and institutions (a path care ethics would quibble with, as we will see): namely, anonymization or, as I wish to phrase it, the veiling of particulars. Fricker tackles the issue of anonymization within the context of a discussion of the fault and responsibilities public servants might have for letting their dealings with citizens be tainted by a negative implicit prejudice (38). For Fricker, the influence that implicit prejudices have on our judgments is exceedingly hard to perceive; they are biases that we are "radically unaware of" (34). Partially for that reason, she believes that we cannot assign moral blame to the employee who has let these biases affect her judgment. Nonetheless, she insists that these situations do not free public servants from the responsibility to do something: there should be concrete acts done to address the harm. And it is here that the remedy of anonymization (the veiling of particulars) comes in. Fricker insists that the responsibility of biased employees in these no-fault situations entails two things: First is an immediate obligation to mend (if possible) the particular case where something went wrong. Fricker's example here concerns the chair of a university appointment process who is alerted to the fact that she has unconsciously evaluated all the writing submissions from male candidates more favorably than women's because of an implicit prejudice. For Fricker, what the "mending" of the case entails is that the chair should withdraw from the committee and have the files reassessed by someone else "under anonymized conditions" (47). Second, the chair also has an *institutional* obligation that goes beyond this case: she must change her workplace practices more generally. Significantly, the concrete example of change offered by Fricker is, here again, the *anonymization* of files; the committee's chair has an "obligation to push institutionally for greater anonymization." Fricker is convinced that "the removal of names at the top of writing samples for long-listing purposes in appointment processes" would be one way to diminish the likelihood of prejudice again slipping in.[2]

Now, Fricker is obviously not the first to suggest that the veiling of names or bodily features (e.g., markers of gender, religious affiliations) might improve hiring practices or employees' judgment in public institutions. There are many studies indicating the effectiveness of such practices: think of the well-known case of orchestras in the United States that started adopting blind audition policies, placing musicians behind a screen during auditions, a veiling practice that led to increased female hires (Goldin and Rouse 1997).

That the anonymization of files can increase impartiality and diminish social marginalization is precisely why some public administration scholars have looked with hope to the increased usage of digital technology in state-citizen interactions—something I wish to consider here as one manner of "veiling" particulars, of hiding bodies. Bovens and Zouridis (2002), for instance, suggest that fewer face-to-face encounters between street-level bureaucrats and citizens could decrease bad discretion/arbitrary treatment. In their study, the authors considered the increased use of information and communication technology (ICT) in the Dutch student loan and scholarship system and in traffic regulations (e.g., cameras for speed ticketing). From one angle, the increased resort to ICT is a positive development since "hardly any margin remains for the arbitrary exercise of power in implementing rules" (181). But the authors do not praise this wholeheartedly: they warn that the discretionary power formally possessed by employees at university desks or police offices has moved elsewhere—namely, into the hands of system designers. These designers may not have "discretion" in the old sense of application of general rules to particulars, but they have something more: discretion over the very "drafting and composing of the *rules themselves*" (181). This is worth underscoring: even if we remove the particular biases at the street level by removing all-too-human, imperfect civil servants, our institutions will not necessarily be free from biases. Discretion may not always be decreased by resorting to "blind" programs; it can also get obscured, rendered *less* amenable to critique. Algorithms can reinforce social categories and prejudices (Origgi and Ciranna 2017) and may thus end up working *against* the creation of more inclusive and caring institutions.

To be clear, there are benefits to having a veiling of particulars and a recourse to nonhuman means of processing cases. We saw above some of these benefits in the case of orchestra auditions, which decreased sexism in hiring; we could also mention the benefits attached to other cases of veiling particulars in institutions like universities. Consider the increasingly prevalent practice of professors having students' work evaluated anonymously to decrease bias. Web-based learning and online university discussion groups could also be regarded as examples of projects that can, by veiling bodies, increase the inclusion of marginalized students and promote unprejudiced assessment by teachers. Online interaction (with cameras off) can sometimes provide an anonymous forum for increasing the participation of students who may lack confidence in an embodied setting because of prejudices tied to their race, weight, or disability. Their participation might thus be increased by allowing them to gain discursive confidence through the bracketing of bodily or cultural markers. Somewhat similarly (albeit in a different setting), some welfare benefit applicants feel that a digital encounter with government minimizes the humiliation entailed in asking for support because the gaze of the bureaucrat is avoided (Hetling, Watson, and Horgan 2014). (One might here retort that better "solutions" to the issue of humiliation would be to *prevent* poverty in the first place and to change societal perceptions of vulnerability—a project to which care ethicists have been actively devoted.)

These are just a few examples of the benefits of veiling particulars and anonymizing encounters between citizens and institutions. What I wish to underscore is that choosing measures of the sort *takes us away* from what was called for earlier in this chapter (e.g., contact, attending to particulars); it runs counter to the previous strategy and presupposes a radically different account of our hermeneutic skills or of our capacity to "listen through the noise of prejudice." For instance, choosing the path of veiling entails trade-offs in terms of the quality of the responsiveness and attentiveness of the institution and its employees (two qualities repeatedly underscored by care ethicists; e.g., Tronto 2010; Stensöta 2010). In their review of research on ICT and discretion, Busch and Henriksen (2018) have concluded that if the benefits of digital discretion are significant in terms of "ethical and democratic values" (integrity, fairness, accountability), the losses are considerable for "*relational* values" (caring, fairness, decency, humanity). What is sacrificed when resorting to anonymous, digital citizen-government encounters is the consideration of *particulars* that may appear at first glance irrelevant for decision making but that are in fact critical. Studies indicate that for now computer systems are unable to process information in a way that takes complex cases into account (Busch and Henriksen 2018). Digital rigidity typically compromises the responsiveness and attentiveness of public service; hence a choice might have to be made between conflicting values. What I suggest is that *the path of anonymization, which tends to compromise attentiveness, is at odds with what care ethics celebrates.*

Obviously, the trade-offs and consequences of veiling particulars vary according to each institution and case. There is an obvious difference between the loss of human contact entailed in renewing a driver's license online instead of in person and that involved in registering a child at a school with a web-based form (instead of in person). In the latter case, interacting with a human being (a teacher or secretary) is of greater significance. Nonetheless, in these efforts to anonymize or digitalize public encounters one sometimes finds a similar logic: to get rid of the frailties and unreliability of human judgment precisely *by removing the human*—by putting on blinders. Some might object that the turn to digital technologies / anonymizing measures is hardly relevant for the institutions care scholars are concerned with (e.g., health care, education, eldercare). But one ought to be cautious here: the domains of education and elderly care have recently been significantly transformed by technology and anonymizing measures (Hartman and Darab 2012; Sharkey 2014). And it is partially for this reason that my chapter considers Fricker's "anonymizing" measures; care ethics offers a timely reminder to consider more closely what sort of losses an increased resort to digital technology in caring institutions might entail.

One of the larger sociopolitical reasons we should think about the losses entailed in resorting to digital or "anonymizing" means in institutions is that we know that responsive listening, contact, and "situational adaptation" can increase legitimacy and trust in communities (see, e.g., Jansson and Erlingsson 2014), which are, in turn, critical for the quality of epistemic exchanges and caring relationships. On the importance of face-to-face contact, Elizabeth Anderson (2012) offers us a pertinent rejoinder. In a piece criticizing Fricker for endorsing overly individual means to epistemic justice, Anderson argues that we ought to resort to structural remedies such as group integration measures (e.g., eliminate segregated schooling along racial or class lines): "When social groups are educated *together* on terms of equality, they share equally in educational resources and thus have access to the same (legitimate) markers of credibility.... Shared inquiry also tends to produce a shared reality, which can help overcome hermeneutical injustice and its attendant testimonial injustices" (Anderson 2012, 171). From a care ethics perspective this is crucial: this production of a shared reality (even if imperfect and crisscrossed by inequalities and tensions) is one significant reason why we might want to hold on to face-to-face encounters wherever possible (and pertinent) and to consider carefully the long-term losses that might be incurred by addressing epistemic marginalization/injustices via "quick-fix" veiling measures.

This section has considered a few of the trade-offs entailed in resorting to anonymization measures and technology. Before concluding, let me note that Fricker (2013) also acknowledges the importance of monitoring measures and incentives (financial, promotion) to help minimize epistemic injustice in institutions. But quite significantly, Fricker (2013, 1326) observes that for some institutions (e.g., social care and education) it may *not* be possible and desirable to adopt these: here, good outcomes depend "not merely on certain things being done, but rather their being done in the right spirit." For these cases, she insists, we ought "to cultivate a driving *ethos* within the institution" (1326). For Fricker, there is "no substitute for the 'ethos,' for a collective value commitment." In many respects, then, we have come full circle: we are back to ethos and to a fairly optimistic perspective on what our hermeneutic/listening skills might accomplish despite their daily dysfunctions. We are back to the main remedy espoused by Fricker in her early work: namely, virtuous hearing or *better listening*.

Now, one might object that in the face of discriminatory treatment in health care and in the judicial system like that encountered by Indigenous women in Canada (see, e.g., Razack 2002; Goodman et al. 2017; Government of Canada 2019a; Government of British Columbia 2020) the language of "virtuous hearing" might be at best naïve, at worst offensive and politically irresponsible. There are, after all, complex but entirely concrete, structural injustices caused by colonialism and patriarchy that urgently need remedying to address the past and ongoing injustices done. But this does not lessen the importance of improving the epistemic quality of exchanges with officials in the *imperfect* condition in which both parties find themselves. And, indeed, from the perspective of some Indigenous women, it is the refusal to acknowledge the importance of attentive listening that might be politically negligent. For some, it is colonialism and patriarchy that are partially at the root of the inability to listen and that ought to be resisted. This thesis speaks to the view of Gayatri Spivak (1990, 59–60), who once observed, "For me, the question 'Who should speak?' is less crucial than 'Who will listen?' 'I will speak for myself as a Third World person' is an important position for political mobilisation today. But the real demand is that, when I speak from that position, I should be listened to seriously."

Nevertheless, the case of missing and murdered Indigenous women in Canada underscores not only the interest of Fricker's work for care ethicists and feminist theorists more generally but also its grave *limitations*. Two of these (there are additional ones) are that Fricker insufficiently considers the importance of structural/ material changes and that she radically downplays the agency and capacity for resistance of subordinated groups in my view. Indeed, Fricker (2007, 2013) focuses much more on the responsibilities of the dominant and privileged as well as *their* virtues, *their* institutional value commitments. In contrast, a care ethics perspective on epistemic justice compels us to pay greater attention to the *relationship* itself as well as to the role of marginalized groups and *their* epistemic virtues, *their* capacities for mobilization, resistance, and solidarity (cf. Medina 2013; in this volume, see most notably the chapters of Koggel; Harris; Doucet, Jewell, and Watts).

Indeed, it is largely in response to *Indigenous* mobilization and solidarity, pushing authorities to address centuries of colonial violence, that the Canadian government finally launched its national inquiry into Missing and Murdered Indigenous Women and Girls (MMIWG). One view expressed by some Indigenous women at the time of this mobilization was that Canadian institutions needed to genuinely *listen*. Many argued that one reason for the tragic fate of many girls and women was that police officers, community workers, and judicial bodies were unable to "listen through the noise of prejudice" (to use Fricker's terms). Partially for this reason, at the pre-inquiry stage, several Indigenous families were angry at Canadian officials' request that the inquiry *not* focus on racism and dysfunctional communications with the police (Tasker 2017). Nonetheless, the interim report (Government of Canada 2017) amply acknowledged this racism and the grave testimonial injustices experienced by the victims' families—e.g., police officers' half listening and scolding (blaming victims for substance abuse, poverty) and their radical failures to document disappearances and investigate in a fair manner (in these matters, police have a high degree of discretion that has been revoltingly abused).

Quite significantly, it is in part also a lack of listening and face-to-face responsiveness that almost made the inquiry itself derail shortly after it began; some people in remote communities who wished to testify were not offered the opportunity to do so *in person* but were instead invited to submit comments online or by phone. These online submissions were deemed by many an insulting and inadequate way to listen to and document people's testimonies (Galloway 2017). Face-to-face encounters were called for; partially as a result of these complaints (and many others of a different nature), some members of the inquiry resigned and some people called for an end to the inquiry. Such calls were not heeded; the commission continued its work and presented its final report to the public in June 2019. Nonetheless, these angry protests are a sober reminder of the need to consider closely the significance of a face-to-face attending to particulars.

Once again, this is absolutely not to suggest that the chief thing required to address the violence and discrimination faced by some racialized groups or some Indigenous women in Canada is for privileged white Canadians (or their institutions) to better listen, although that would be a feat. Any serious effort toward epistemic justice will definitely require *massive* structural, cultural, and material changes, radical reforms of the legal and policing systems, the repatriation of land (Tuck and Yang 2012), a meaningful Indigenization of research, universities, and other institutions (without succumbing to epistemic extractivism), a profound challenging of settler ignorance, and so much more (Simpson 2017; Cook 2018; Starblanket 2018; see also Doucet, Jewell, and Watts in this volume). The simple fact that the MMIWG final report contains a total of 231 recommendations (most of which have not been acted upon) is a clear indication of the very wide range of changes required in order to work our way to something even remotely akin to (epistemic) repair.

CONCLUSION

This chapter has suggested that there is a tension between some of the remedies proposed by Fricker to alleviate epistemic injustices—a tension between the veiling and the unveiling of particulars. My modest aim here was to underscore the basic ambivalence located in efforts to make institutions more inclusive, caring, and responsive. I have indicated that when one seeks to veil particulars in an attempt to mitigate for epistemic injustice, one faces a conflict with another principle. Indeed, one cannot *simultaneously* seek both the unveiling and the veiling of particulars: in any given situation, one will have to choose which policy one wishes to pursue—and each choice will face significant trade-offs.

If bodily presence can cause prejudicial treatment, bodily absence can entail the loss of recognition and of something distinctively human and desirable for (caring) institutions. The bodily absence entailed in the institutional recourse to digital service delivery might—paradoxically—lead to the loss of significant means to undercut negative prejudices in the long term. Direct contact and *familiarity* with difference—which entails significant temporal and financial commitments— might help mitigate identity-based prejudice (though, as we noted, the devil is in the details). To give up on the human capacity to correct for some of our epistemic difficulties by resorting to more reliable, impartial "technological" means or to anonymizing measures might in the long run increase some of our discursive and epistemic failures.

This is not to suggest that we ought to—or *can*—completely put aside ICT (and other "blinding" measures) in institutional life. This essay is not a Luddite manifesto. But it is a *concerned* reminder, voiced from a care ethics perspective, about the ethical and political importance of face-to-face contact and of listening. It is also an invitation to carefully consider some of the difficult trade-offs and dissonances entailed in the choosing of veiling or unveiling measures—a timely invitation, I think, as we witness the massive entry of digital tools in institutions, including those scholars considered largely immune to algorithms or disembodied technology (i.e., education, health).

ACKNOWLEDGMENTS

This is a shortened and modified version of an article previously published in the *International Journal of Care and Caring* (2020). Thanks to Bristol University Press for the permission to reprint. I also wish to thank Petr Urban, Fiona Robinson, and Rob Sparling for helpful comments on an earlier version of this text.

NOTES

1. Fricker (2007) uses the term "listening" widely—it can include the reading of written documents and observations of artwork. Nonetheless, most cases she examines involve face-to-face attending to *someone's speech*.
2. Fricker (2016) briefly acknowledges that anonymizing files in hiring might have some undesirable consequences. In the case of a university hiring committee, she observes that the veiling of information such as age might disadvantage young PhDs and favor senior scholars—and this in turn is likely to *disfavor* members of groups who are underrepresented in academia. She is aware of the trade-offs.

REFERENCES

Anderson, Elizabeth. 2012. "Epistemic Justice as a Virtue of Social Institutions." *Social Epistemology* 26 (2): 163–173.

Barnes, Marian, Tula Brannelly, Lizzie Ward, and Nicki Ward, eds. 2015. *Ethics of Care: Critical Advances in International Perspective*. Bristol: Policy Press.

Bilodeau, Antoine, and Luc Turgeon. 2014. "L'immigration: Une menace pour la culture québécoise?" *Canadian Journal of Political Science* 47 (2): 281–305.

Bourgault, Sophie. 2016. "Attentive Listening and Care in a Neoliberal Era: Weilian Insights for Hurried Times." *Ethics and Politics* 18 (3): 311–377.

Bovens, Mark, and Stavros Zouridis. 2002. "From Street-Level to System-Level Bureaucracies: How Information and Communication Technology Is Transforming Administrative Discretion and Constitutional Control." *Public Administration Review* 62 (2): 174–183.

Busch, Peter A., and Helle Z. Henriksen. 2018. "Digital Discretion: A Systematic Literature Review of ICT and Street-Level Discretion." *Information Polity* 23 (1): 3–28.

Brugère, Fabienne. 2011. *L'éthique du 'care'*. Paris: Presses Universitaires de France.

Cook, Anna. 2018. "Recognizing Settler Ignorance in the Canadian Truth and Reconciliation Commission." *Feminist Philosophy Quarterly* 4 (4): article 6.

Dalmiya, Vrinda. 2016. *Caring to Know: Comparative Care Ethics, Feminist Epistemology, and the Mahabharata*. Oxford: Oxford University Press.

Damamme, Aurélie, and Patricia Paperman. 2009. "Temps du care et organisation sociale du travail en famille." *Temporalités* 1036:1–13.

Dotson, Kristie. 2012. "A Cautionary Tale: On Limiting Epistemic Oppression." *Frontiers: A Journal of Women Studies* 33 (1): 24–47.

Dovidio, John F., Louis A. Penner, Terrance L. Albrecht, Wynne E. Norton, Samuel L. Gaertner, and Josette Nicole Shelton. 2008. "Disparities and Distrust: The Implications of Psychological Processes for Understanding Racial Disparities in Health and Health Care." *Social Science & Medicine* 67 (3): 478–486.

Engster, Daniel. 2020. "A Public Ethics of Care for Policy Implementation." *American Journal of Political Science* 64:621–633.

Fricker, Miranda. 2007. *Epistemic Injustice: Power and the Ethics of Knowing*. Oxford: Oxford University Press.

———. 2012. "Silence and Institutional Prejudice." In *Out from the Shadows: Analytical Feminist Contributions to Traditional Philosophy*, edited by Sharon L. Crasnow and Anita M. Superson, 287–306. Oxford: Oxford University Press.

———. 2013. "Epistemic Justice as a Condition of Political Freedom." *Synthese* 190 (7): 1317–1332.

———. 2016. "Fault and No-Fault Responsibility for Implicit Prejudice." In *The Epistemic Life of Groups: Essays in the Epistemology of Collectives*, edited by Michael S. Brady and Miranda Fricker, 33–50. Oxford: Oxford University Press.

Galloway, Gloria. 2017. "Inquiry into Missing and Murdered Women a Failure: Indigenous Group." *Globe and Mail*, May 16, 2017. https://www.theglobeandmail.com/news/politics/inquiry-into-missing-and-murdered-women-a-failure-indigenous-group-says/article35003027/.

Glenn, Evelyn Nakano. 2000. "Creating a Caring Society." *Contemporary Sociology* 29 (1): 84–94.

Goldin, Claudia, and Cecilia Rouse. 1997. "Orchestrating Impartiality: The Impact of 'Blind' Auditions on Female Musicians." NBER working paper no. 5903. https://www.nber.org/papers/w5903.

Goodman, Ashley, et al. 2017. "'They Treated Me Like Crap and I Know It Was Because I Was Native': The Healthcare Experiences of Aboriginal Peoples Living in Vancouver's Inner City." *Social Science & Medicine* 178:87–94.

Government of British Columbia. 2020. "In Plain Sight: Addressing Indigenous-Specific Racism and Discrimination in B.C. Health Care." https://www.bcchr.ca/sites/default/files/group-opsei/in-plain-sight-full-report.pdf.

Government of Canada. 2017. "Our Women and Girls Are Sacred: National Inquiry into Missing and Murdered Indigenous Women and Girls." Interim report. http://www.mmiwg-ffada.ca/wp-content/uploads/2018/03/ni-mmiwg-interim-report.pdf.

———. 2019a. "Inquiry into Missing and Murdered Indigenous Women and Girls." Final report. https://www.mmiwg-ffada.ca/.

———. 2019b. "Towards a More Inclusive Health System." Chief Public Health Officer's Report on the State of Public Health in Canada. https://www.canada.ca/content/dam/phac-aspc/documents/corporate/publications/chief-public-health-officer-reports-state-public-health-canada/addressing-stigma-what-we-heard/stigma-eng.pdf.

Hamington, Maurice. 2004. *Embodied Care: Jane Addams, Maurice Merleau-Ponty, and Feminist Ethics*. Urbana: University of Illinois Press.

Hartman, Yvonne, and Sandy Darab. 2012. "A Call for Slow Scholarship." *Review of Education, Pedagogy and Cultural Studies* 34:49–60.

Hastings, Annette. 2009. "Poor Neighbourhoods and Poor Services: Evidence on the 'Rationing' of Environmental Service Provision to Deprived Neighbourhoods." *Urban Studies* 46 (13): 2907–2927.

Hetling, Andrea, Stevie Watson, and Meghan Horgan. 2014. "'We Live in a Technological Era, Whether You Like It or Not': Client Perspectives and Online Welfare Applicants." *Administration and Society* 46 (5): 519–547.

Jansson, Gabriella, and Gissur Erlingsson. 2014. "More E-government, Less Street-Level Bureaucracy?" *Journal of Information Technology & Politics* 11 (3): 291–308.

Kidd, Ian, and Havi Carel. 2017. "Epistemic Injustice and Illness." *Journal of Applied Philosophy* 34 (2): 172–190.

Kidd, Ian, José Medina, and Gaile Pohlhaus Jr., eds. 2017. *The Routledge Handbook of Epistemic Injustice*. New York: Routledge.

Koggel, Christine. 2018. "Epistemic Injustice in a Settle Nation: Canada's History of Erasing, Silencing, Marginalizing." *Journal of Global Ethics* 14 (2): 240–251.

Lipsky, Michael. 1990. *Street-Level Bureaucracy: Dilemmas of the Individual in Public Services*. New York: Russell Sage.

Medina, José. 2011. "The Relevance of Credibility Excess in a Proportional View of Epistemic Injustice." *Social Epistemology* 25 (1): 15–35.

Medina, José. 2013. *The Epistemology of Resistance: Gender and Racial Oppression, Epistemic Injustice, and Resistance Imaginations*. Oxford: Oxford University Press.

Origgi, Gloria, and Serena Ciranna. 2017. "Epistemic Injustice: The Case of Digital Environments." In *The Routledge Handbook of Epistemic Injustice*, edited by Ian J. Kidd, José Medina, and Gaile Pohlhaus Jr., 303–312. New York: Routledge.

Penner, Louis A., Susan Eggly, Jennifer J. Griggs, Willie Underwood III, Heather Orom, and Terrance L. Albrecht. 2012. "Life-Threatening Disparities: The Treatment of Black and White Cancer Patients." *Journal of Social Issues* 68 (2): 1–25.

Razack, Sherene. 2002. "Gendered Racial Violence and Spatialized Justice: The Murder of Pamela George." In *Race, Space and the Law: Unmapping a White Settler Society*, edited by Sherene Razack, 121–156. Toronto: Between the Lines.

Robinson, Fiona. 2011. "Stop Talking and Listen: Discourse Ethics and Feminist Care Ethics in International Political Theory." *Millennium* 39 (3): 845–860.

Sharkey, Amanda. 2014. "Robots and Human Dignity: A Consideration of the Effects of Robot Care on the Dignity of Older People." *Ethics and Information Technology* 16:63–75.

Simpson, Leanne Betasamosake. 2017. *As We Have Always Done: Indigenous Freedom through Radical Resistance*. Minneapolis: University of Minnesota Press.

Spivak, Gayatri Chakravorty. 1990. *The Post-colonial Critic*. New York: Routledge.

Starblanket, Gina. 2018. "Complex Accountabilities: Deconstructing 'the Community' and Engaging Indigenous Feminist Research Methods." *American Indian Culture and Research Journal* 42 (4): 1–20.

Stensöta, Helena O. 2010. "The Conditions of Care: Reframing the Debate about Public Sector Ethics." *Public Administration Review* 70 (2): 295–303.

Tasker, John Paul. 2017. "'We're Very Much Aware of the Impatience': MMIW Commissioners Reassure Families at 1st Press Conference." CBC News. February 7.

Tronto, Joan C. 2003. "Time's Place." *Feminist Theory* 4 (2): 119–138.

———. 2010. "Creating Caring Institutions: Politics, Plurality and Purpose." *Ethics and Social Welfare* 4 (2): 158–171.

———. 2013. *Caring Democracy: Markets, Equality, and Justice*. New York: New York University Press.

Tuck, Eve, and K. Wayne Yang. 2012. "Decolonization Is Not a Metaphor." *Decolonization: Indigeneity, Education & Society* 1 (1): 1–40.

Vezzali, Loris, and Sofia Stathi. 2016. *Intergroup Contact Theory*. New York: Routledge.

3 · PRIVILEGE AND THE DENIAL OF VULNERABILITY

When Care Ethics Meets Epistemologies of Ignorance

MARIE GARRAU

The starting point of this text lies in what at first sight appears to be a paradox—one that concerns the acknowledgment of vulnerability, most notably in the work of care theorists. It could be stated as follows. On the one hand, the acknowledgment of vulnerability seems to be a necessary condition for the establishment of a "caring society," as envisaged by the likes of Evelyn Nakano Glenn (2000) and Joan Tronto (2013).[1] The idea here is that it is only if we all recognize ourselves as vulnerable will we be able to recognize the social and moral importance of care in our lives as well as the value of the work done by care workers daily. On the other hand, this recognition constitutes a problem that is never really studied for its own sake. Take, for instance, Tronto's call (2013) that all of us consider ourselves as care *recipients*. As Tronto shows, we generally don't see ourselves in this way, which has problematic implications: we tend to presume that "the vulnerable" are *others*, and that is why we do not feel concerned by care work and do not take the measure of what is at stake in it.[2] And yet this difficulty in acknowledging vulnerability is never analyzed extensively. As a result, the acknowledgment of vulnerability appears to be the object of a moral injunction whose conditions of effectiveness are never elucidated—an empty injunction, therefore, or even a pious wish that seems to constitute an aporia on which theoretical reflection stumbles.

This situation seems problematic to me because I share with care theorists the view that the acknowledgment of vulnerability constitutes an epistemic and ethical *condition* for the establishment of a just society. Differently put, a just society is both a society whose institutions see citizens as both "vulnerable and capable," to use Martha Nussbaum's (2000) expression, and a society whose members see themselves and each other as "vulnerable and capable." I further believe that there is a link between acknowledging one's own vulnerability (i.e., recognizing oneself as vulnerable and, as such, dependent on the attention and care of others) and recognizing the vulnerability of others as normatively significant (i.e., as calling for an ethical attitude and conduct based on care and respect). In this perspective, the ability to treat others with care would be based on a particular type of relationship to oneself. It is this kind of relationship that is reflected in the idea of "acknowledgment of vulnerability," which must be understood in a twofold sense: in an epistemic sense, as the ability to perceive and become aware of one's own vulnerability; and in an ethical sense, as the ability to consent to its normative implications. Conversely, the inability to consider and treat others ethically—which manifests itself through contempt, disqualification, stigmatization, or violence—would express among other things the inability to relate to oneself as a vulnerable being and to see oneself as belonging to the same existential and moral community as others.

If these ideas are correct, the recognition of vulnerability is undoubtedly not only a moral but also a political issue. The question then is to figure out how to foster it. Is it enough to *want* to acknowledge one's vulnerability in order to become capable of doing so? But even prior to that, is it really that simple to want to acknowledge one's vulnerability?

Through her calls to consider ourselves as recipients of care, Tronto suggests that the acknowledgment of vulnerability is a problem and offers two ways to approach it.[3] The first is as a matter of cultural critique and consists in underlining the fact that contemporary liberal societies have been constructed with reference to an imaginary of autonomy, wrongly understood as independence, in the light of which vulnerability can appear only as a defect or a deficiency that must be overcome or hidden. If this idea is present in *Moral Boundaries* (1993), it takes on a new scope in *Caring Democracy* (2013), where Tronto analyzes the rise of neoliberal discourse. Here, she returns to the conception of the subject as self-entrepreneur that underlies this discourse and shows how it is linked to a specific, narrow understanding of responsibility—namely, *individual* responsibility and responsibility for oneself.

In this first explanation of Tronto, the idea is that there are discourses and social norms that favor the concealment or denial of vulnerability. This view is echoed by Martha Fineman (2004), who analyzes and criticizes the "myth of autonomy," and more recently by Erinn Gilson (2011), who insists on the "myth" of invulnerability's role in perpetuating the ignorance of our vulnerability. For these authors, promoting vulnerability's acknowledgment would require deconstructing these discourses and the myths they convey and countering them with alternative representations and norms (e.g., different conceptions of autonomy, responsibility, and vulnerability). Such a line of analysis is promising and the practical perspectives it opens are important. But it seems insufficient in some respects, particularly because it does not ask the question of the reception of the discourses at the origin of the problem, nor that of the differentiated relationship agents have with norms according to the position they occupy in social space. As such, this perspective portrays the denial of vulnerability as a common and ordinary phenomenon and as a homogeneous one insofar as we are all *equally exposed* to it. But as I will show later, things may not be that straightforward.

However, Tronto's work also offers a second analytical lead to account for the denial of vulnerability, which I wish to consider closely below. This explanation is tied to the concept of privileged irresponsibility (Tronto 1993, 2013), which refers to the tendency of members of dominant groups to transfer the work of care to members of dominated groups. As many have shown (e.g., Glenn 2010; Hirata 2021), care work is mostly taken on by working-class and racialized women. Conversely, men, but also and to a lesser extent white women from the upper classes, manage to exempt themselves totally or partially from care work (Riikka Prattes's chapter in this volume [chapter 4] is pertinent here). Tronto suggests that such a transfer has first and foremost a social function, in that it allows the dominant to free themselves from care responsibilities and thus to engage in more socially valued activities. But we can also suggest that it has a psychological function: by allowing the dominant to keep their distance from taking charge of others' vulnerability and to avoid feeling concerned by it, this protects them from being confronted by their own vulnerability. This encourages the reproduction of a symbolic frontier between individuals deemed to be autonomous and successful on the one hand, and individuals deemed to be vulnerable on the other. And with all this comes the reinforcement of a truncated, univocal, and stigmatizing vision of vulnerability.

This second line of analysis therefore offers a slightly different explanation of the denial of vulnerability than the first: the problem does not, or at least not only, come from the discourses, representations, and norms that circulate indifferently in the social space and that structure the dominant collective imaginary; it comes from various social positions of domination, which can be defined as positions of privilege insofar as they give access to material, symbolic, and psychological advantages that are denied to others. This is why, in the same society, not everyone will be affected in the same way by the denial of vulnerability, even if the dominant ideology and dominant norms encourage this denial.

The chief uptake from Tronto's discussion of privileged irresponsibility is, then, that certain social positions offer those who occupy them the possibility of not confronting the vulnerability of others and of not thinking of themselves as vulnerable. This is what make such positions both socially and psychologically attractive, and morally and politically problematic. In what follows, I would like to explore this idea in greater depth, by returning to what we can identify as obstacles to the acknowledgment of vulnerability. We will see that this acknowledgment is a complex process that relies on particular psychological and social conditions, which may be lacking or hindered. The hypothesis I propose is that social relationships of domination, and more particularly the construction of dominant positions or positions of privilege, constitute one major obstacle to such acknowledgment.[4] The general idea underlying this hypothesis is that social relations of domination produce differentiated affective, epistemic, and moral effects on the dominant and on the dominated, effects that are essential to their maintenance. And among them, one finds, on the side of the dominant, a double tendency:[5] first, to deny one's own vulnerability and, second, to project this vulnerability onto others.

In what follows, I will first return to the definition of vulnerability with which I work; then I will address the concept of denial and show that the denial of vulnerability cannot be understood simply in light of a psychoanalytic explanation. I will then reflect on the social factors behind the denial of vulnerability, drawing on both the contributions of care theories and the epistemologies of ignorance.

DEFINING VULNERABILITY AS A COMMON AND PARADOXICAL EXISTENTIAL CONDITION

In my perspective, vulnerability refers to a common existential condition that results from the situation of exposure and dependence in which human subjects find themselves with respect to an otherness that they never fully master, with which they are necessarily in relation and which is likely to affect them (Garrau 2018). To be vulnerable in this sense is therefore to be open—in a constitutive way—to the possibility of being affected by an otherness on which one depends. Vulnerability hence presupposes an essential passivity and an absence of self-sufficiency and self-mastery that are profoundly ambivalent (Gilson 2013), since they open us up as much to the possibility of suffering as to that of attachment.

This vulnerability is rooted in the very nature of human existence, and first of all in the fact that we are embodied beings: bearers of needs that, initially, we cannot satisfy on our own; endowed with capacities that are not immediately functional and that will not be so indefinitely; subject to the passage of time, to the experience of pain and illness; living under the horizon of death. The body, however, is only one of the foundations of vulnerability, which is also rooted in the relational dimension of human existence and the fact that we depend on others to become ourselves.[6] We are first dependent on others: on their care, love, respect, esteem. Others mediate the satisfaction of our physiological needs, but beyond that, they give us access to "relational goods" (Nussbaum 2001) and to social goods without which we could neither form a positive relationship with ourselves nor engage in projects to which we attach value. In turn, this interpersonal dependence exposes us to the possibility of neglect, violence, contempt, isolation. We are also dependent on the organization of the society in which we live—especially political and economic institutions, which distribute a certain number of rights and goods, and which form the context of the interpersonal relationships we establish with those we meet. In turn, this social dependence exposes us to the possibility of poverty, disaffiliation, social disqualification, domination, and exploitation. Finally, we are dependent on the natural environment where we find the resources needed to meet our collective needs, and which we transform for this purpose. This ecological dependence exposes us to the possibility of scarcity, disease, and the destruction of our communities. Thus, our vulnerability stems as much from the fact that we are bodies, marked by finitude and need, as from the fact that we are from the outset caught up in relations on which depends the possibility of living meaningful lives. If we are vulnerable, it is therefore because we are relational beings. Our dependence and openness allow us to experience love, surprise, joy, and wonder; but they also expose us to suffering, privations, neglect, and violence.

To speak of a fundamental vulnerability is to suggest that this vulnerability is a common and universally shared existential condition that cannot be overcome, suppressed, or eradicated. Vulnerability is given with human existence and is consubstantial with it. This entanglement of vulnerability and existence accounts for the first paradox of vulnerability: inherent to human existence and constitutive of the form this existence takes, vulnerability can go unnoticed, operating in the background as the basis around which existence unfolds and subjectivity, capacities, and life projects develop. However, it becomes manifest in experiences that attest to the limits of our power to act and that allow us to understand that this power—and even more so the autonomy with which we identify cognitive and moral maturity—is a fragile achievement because it is conditioned by a set of elements that are impossible to fully master. Through loss, powerlessness, suffering, illness, death, the subject discovers herself vulnerable: she experiences the limits of her power to act and the impossibility of escaping exposure and dependence to the world. This ordeal is however lived by each one in a singular manner. This is the second paradox of vulnerability: common and universally shared, vulnerability is nevertheless always experienced in a unique way. To account for this paradoxical status, we may distinguish fundamental vulnerability from its situational variations (Mackenzie, Rogers, and Dodds 2013; Garrau 2018). This distinction helps us grasp that fundamental vulnerability only ever manifests itself in differentiated ways and with varying intensities, which then help define the situation in which the subjects find themselves and the way in which they relate to this situation. It thus elucidates the view that although we are all fundamentally vulnerable, we are not all equally so.

The fact that vulnerability both is constitutive and sometimes operates in the background of human existence, both universal and singularly experienced, may explain our difficulty in acknowledging it. The paradoxes of vulnerability are undoubtedly parts of the explanation for the fact that it is the object of an ordinary forgetfulness or even denial—that is, the fact that most of the time we live as if we are not vulnerable. In order to understand this phenomenon, however, we must go further and point to the role of psychological and social factors.

DENIAL AND ITS FACTORS: THE INTERWEAVING OF PSYCHOLOGICAL AND SOCIAL PROCESSES

To understand the phenomenon of the denial of vulnerability, we can turn to psychoanalysis. Indeed, psychoanalysis distinguishes three defense mechanisms (Laplanche and Pontalis 2018), which can shed light on what I have referred to by the generic term "denial of vulnerability." First, disavowal (*Verleugnung*) designates the action of refusing the reality of a perception experienced as dangerous or painful for the subject, which results in the appearance of a localized form of unconsciousness. The object of disavowal is thus simply negated as such: it does not exist. Second, denial (*Verneinung*) designates the action of refusing as one's own (after having formulated them) a thought, a desire, or a feeling that are sources of conflict. Contrary to disavowal, denial presupposes the recognition of negative feelings or thoughts, which are then put at a distance from the subject as not concerning him. The object of denial is thus recognized before it is denied. Third and finally, projection (*Projektion*) designates the operation by which the subject expels from herself and localizes in the other qualities, feelings, or desires that she refuses in herself. Here the object is unrecognized because dissociated from oneself and associated with another.

This typology can be compared to another one proposed by sociologist Stanley Cohen (2001). In *States of Denial*, Cohen analyzes the different meanings of the term "denial," including the one developed by psychoanalysis, and proposes to distinguish three figures of denial: (1) literal denial, which consists in purely and simply denying the facts and which is thus close to disavowal; (2) interpretive denial, which consists in recognizing what one wishes to deny but neutralizing its meaning by proposing a particular interpretation of it, which is close to what psychoanalysis calls denial; and (3) implicatory denial, which consists in recognizing a fact without, however, drawing any practical consequences from it, as if this fact did not have any consequences or at least none that concerns you.

Cohen points out that, whatever its form, denial is always paradoxical in that the subject knows and, at the same time, does not know something. In the psychoanalytical perspective, the concepts of unconscious and repression help illuminate this paradox. Psychoanalysis is also interesting because it offers an explanation for denial: it suggests that denial serves to protect the psychic subject by putting her at a distance or even by isolating her from that which produces her anguish. As Laplanche and Pontalis (2018) point out, the purpose of these defense mechanisms is to "reduce or suppress any modification that might endanger the integrity and constancy of the biopsychological individual"—a finality that is reached by an unconscious reshuffling of the internal or external realities. If defense mechanisms can be pathological and are classically associated with specific mental pathologies, it is important to note that they are part of the normal functioning of psychic life. According to psychoanalysis, it is when they become rigid or invasive that they are deemed pathological, for mental functioning's flexibility and adaptability is hereby hindered.

At an individual level, it seems difficult to dispute that vulnerability is subject to denial in the broadest sense of the term or to various forms of negation. Most of us live as if those we care about would never get sick or disappear, as if men, women, and children like us did not live in conditions of absolute destitution in the cities we travel through every day to go to work; as if the planet was not undergoing irreversible transformations that could eventually compromise human life and that already threaten human communities all around the world. To stop thinking; to look away; to change sidewalk; to turn off the radio; to absorb ourselves in work, consumption, or play; to tell ourselves that it is about others, but not us; that we are different, that we are safe ... all these behaviors through which we put the others' vulnerability and our own at a distance seem to be commonplace. Their banality should not, however, mask the epistemic and moral problems they raise: if it is neither possible nor desirable to live with our eyes permanently riveted on the most salient, tragic, or revolting manifestations of our vulnerability, the inability and refusal to recognize it are at least as problematic, if only because they prevent us from asking crucial political questions about collective ways of dealing with our vulnerability. This observation thus opens epistemological questions that a moral and political reflection on vulnerability cannot avoid: What knowledge of vulnerability do we need? How can such knowledge be acquired? What obstacles are likely to thwart the acquisition of such knowledge?

From an individual point of view, it seems easy to understand why we are inclined to deny our vulnerability as well as others'. The discovery of one's own vulnerability first takes place in an affective mode before becoming the object of a cognitive elaboration: one experiences one's vulnerability sensitively before *thinking* oneself vulnerable. Now, whether it is provoked by the experience of suffering, by that of separation, or by that of loss, such an experience reminds subjects of their initial powerlessness and confronts them with the possibility of their own disappearance. This is why it arouses anguish. The same is true when others' vulnerability is at stake. As psychologist Pascale Molinier (2009) points out, the experience of others' vulnerability first of all seizes the body. It awakens ambivalent affects in the subject, in which solicitude vies with anxiety and irritation. The confrontation with others' vulnerability constitutes a test for the subject, to whom it recalls her own vulnerability, and whose psychological balance it threatens to undo. Disavowal, denial, and projection are therefore psychically expected reactions in such a situation.

Molinier emphasizes, however, that these are not the only possible reactions to the experience of vulnerability. She also notes that social and not only psychological processes are at work to account for the differentiated reactions of subjects to this experience. Care workers, for example, cannot in principle deny the vulnerability of their patients. Their work consists in responding to this vulnerability: in order to work well, they must therefore perceive it and, to do so, must be attentive to their own affective life and symbolize the affects that the confrontation with the patients arouses in them. Molinier (2006) shows that, when care institutions allow it, caregivers create "collective defense strategies" that have a dual purpose: to preserve their sensitivity to vulnerability (in the other and themselves) and to domesticate the anguish produced by the perception of vulnerability. The recounting of difficult experiences with patients as well as humor are part of such strategies, which allow the experience of vulnerability to be grasped rather than distanced, so that it becomes possible to respond to it.

Molinier's (2006) work thus underscores that psychic postures and the ethical dispositions they help nourish are shaped by our social positions and the social institutions we are situated in: they depend on the activities we engage in, the identities associated with them, and the social relations and institutional rules in which we are caught. They thus give substance to the idea that denial as a defense mechanism is not inevitable and that the psychological processes triggered by the experience of vulnerability are mediated by social positions and trajectories. For care workers, this denial is not necessary; it becomes an option only when their suffering, because it is not acknowledged and addressed collectively, becomes unbearable. When the activity is framed in terms of cost-efficiency, when work teams are destabilized by workers' turnover, when resources in time are shortened,[7] it becomes difficult for them to acknowledge their vulnerability and to respond to that of the care receivers.[8] The forms of abuse observed in many healthcare institutions can thus be understood in terms of a collapse of the collective defense strategies that allow caregivers to accept patients' vulnerability. They indicate the setting up and rigidification of individual defense mechanisms against vulnerability—mechanisms that foster insensitivity in caregivers and make violence possible. But this happens only as the result of an institutional failure. From Molinier's analysis, we can conclude that social circumstances and institutional contexts play a central role in the acknowledgment or denial of vulnerability and that certain contexts foster the acknowledgment of vulnerability while others encourage denial. It is this last hypothesis that I would like to explore further in the last section.

A DIVERSELY DISTRIBUTED DENIAL? POSITIONS OF PRIVILEGE AND DENIAL OF VULNERABILITY

In her book *L'Énigme de la femme active* (2003), Molinier suggests that certain social positions predispose those who occupy them to denying vulnerability by encouraging the development of various psychological mechanisms. She shows that gender, understood as a transversal social structure attaching differentiated and differently valued qualities to individuals and activities, plays a central role in individuals' ability to recognize and accept their own and others' vulnerability. While the activities and positions considered feminine are usually defined in reference to emotions and care, activities and positions considered masculine are typically defined in reference to reason and control. As such, they imply the distancing of emotions and relationships. The learning of hegemonic masculinity (Connell 1995), mediated chiefly by work activities according to Molinier, would thus require men to close themselves off from their emotions and to turn away from a vulnerability perceived as the prerogative of femininity and therefore as a threat to their identity. Such a psychic posture, encouraged by dominant gender norms, would then account for the particular relationship that men may have with violence—both acted and suffered. It would make it possible to understand the tendency of some men to use violence on others, but also the tendency of some men to expose themselves physically and to put themselves in danger—two types of behavior that can be seen as vulnerability denial and are considered normal, even desirable, within a certain conception of masculinity, as Bourdieu showed in *Masculine Domination* (2002).

Molinier's analysis of the relationship between masculinity and denial of vulnerability echoes that of moral developmental psychologists Carol Gilligan and Naomi Snider in *Why Does Patriarchy Persist?* (2018). In this book, the authors defend the idea that gender initiation functions as a trauma: patriarchal norms require women to silence their attempts at self-expression in order to devote themselves to the care of others and encourage men to renounce relationship in exchange for a fantasized invulnerability. In patriarchal societies, invulnerability is thus prescribed to men (vulnerability being regarded as what one must guard against in order to assert oneself and be recognized as a man) and as the prerogative of others: non-men and sub-men. For, as the authors point out, patriarchy is based on not simply the domination of men over women but also the hierarchy of men among themselves, according to their ability to embody the dominant norms of masculinity. If, therefore, the denial of vulnerability is constitutive of patriarchal masculinity, not all men conform equally to such a norm and their position within the group depends on their greater or lesser conformity to it.

Molinier's (2003) and Gilligan and Snider's (2018) works thus underscore that certain social groups have a specific relationship with vulnerability. In particular, they point to a differentiated relationship to vulnerability according to gender and a strong correlation between masculinity and denial of vulnerability, although it is important to bear in mind the plurality of the male group (partially tied to the interweaving of gender, race, and class relations). Their work deserves to be pushed further, by investigating the particular relationships to vulnerability that racialized men, men from working-class backgrounds, but also white women and women from the upper classes, have. Shannon Sullivan's work on white privilege could be useful here. Sullivan shows that white privilege, inscribed in bodies in the form of unconscious habits, is reflected in a particular relationship to the body and to space. While the white body is experienced as transparent and as a tool for taking hold of the world (Sullivan 2006, 10, 51, 103), white space is understood as a field of possibility within which it is possible to move freely, so that whiteness is characterized by "ontological expansiveness" (Sullivan 2006, 144–166).[9]

What one can gather from Sullivan's work is that the claim that vulnerability remains mostly in the background of existence must be qualified, or rather situated. It could be that this particular experience of vulnerability, which is characterized by the ease with which it can be put at a distance and forgotten, is the product of a particular social position in gender, race, and class relations. When one is subjected to regular forms of harassment, exposed to repeated and arbitrary police checks, or deprived of the ability to eat every day, vulnerability is more difficult to deny.

This leads me to the last work I wish to draw on in order to defend the view that our relationship to vulnerability, and our greater or lesser propensity to deny or acknowledge it, is strongly linked to our social positions. This is José Medina's *Epistemology of Resistance* (2013), which builds on Miranda Fricker's (2007) work on epistemic injustice and the epistemologies of ignorance initiated by Charles Mills (1997). As suggested by Christine Koggel and Sophie Bourgault in this volume, I think care ethics and more generally ethical and political theories of vulnerability can greatly benefit from the insights of theorists of epistemic injustice and epistemologists of ignorance, who bring to the fore the question of the epistemic effects of social relations of domination.

Starting from the presupposition that social relations of domination position subjects differently in relation to knowledge and produce differentiated forms of knowledge and ignorance, Medina argues that members of dominant groups develop, as a result of their position in social space, particular epistemic vices, which make them insensitive to certain realities concerning the world, others, and themselves. Among these vices are epistemic arrogance, epistemic laziness, and closed-mindedness (Medina 2013, 30–35). These are created by the habit of being seen as knowing or as legitimate to give one's point of view, by being listened to, and rarely being challenged or questioned. According to Medina, these vices function as unconscious defense mechanisms or forms of "cognitive self-protection" that allow the dominants to live in ignorance of certain social realities. They are responsible for what he calls active ignorance, which he defines as "an ignorance that occurs with the active participation of the subject and via a battery of defense mechanisms, an ignorance that is not easy to undo and combat, as it requires re-education—the reconfiguration of attitudes and epistemic habits—and social change" (Medina 2013, 39).

Active ignorance refers, like denial, to a substantial form of ignorance: it is not simply the absence of true representations but the presence of false representations, which function both as screens and as protections against realities that might challenge one's privileged position in social space. As Medina (2013, 33) notes, the ignorance surrounding care work's materiality—an ignorance socially organized by the invisibilization of care work and of care workers, and by the unequal distribution of this work along gender, race, and class lines—provides an example of such ignorance. The ignorance that surrounds the daily difficulties, but also the forms of resistance enacted by single women, by people with disabilities or by precarious individuals, would provide another.

These forms of ignorance are not accidental: they are systemic and participate in the reproduction of an inegalitarian social structure by allowing those who occupy privileged positions in this structure not to question, because they do not perceive them, the conditions under which they can effectively enjoy the privileges they hold, and the cost of these privileges for others. These forms of active ignorance are thus similar to forms of denial—but the denial here is about others' vulnerability. Medina notes, however, that these forms of ignorance are rooted as much in an unequal social structure as in a certain type of relationship to the self, characterized by what he calls a "blindness to relationality" (2013, 154–155). This blindness is defined by Medina in part as a lack of capacity to see how we are connected to others and how their lives (and histories) affect ours. Such a blindness translates into the tendency, on the one hand, to think of oneself as a self-sufficient being and, on the other hand, to absolutize one's point of view on the world, so that this point of view constitutes the implicit reference or standard for all judgment. Ignorance or insensitivity to the vulnerability of others would thus be based on an ignorance of the self, and more precisely on a denial of our existential and social situation, and of what we owe to others—in other words, on a denial of our vulnerability. Such a denial should then be understood as the product of different but intertwined factors: psychological (the anguish produced by the experience of vulnerability), ideological (the social value given to invulnerability and its avatars), material (the division of care labor), but also social (relations of power and domination) and epistemological (ways of seeing and ignoring oneself and others as shaped by epistemological attitudes, virtues, and vices).

CONCLUSION: GETTING OUT OF DENIAL?

To be considered fully convincing, the hypothesis formulated here of a close link between the denial of vulnerability and dominant social positions would require an in-depth study of scholarship on social epistemology and social psychology that would take as its object the dominants' point of view in their different declinations (according to gender, race, class, disability, age). Although we did not undertake this work here, it seems possible at this stage to make the following points as a tentative conclusion.

First, the experience of vulnerability, whether of others or of oneself, is an ordeal from which the subject may seek to protect herself, notably by means of denial. Second, whether it concerns one's own vulnerability or that of others, this denial is problematic for moral reasons, insofar as it can inhibit the agent's moral capacity to respond to the vulnerability of others, and for epistemic reasons, insofar as it produces ignorance: about oneself and about the social world. Third, this denial is supported by certain social norms and positions: gender, race, and class norms produce differentiated relations to vulnerability, and more precisely a differentiated capacity to deny or acknowledge it. Occupying a dominant position can thus encourage subjects to develop a form of ignorance or denial with regard to the vulnerability of others and their own, the two phenomena being linked by a feedback loop. Because these positions are associated with material and social advantages that allow self-protection from certain forms of vulnerability and because these positions are defined in reference to identities that symbolically exclude vulnerability and associate it with other identities, being male, being white, and belonging to a high social class would mean (albeit in different ways) not being vulnerable. Vulnerability, and its connotations of passivity, dependence, and weakness, can thus be considered the prerogative of others, that is, of the dominated: women, racialized individuals, members of the working class, but also sick people, people with disabilities, the elderly, children, and so forth.

Although these results are still at the stage of hypothesis, they are not without interest from a practical and more explicitly political point of view. They indicate, first of all, that the creation of a "caring society," and the recognition of care's importance for social reproduction and citizens' daily lives, will probably not be possible in a social context marked by massive inequalities and the social relations of domination that produce them. If recognizing care implies acknowledging vulnerability, it also implies working toward the abolition of the social relations of domination that currently structure our societies. This conclusion demonstrates once again, albeit via a different route, the political radicality of care ethics or the radicality of care ethics understood as a "critical political theory," to use Fiona Robinson's (2019) term.

These results then indicate a possible way out of the denial, or rather they allow us to highlight a lever for doing so. One of the contributions offered by Molinier, Gilligan and Snider, and Medina is thus to have shown—thanks to the psychological and epistemic angle they take—that the positions of the dominant and the dominated are more complex than they appear. The dominated have, in fact, because of their material conditions of existence, the social division of labor, and the dominant social norms and identity injunctions that weigh on them, more chance of developing a lucid knowledge of vulnerability, whether it be that of others or their own. Of course, such knowledge does not come without suffering. First, because the discovery of one's vulnerability, as soon as it implies the recognition of one's finitude and the multiple forms of one's exposure and dependence on the human and nonhuman world, always constitutes for the subject a destabilizing experience. But this is, above all, also because for the members of dominated groups, the understanding of one's vulnerability always rhymes with the discovery of an injustice inflicted upon oneself and one's group—that of having been and being the object of a structural, lasting and arbitrary violence. As Audre Lorde (1984) pointed out, it can give rise to a sadness and anger that are particularly difficult to overcome. But the acknowledgment of one's vulnerability can also foster an understanding of one's situation in the world and one's power to act, create joy, and arouse gratitude for those to whom we owe our survival. Its counterpart can be the development of a practical and moral knowledge essential to life's maintenance, as well as the development of positive epistemic and ethical dispositions, such as sensitivity, attention, or epistemic humility (see Dalmiya in this volume [chapter 5]). Indeed, it is only by recognizing and knowing the vulnerability in oneself and in others that one can take care of oneself, others, and the common world.[10]

This potential increased lucidity of the dominated, which goes hand in hand with an increased power to act, is mirrored in the potential blindness of the dominant, who can be caught in the clutches of a denial that, while it protects them from painful realities, also locks them into a world, a relationship with themselves and a relationship with others that are truncated and cannot but diminish their agency. Privilege therefore has its flip side, or domination has a cost, as Bourdieu (2002) pointed out. From an epistemic and ethical point of view, privilege can paradoxically prove disabling, hindering the development of a lucid relationship with oneself, as Medina points out, and of authentic relationships with others, as Gilligan and Snider argue. To emphasize this cost is neither to reintroduce between the dominant and the dominated a symmetry that domination de facto denies, nor to place the members of the dominant groups in the paradoxical position of victims of the domination they benefit from.[11] The issue is to see that the analysis of the dominant position in terms of epistemic and moral losses or deficits can be practically and politically fruitful, for it can contribute to making change desirable for those who have no material interest in it. It can help convince the dominant, or at least those among them who feel confusedly that they are living a "false life," to use Adorno's expression (2020), that they too have something to gain from social transformation. Such a suggestion may seem idealistic: it supposes indeed to grant a value to knowledge and an efficiency to the desire for knowledge; it rests moreover on the presupposition that relations of domination neither compromise the possibility of accessing true knowledge, nor irreversibly alter the desire for truth that drives human subjects. As long as we have to live with each other, however, it seems that we cannot do without such an idealism, or without such a hope. Finally, the idea that the fight against the epistemic effects of privilege should be a central part of the fight for social justice does not by itself rule out any other strategy for social change. In particular, as Medina (2013) makes clear with his concept of epistemic friction, it is compatible with the recognition of the value of conflict in the political realm, although it implies to locate conflict first in the realm of discursivity. For all these reasons, those who care for care and vulnerability should definitely try to explore further the epistemic effects of privilege, which implies to dig deeper into the mechanisms of the ignorance of the dominant and to ask how they can be fought effectively.

ACKNOWLEDGMENTS

I wish to thank Sophie Bourgault and Maggie FitzGerald for their help and precious remarks on an earlier version of this text. I hope the conversation will continue.

NOTES

1. The idea of a caring society can be understood with reference to three dimensions: it refers to (1) a society that publicly promotes the values of care, such as attention, responsibility, and solicitude; (2) a society that recognizes the importance of care work for its own reproduction

and therefore materially and symbolically recognizes the value of those who perform it; (3) a society that makes the organization of this work a major issue in public discussion. See Garrau (2020).
2. See Paperman (2005).
3. See Tronto (2013, 29, 146).
4. Classically, privilege refers to a set of advantages that members of a group enjoy in an exclusive way and that ensure them a lasting position of dominance. In her work on white privilege, however, Sullivan (2006) convincingly shows that, insofar as it is inscribed in the body and the psyche through the development of certain habits, privilege also engages a specific relationship to the self and the world: a way of feeling, seeing (or not seeing), and sensing. Based on a double reference to Dewey's pragmatism and Freudian psychoanalysis, this approach resonates with that of Pierre Bourdieu, who also insists on the incorporation of social structures in the form of mental structures determining in a nonconscious way the conduct of agents, and this in a differentiated way according to class membership. See Bourdieu (1984).
5. I argue not that individuals' capacity for social and moral perception is determined by their social position but that occupying a social position increases the likelihood of being sensitive or insensitive to certain inner experiences and social phenomena. See Medina (2013, 40).
6. That is why vulnerability should not be reduced to physical vulnerability, as rightly emphasized in Vrinda Dalmiya's chapter in this volume (chapter 5).
7. On the importance of time for care, see Sophie Bourgault's contribution to this volume (chapter 2).
8. On this, see Molinier (2009) and Dujarier (2002).
9. On whiteness as a mode of inhabiting the world that goes unnoticed, see also Sara Ahmed (2007). I thank Sophie Bourgault for drawing my attention to this text.
10. See Dalmiya in this volume (chapter 5).
11. This objection was addressed to Bourdieu by Nicole-Claude Mathieu. See Mathieu (1999).

REFERENCES

Adorno, Theodor. 2020. *Minima Moralia: Reflections from Damaged Life*. Translated by E. F. N. Jephcott. New York: Verso.

Ahmed, Sara. 2007. "A Phenomenology of Whiteness." *Feminist Studies* 8 (2): 149–168. https://doi.org/10.1177/1464700107078139.

Bourdieu, Pierre. 1984. *Distinction. A Social Critique of the Judgement of Taste*. Translated by Richard Nice. Oxon: Routledge.

———. 2002. *Masculine Domination*. Translated by Richard Nice. Stanford, CA: Stanford University Press.

Butler, Judith. 2004. *Precarious Life: The Power of Mourning and Violence*. New York: Verso.

Cohen, Stanley. 2001. *States of Denial: Knowing about Atrocities and Suffering*. Cambridge: Polity.

Connell, Raewyn. 1995. *Masculinities*. Berkeley: University of California Press.

Dujarier, Marie-Anne. 2002. "Comprendre l'inacceptable. Le cas de la maltraitance en gériatrie." *Revue Internationale de Psychosociologie* 8 (19): 111–124.

Fineman, Martha. 2004. *The Autonomy Myth: A Theory of Dependency*. New York: New Press.

Fricker, Miranda. 2007. *Epistemic Injustice: Power and the Ethics of Knowing*. New York: Oxford University Press.

Garrau, Marie. 2018. *Politiques de la vulnérabilité*. Paris: CNRS Éditions.

———. 2020. "Care between Dependence and Domination: The Appeal of Neo-Republican Theory for Envisioning a 'Caring Society.'" In *Care Ethics in Yet a Different Voice: Franco-*

phone Contributions, edited by Sophie Bourgault and Franz Vosman, 163–195. Leuven: Peeters.
Gilligan, Carol, and Naomi Snider. 2018. *Why Does Patriarchy Persist?* Cambridge: Polity.
Gilson, Erinn. 2011. "Vulnerability, Ignorance and Oppression." *Hypatia* 26 (2): 308–332. https://doi.org/10.1111/j.1527-2001.2010.01158.x.
———. 2013. *The Ethics of Vulnerability*. New York: Routledge.
Glenn, Evelyn Nakano. 2000. "Creating a Caring Society." *Contemporary Sociologies* 29 (1): 84–94.
———. 2010. *Forced to Care: Coercion and Caregiving in America*. Cambridge, MA: Harvard University Press.
Hirata, Helena. 2021. *Le care. Théories et pratiques*. Paris: La Dispute.
Laplanche, Jean, and Jean-Bertrand Pontalis. 2018. *The Language of Psychoanalysis*. Translated by Donald Nicholson-Smith. New York: Routledge.
Lorde, Audre. 1984. *Sister Outsider. Essays and Speeches*. New York: Random House.
Mackenzie, Catriona, Wendy Rogers, and Susan Dodds, eds. 2013. *Vulnerability: New Essays in Ethics and Feminist Theory*. Oxford: Oxford University Press.
Mathieu, Nicole-Claude. 1999. "Bourdieu ou le pouvoir auto-hypnotique de la domination masculine." *Les Temps Modernes*, no. 604: 286–324.
Medina, José. 2013. *The Epistemology of Resistance: Gender and Racial Oppression, Epistemic Injustice and Resistant Imaginations*. New York: Oxford University Press.
Mills, Charles. 1997. *The Racial Contract*. Ithaca, NY: Cornell University Press.
Molinier, Pascale. 2003. *L'Énigme de la femme active. Égoïsme, sexe et compassion*. Paris: Payot.
———. 2006. *Les Enjeux psychiques du travail*. Paris: Payot.
———. 2009. "Vulnérabilité et dépendance: de la maltraitance en régime de gestion hospitalière." In *Comment penser l'autonomie?*, edited by Marlène Jouan and Sandra Laugier, 433–458. Paris: Vrin.
Nussbaum, Martha. 2000. *Women and Human Development: The Capability Approach*. Cambridge, MA: Cambridge University Press.
———. 2001. *The Fragility of Goodness: Luck and Ethics in Greek Tragedy and Philosophy*. Cambridge: Cambridge University Press.
Paperman, Patricia. 2005. "Les gens vulnérables n'ont rien d'exceptionnel." In *Le souci des autres. Ethique et politique du care*, edited by Sandra Laugier and Patricia Paperman, 321–337. Paris: EHESS.
Robinson, Fiona. 2019. "Resisting Hierarchies through Relationality in the Ethics of Care." *International Journal of Care and Caring* 2 (3): 11–23. https://doi.org/10.1332/239788219X 15659215344772.
Sullivan, Shannon. 2006. *Revealing Whiteness: The Unconscious Habits of Racial Privilege*. Bloomington: Indiana University Press.
Tronto, Joan C. 1993. *Moral Boundaries. A Political Argument for an Ethic of Care*. New York, Routledge.
———. 2006. "Vicious Circles of Privatized Caring." In *Socializing Care*, edited by Maurice Hamington and Dorothy Miller Boulder, 3–27. Lanham, MD: Rowman & Littlefield.
———. 2013. *Caring Democracy: Markets, Equality, and Justice*. New York: New York University Press.

4 · LEARNING THROUGH CARE

Decentering an Epistemology of Domination to Theorize Caring Men at the "Center"

RIIKKA PRATTES

In 2014, as a precursor to my current project, I worked on an empirical study that dealt with the "outsourcing" of domestic cleaning from Viennese middle-class households to migrant women in the informal market. My focus, then, was particularly on the perspectives and practices of men in these households, which are rarely researched in scholarship on the international division of reproductive labor. Yet failing to examine men's role in care work (however marginal that might be) reinforces the dominant perception that domestic and care work is "women's work" and not crucial societal labor. Doing research with white, German-speaking, middle-class, cisgender, able-bodied, and well-educated men, I investigated how they took care of their apartments, took care of their places. I was interested in what they did and did not do, what they knew or did not know about the work of care. I was, and continue to be, interested in embodiment and practices of care, especially as they relate to epistemology. How and what do people learn from doing care work? Connected to this epistemological question is another political question about the distribution of caring labors. As I have argued (Prattes 2017), mundane, everyday care practices are important, and it is through them that worlds are made and knowledge produced. It matters—to paraphrase Françoise Vergès (2021)—who cleans the world.

In my 2014 project, in a conversation with Michael, one of the participants in Vienna, my focus on embodied practice as a locus of learning about care work was confronted head-on.[1] Michael reported that he often said to his woman partner as a sort of standing joke between them that "actually I clean the whole of the flat because I pay for [the domestic worker]" (Michael, individual interview). I was baffled by his conflation of paying for and doing the work of cleaning. Such a blatant denial that reproductive labor has any value in its noncommodified form makes it difficult to engage with the question of what and how we learn through the work of care. It becomes difficult to trace the epistemic consequences of embodied practices of care when their existence is negated in this way. Paying for cleaning, for Michael, has the same impact (epistemic or otherwise) as doing the cleaning. The process, the practice, loses all significance—except for leading to a goal: a clean apartment, which is important to Michael and the other men interviewed. However, this goal-orientedness has no appreciation for practice, for the path leading to this goal. Starting with this anecdote, I want to think about the possibility of taking care of a place (broadly defined) in the absence of embodied practice—and whether that is possible at all.

This chapter engages with two crucial aspects of knowledge formation: embodiment and place. I am thinking of being placed here not only in the sense of positionality and social situatedness (as has been highlighted by feminist and social epistemologists over the past four decades); I am thinking of place as an active agent and knowing collaborator for human knowledge making (as highlighted in many Indigenous epistemologies—since time immemorial).[2]

I thereby hope to contribute to the ongoing challenges to what I call an epistemology of domination—a particular, Western epistemology others have variously termed an "epistemology of separation" (Collins 1991), "epistemology of mastery" (Code 2006), or "epistemology of control" (Cheney 2002). I aim to work against the violent core of the dominant Western/colonial tradition of knowledge "production," which is always connected to a history of extraction and exhaustion (Vergès 2021), by highlighting other ways of knowing that exist—the many epistemologies that do recognize the primary significance of connection, relationality, and interdependence, as well as embodiment, place, and practice.

The first section of the chapter, "Decentering the Center," builds on critiques of an epistemology of domination to show that this Western paradigm of epistemology cannot grasp some of the ways of knowing that are central to care. I specifically draw on feminist (and) First Nations scholarship that highlights the importance of embodiment and place for knowledge formation. The section closes by posing the question of "how" learning from Indigenous place-based epistemologies can be achieved without this being epistemic extractivism—without it being yet another iteration of relations of coloniality. The term "epistemic extractivism" was coined by Ramón Grosfoguel (2019), who draws on Leanne Betasamosake Simpson's and Silvia Rivera Cusicanqui's challenges to how information (especially Indigenous knowledges) is being extracted in the Global South and used in the Global North, in and beyond academia (see also Alcoff 2022). Epistemic extractivism names a colonial move that, instead of understanding Indigenous knowledge on its own terms, "aims to extract ideas to colonize them, subsuming them within Western cultural parameters and episteme" (Grosfoguel 2019, 208). Simpson calls for non-Indigenous folks like me and others to *extract ourselves from extractivist thinking* (in Klein 2013). This is to be done by entering sustainable (caring) relationships because the alternative to extractivism, according to Simpson, is responsibility and "deep reciprocity. It's respect, it's relationship, it's responsibility, and it's local" (in Klein 2013). Trying to "locate" a starting point from which reciprocal and responsive relationality might emerge, section 2, "Practice," suggests we look to practices—in my case, men's practices of care work—in an effort to go beyond the colonial trajectory. Care practices are both embodied and located in specific places—*in all worlds*. Thus, focusing on practices could allow Western subjects to mobilize embodied and place-based epistemologies in ways that, while learning from Indigenous frameworks, do not extract from Indigenous worlding practices. Rather than appropriating from "other" worlds, such learning from Indigenous epistemologies in their diversity could help Western subjects to develop more responsive epistemic practices connected to place—in ways that do not harm others. In this way, I aim to break away from the dominant—and often dominating—paradigm of epistemology.

DECENTERING THE CENTER

The epistemology of domination cannot easily grasp the kinds of knowledges and the ways of knowing related to care in which I am interested. Operating from a—supposedly—neutral and value-free place, this dominating epistemology lacks an ethical dimension;[3] it lacks accountability. As Deva Woodly (2020) puts it, accountability is the flip side of recognizing interdependence "as a plain fact." Which is to say, because we depend on one another, we ought to be accountable to these others we are interwoven with in our knowledge formation practices. However, an "epistemology of separation" (Collins 1991) that is based on independence tends to be "unbounded" in its limitless endeavor to know everything and anything. The epistemology of domination rarely asks questions of what is appropriate to know and under which circumstances (see Smith 2002). Scholars such as Patricia Hill Collins (1991) and Linda Tuhiwai Smith (2002)—writing on Afrocentric feminist and Māori feminist ways of knowing, respectively—engage with knowledge systems in which the personal accountability of knowers is a crucial part of knowledge formation. Smith (2002, 173) challenges those located within the Western paradigm to "question that most fundamental belief of all, that individual researchers have an inherent right to knowledge and truth." Collins (1991) argues that within the Afrocentric epistemology she outlines, an ethics of care as well as personal accountability and assuming responsibility for arguing validity (218) are key, in that "truth emerges through care" (217). While there are many more critiques from feminist, Indigenous, and feminist Indigenous scholars that reveal the harms of an epistemology of domination, I focus on two in particular: the ways in which this epistemology is ignorant of the importance of embodiment and of place.

Bodies of Knowledge

While I have previously written about how epistemic ignorance shapes and reproduces unjust structures in the international division of reproductive labor

(Prattes 2020), I am here interested in a different kind of relationship between knowledge and ignorance. Engaging with the positive epistemic implications that (can) arise out of performing caring labor evinces how difficult it is to grasp this kind of knowledge as knowledge under the dominant Western paradigm of epistemology. As "knowledge that is ignored," it points to ways of knowing that do not register within a framework that is narrowly trained on the cognitive and propositional form. Central knowledges about care are held in bodies; they emerge out of and are transmitted through embodied practices, such as the performance of domestic and care work.

The term "bodies of knowledge" emphasizes that knowledge is located and embodied. In contrast to the view from nowhere, knowledge emerges somewhere; it emerges in a specific place, in the interactions of human and more-than-human bodies.[4] These bodies are not to be imagined as bounded, discrete, and isolated. On the contrary, the bodies I seek to describe here have fuzzy edges; they are interdependent, interwoven through knowing practice (taking a cue here from anthropological work on socially embedded, plural, and composite, thus, partible, "dividuals"; i.e., Marriott 1976; Strathern 1988). They move through dynamic interactions of knowledge making and need to be grasped beyond an either-or binary framing of knower "versus" known. Knowing emerges through interactions. It is located in bodies and placed in world/s. While knowledge might be "held" in bodies, as spaces, this holding is not static or fixed but a dynamic process between moving and changing bodies.

Bodies of knowledge do not need to be human bodies. Learning from Indigenous epistemologies, bodies of water are bodies of knowledge. Nonhuman animals, stones, and the land itself (as a complex interweaving and coming together of diverse, integral parts) engage with one another in producing knowledge and "hold" knowledge. Practice and movement are, thus, critical in knowledge-formation processes within such a framework—as is (respectful) interaction. Knowledge decidedly does not emerge through the investigation of a disjointed and isolated object of study by a neutral, detached, isolated, independent knower under "pure" conditions uncontaminated by its world. On the contrary, knowing emerges through interdependence, through intermingling parts in dynamic processes that are very much part of their respective world/s (de la Cadena and Blaser 2018; Escobar 2018; FitzGerald 2021).

Standpoint theorists (Haraway 1988; Harding 1991, 1993) advocate for considering the specificity not only of individual embodiment but of social location and the epistemological relevance of positionality. They mobilize a relational understanding of knowledge and knowing that can capture structures of differential power that accrue to groups of knowers. Beyond the importance of human embodiment and social location that these theorists have highlighted, Indigenous onto-epistemologies (Bawaka Country et al. 2013, 2022; Coulthard 2010; Moreton-Robinson 2013; Rey 2021; Simpson 2014, 2017, 2021; Tuck and McKenzie 2015; Welch 2019) go further than the Western feminist conceptions of positionality and unfold a more substantial theory of location, in which human persons know and care with (and as) Country (Bawaka Country et al. 2013). These accounts are more encompassing in that they not only challenge the supposed neutrality of universal knowers and their detachment from the known but transcend some fundamental Western oppositions, such as human/earth, animate/inanimate, and living/dead. The Aboriginal[5] epistemology Aileen Moreton-Robinson puts forward, for instance, is based on an ontological relationship that "occurs through the inter-substantiation of ancestral beings, humans and country; it is a form of *embodiment* based on blood line to country" (Moreton-Robinson 2013, 341, emphasis added). In Nishnaabeg knowledge too, Leanne Betasamosake Simpson (2014, 7, emphasis original) writes that learning comes "both *from* the land and *with* the land."

Caring for and in Place

Feminist care ethics—marginalized within the Western paradigm—have points of contact and overlap with Indigenous and other relational epistemologies.[6] Yet it bears repeating that most people working with care ethics from Western locations (myself included), even if marginalized therein, remain embedded within Western ontologies—and a conceptual human/Country split (see also Doucet, Jewell, and Watts in this volume [chapter 7]). Consequently, they mostly remain human-centered.[7] Glen Coulthard (2010) distinguishes between land-based epistemologies and time-based (colonial) frameworks and underlines the ontological (and epistemological) importance of land for his people, the Dene Nations, in the settler-colonial context of Canada: "Place is a way of knowing, experiencing, and relating with the world—and these ways of knowing often guide forms of resistance to power relations that threaten to erase or destroy our sense of place" (80). In Australia, the Aboriginal and settler collective writing as Bawaka Country (2022) emphasizes how in Yolŋu epistemology, human and more-than-human beings hold knowledge and depend on each other's knowledge and care for their continued existence/creation and flourishing (4).[8] Knowledge can be held by individuals as well as by collectives (see also Welch 2019, 7) and is not limited to human knowers. Many Indigenous epistemologies differ from the "epistemology of mastery" (Code 2006) in that they do not center or prioritize human knowledges; they include nonhuman animals and other more-than-human teachers (Simpson 2014, 12). Relational epistemologies of interdependence usually start from the assumption that all knowledges and all beings depend on each other.

Among the many epistemologies that consider not only embodied practice but also place, as well as care and accountability, Aboriginal Australian onto-epistemologies evince more elaborate understandings of the importance of place in knowledge-formation processes than the epistemology of domination does. Take the existence of songlines (or songspirals) (see Bawaka Country et al. 2022; Australian Institute of Aboriginal and Torres Strait Islander Studies [AIATSIS] 2021). These are paths across land—and sometimes the sky—that mark the routes of ancestral creators of Aboriginal Australia. They are navigational routes—geographical, cultural, and spiritual—that trace places of significance. They connect humans to Country.[9]

The Marlaloo songline project aims to record, map, and maintain the ceremony of this songline that runs from Balginjirr to Marlaloo in Western Australia and covers a significant part of the Martuwarra (Fitzroy River). In the context of that songline project, scholar and Nyikina Warrwa traditional owner Anne Poelina says that songlines "are profound, they are still alive, because one of the things... Indigenous people [say] is, the land is alive, the rivers are alive, the Country is alive, *because it holds memory*" (AIATSIS 2021, emphasis added). Poelina explains how, in order for the important knowledge about this songline to be shared, the community had been waiting "in a circle of time" (AIATSIS 2021) for the right moment, for the opportunity to pass on the knowledge in an appropriate manner that was "respectful to the land, but importantly, the songlines" (AIATSIS 2021). The actualization and transmission of this knowledge required embodied performance (dancing and singing). However, first it required being in a specific place: the dancers and new knowledge holders had to be on Nyikina Country and be with the elders, to travel through the landscapes, and do ceremony at each significant place. As Poelina puts it, "So we had to go to Countries, so Countries could see that we were legitimate, and that the transfer and [t]his knowledge and wisdom, were going to Nginarr men who were ready to carry the songline into the future, by learning and... engaging Country now" (AIATSIS 2021). Respect, legitimacy, reciprocity, responsibility, and care are necessary here to hold and share knowledge. Practice and performance are key to knowledge production and transmission. Accountability and care are crucial, as is the specificity of place. Knowledge comes into existence through a collaborative effort of human and more-than-human people (such as the ancestral serpents in this songline) with Country. In this framework, knowledge emerges not only "in" place but with and "as" Country.

I recognize the specificity of this epistemology on Nyikina Country as rooted in and significant to that particular Country. It cannot simply be transferred to other places. Still, certain features of that epistemology stand out to me as relevant in other contexts, such as the importance assigned to place, embodiment and performance, and accountability and care.

Learning from Place-Based Epistemologies

Such co-becoming of Country, alongside or with human and nonhuman persons, is a central part of caring for Country in different Aboriginal Australian contexts—and First Nations elsewhere (Coulthard 2010; Simpson 2017, 2021). Caring with Country or, as Bawaka Country have called it on Yolŋu Country in North East Arnhem Land, "caring-as-country" (Bawaka Country et al. 2013) is crucial in Aboriginal onto-epistemologies. Here, embodiment is "based on blood line to country" (Moreton-Robinson 2013, 341). This kind of relationality, such interdependent embodiment with place, is unfamiliar to most non-Indigenous people, as we lack this kind or level of place-centeredness. As Welch poignantly puts it, "Western frameworks, because grounded in universality, atomistic individualism, and hierarchy, do not recognize the importance of place since the recognition of relations of space and place would have precluded or, at least, most certainly caused great cognitive difficulty and dissonance for their colonial ventures" (Welch 2019, 20). How can those of us who are not embedded within them learn from place-based epistemologies? Or is my aim—to "use" Indigenous epistemic wealth to solve problems of the North—itself an extractivist project, which removes such knowledges from the very places that give them meaning?

PRACTICE

> [To] set this idea of caring—having the proper attitude as originary—misses the ways in which caring attitudes themselves arise out of caring practices. It ignores the fact… that attentiveness to needs can and must itself be trained. Care-giving is not (only?) natural and innate, one can become attuned to it.
>
> —Tronto (2013, 48–49)
>
> Doing care work helps men develop caring forms of masculinities and more nurturing identities.
>
> —Elliott (2016, 255)

The two above quotes speak to the connections between practices of care work and distinct ways of learning. I suggest that diverse "knowledges" can emerge through the performance of embodied caring practices: know-how and caring skills; caring attitudes and dispositions; and more abstract knowledge that can emerge for changed selves—such as knowledge about the value of care or about the general devaluation and the abysmal conditions in which caring work is often expected to be performed.

As feminist epistemologists argue (Code 1991, 1993; Dalmiya 2001, 2016; Shotwell 2011, 2014), the framing of propositional knowledge as the only game in town is problematic. Vrinda Dalmiya and Linda Martín Alcoff (1993) challenge the primacy of propositional knowledge and the disregard for "knowing how" and "experiential knowledge," two key aspects of knowledge through care. Their critique, and Dalmiya's later work (2001, 2016), is central to my focus on practice. Dalmiya (2016) develops a "care-based epistemology" in which the experience of concrete situations is central to knowledge formation and knowers are understood as embodied beings embedded in webs of relations. In *Caring to Know* (2016), Dalmiya argues that good knowing practices and good caring practices are to be regarded not as separate from each other but as connected to each other. Shay Welch's (2019) work on Native American epistemology as a performative knowledge system highlights the fundamental centrality of praxis and performance to knowledge formation and transmission in the Native epistemology she discusses.

Welch analyzes the Native American philosophical definition of Truth, which is purely procedural and action-centered.[10] Using Native dancing as her prime example of "Native Truthing," Welch shows "what it means and how it is for Truth to be constituted by the performance of an action rather than by content or nature of statements" (6). She writes, "Knowledge consists in knowing *how* to P, not *that* P. One typically cannot know how to P without 'knowing that P' but one can easily 'know that P' without knowing how to P, and thus makes a propositional construal of knowledge and Truth relatively useless in the practical sense on which Native epistemology focuses" (Welch 2019, 39, emphasis original).

I have previously written about my Viennese study's findings in terms of (gendered and racialized) practices of epistemic ignorance or "active unknowing" in domestic cleaning (Prattes 2020). Unknowing, among my research participants, was gendered, particularly pronounced among men, and connected to "privileged irresponsibility" (Tronto 1993, 120–121). As I discuss in this section, what I also found—among and between practices of active unknowing—were nascent potentials of an epistemology of care[11] that emerged out of the men's embodied practices.

Building on and weaving together the theoretical insights from the Indigenous embodied and place-based epistemologies cited above, this section speaks about privileged subjects who do little caring labor. Emphasizing the centrality of experiential knowledge and knowing how for knowledge formation, I seek to develop an embodied epistemology rooted in these men's "places" that is mobilized through their practices of care work.

(Privileged) "Man-Knowers" Doing Care Work

In critical studies on men and masculinities (CSMM) we currently find a renewed attention to men and care. Scholars have highlighted that men can be competent caregivers and that men do perform care work (Doucet 2006; Elliott 2016, 2019, 2020; Hamington 2002; Hanlon 2012; Jackson 2021; Ranson 2015). Still, structurally privileged men (who are white, cisgender, heterosexual, middle-class, able-bodied) perform care work in much lower numbers than Black, Indigenous, and other People of Color, as well as white women and nonbinary and gender-nonconforming people.

CSMM scholars from the social sciences have identified the importance of men's embodiment to care, though not all are interested in its epistemological implications.[12] Gillian Ranson (2015) emphasizes that embodiment is crucial for fathers' caregiving for their babies. Ranson argues that fathers learn to care, that this learning makes care work visible to them as work, and that finally, by performing the work of care, men are transformed as people (see also Hanlon 2012).

The vast majority of studies on men doing the work of care focus on fathering. Within the hierarchy of domestic and caring labor fathering is currently the most visible and most valued work for men. By contrast, I am especially interested in the less valued caring work of domestic cleaning, which is hardly investigated—especially concerning men.[13] It is important to note that the care work of fathering again emphasizes a human-to-human relationship, whereas the work of cleaning—while also directed toward the well-being of human persons—necessarily engages with place. Therefore, it is more readily related to the more-than-human parts that make up place and the in/attentive practices to emerge from these interactions.

In the study in Vienna (Prattes 2017), I did research with white, well-educated, cisgender men and their women partners who paid migrant women for domestic cleaning services in the informal market. The men in my sample performed little reproductive labor, as most of it was done either by women domestic workers or by the women partners who lived with them (Prattes 2020). Still, as shown in this section, I found glimpses of knowledge that emerged through their embodied domestic practices in these privileged men's narratives. And it was here that my interest in the relationship between knowledge formation and embodied (care) practices was amplified.

I used a mix of different empirical methods (for details, see Prattes 2017, 2020). One of these methods was so-called go-alongs (see Kusenbach 2003), in which I accompanied the men in my sample in a routine domestic work task of their choosing. Like other participants in the study, Jakob generally found the enjoyment of cleaning to be a bit weird. He strongly associated what he called a "mania for cleaning" (Jakob, individual interview) with women, thus setting himself and his masculine performance apart from devalued, ostensibly "feminine" work. Jakob also told me that generally he was more interested in the "gadget" side of household cleaning and connected the fact that he favored tasks involving electrical appliances (such as vacuum cleaning) over mopping or wiping with masculinity.

There were several points in my interactions with Jakob where he was attentive toward his domestic space and dirty matter in that space. This embodied attentiveness was most strikingly brought to the fore by Jakob's detailed description of using a steam broom, an appliance for cleaning tiles. In his go-along, Jakob mentioned to me the little speckles of toothpaste clinging to the bathroom floor that just by "mopping the floor wet often cannot be removed" (Jakob, go-along). Without the steam broom, Jakob asserted, "yes, you often have to scratch them off the floor" (Jakob, go-along).

This intimate knowledge of what domestic work his household requires and the necessary skills involved in cleaning the floors, I argue, stem from Jakob's embodied performance of engaging in reproductive labor: actually doing some of the cleaning himself. Attentiveness, as an embodied skill that is critically important for caring labor, is honed in the practices of performing care work. In the go-along, Jakob's attentiveness toward the specificity of different kinds of dirt (besides the toothpaste on the bathroom floor, he also mentioned splatters of food on the kitchen floor, the dirt from pets, and dirt brought in from the streets) became very tangible. Distinct forms of attentiveness to dirt and the knowledge and skills needed to clean the dirt away are facilitated by, or emerge out of, the embodied practices of cleaning themselves. This knowledge is held in his body—although, significantly, it does not emerge spontaneously "out of his body," disconnected from his surroundings. Instead, the knowledge emerges through an interactive process that he engages in "through his body" with the specific place of his apartment. What is more, apart from this place (the apartment), his knowledge emerges within a sociopolitical-socioeconomic space in which Jakob is located; and it is this latter location or situatedness that makes paid domestic cleaning accessible to him. In this process, Jakob's human body comes into contact—through a domestic practice—with other "parts" (Strathern 1988) that are crucial for the emerging knowledge. I suggest that knowledge here is relationally co-constituted between Jakob's human body, the materiality of "dirt" (that is itself always socially, culturally, and politically produced as dirt; Douglas 1996), the electrical appliance of the steam broom, the very space of his home, and his social and geopolitical positioning. Which is to say, Jakob's embodied knowledge is shaped by the larger context within which he is performing this work. Jakob is doing this task within a context in which reproductive labor is racialized and feminized and typically not assigned to subjects like him. This context frames why Jakob and other structurally privileged men typically engage in domestic and care work to such a limited degree. It is widely accepted that subjects like him are entitled to receiving copious amounts of care—in contrast, say, to the women of Haitian ancestry employed as domestic workers in the Dominican Republic whom Masaya Llavaneras Blanco writes about (see chapter 10). Indeed, at the time of the interview, Jakob was hardly engaging in his practice with the steam-broom since his household had (after a break in which Jakob and his partner cleaned their apartment themselves) started to pay a migrant woman to do this work again. By "outsourcing" domestic work, I argue, Jakob and his partner have less opportunity to themselves engage in this embodied, located performances of care—they are less likely to learn the specific knowledges that emerge from these care practices.

The Importance of Practice for Knowing

The empirical vignette above from my research with Jakob registers as relatively unremarkable—epistemologically speaking—within the epistemology of domination. By contrast, epistemologies that give more weight to practice and performance have fewer difficulties grasping experiential knowledge and know-how and provide opportunities to perceive the central knowledges of care and ways of knowing through caring that I am interested in. The Native American epistemology that Welch elucidates posits Truth not as a function of proposition—as the dominant Western paradigm does—but as a function of action (Welch 2019, 23), as a social, relational, and ethical practice that is always grounded in land/water, always grounded in place. The epistemology that Michael, Jakob, and I have access to in Vienna is decidedly not a procedural one in Welch's sense—which is to say, embodied performance and practice are not crucial within it. What is more, it is not rooted in place in any way comparable to the Indigenous epistemologies

I have drawn on. Nonetheless, ways of knowing that are better emplaced—situated more deeply and grounded in materiality and embodiment—can be cultivated in part through practices of care, as I have shown here. And indeed, within the domestic caring practices of the men in Vienna I did research with, we could identify glimmers or starting points of knowledge that is taking shape in ways that are relational and responsive—knowledge that is emerging through embodied practices within a specific place. I have tried to focus our attention on these aspects to construct an epistemology that goes beyond separation, mastery, control, or domination and toward relationality with the more-than-human that is of this particular place.[14]

CONCLUDING REMARKS: BEYOND EPISTEMIC EXTRACTIVISM?

This chapter adds to the ongoing efforts to decenter the epistemology of domination. It does so by centering the importance of practices (of men's care work) to knowledge formation. I argue that certain kinds of knowledges and some ways of knowing are accessed and acquired, actualized, and transmitted chiefly through embodied practices. Next, I connected embodied practices of care work with the importance of place to epistemology. The domestic practice of Jakob, just as Michael's equation of paying "as" cleaning that I started this chapter with, took "place" somewhere. Yet they are rooted in an epistemology that lacks a nuanced understanding of the relevance of embodiment, place, and practice for knowledge formation. Still, Jakob has acquired some knowledge through his care work. He knows of the toothpaste, the splatters of food, and the other kinds of dirt he recognizes because he has engaged in cleaning them away in the specificity of his place. He has developed attentive practices that consider what is needed for his—this—home environment to be a livable space. And though Jakob has (some) embodied and cognitive knowledge about cleaning his home, this knowledge does not register as "knowledge" within the epistemology of domination.

Drawing on feminist and, specifically, Indigenous scholarship that sees this embodied, place-based knowledge as knowledge, my effort to decenter the dominant paradigm has led me to the question of "how" to learn from epistemological frameworks such as the nondominating ones considered in this chapter in a way that is relationally humble (Dalmiya 2016) and respectful. To do so is no small feat, given the power asymmetries among and between the worlds we live in—the concepts of "epistemic extractivism" and "epistemic appropriation" highlight common, violent pitfalls.[15] I have already mentioned the concept of epistemic extractivism (Grosfoguel 2019; Alcoff 2022) to name how knowledge is taken and transferred elsewhere, disregarding the epistemic communities that have produced it, decontextualizing and depoliticizing knowledge. By "subsuming these forms of indigenous knowledge within Western knowledge, the radical politics and 'alternative' critique of cosmogony are stripped away to make them more acceptable, or else simply extracted from a more radical epistemic matrix in order to depoliticize them" (Grosfoguel 2019, 208). Epistemic extractivism is not a horizontal dialogue but a vertical/hierarchical taking—an extraction of knowledge that is violent. As Simpson puts it, "Extracting is stealing. It is taking without consent" (quoted in Klein 2013)—without care for the interdependent human-more-than-human relations within which knowledge is produced. In a similar vein, Emmalon Davis (2018) talks about epistemic appropriation, which she defines as composed of two distinct but connected features: first, epistemic detachment and, second, epistemic misdirection. On the first point, Davis maintains that while the harm of epistemic appropriation does not hinder targets of epistemic appropriation "from putting knowledge into the public domain . . . , members of marginalized groups are never *acknowledged as contributors* [which] is essential to the perpetuation of their epistemic marginalization" (28–29, emphasis original). While I have tried not to detach the epistemologies from their worlds and recognize and reference authors, collectives, and places connected to the epistemologies I draw on, the project could be read as unable to avoid the second epistemic harm Davis outlines—that of misdirection. This is so because my aim of learning from relational epistemologies (that recognize embodied practice and place, care and accountability) is connected to an investigation of men in the Global North. In other words, I "use" the epistemic wealth that comes out of marginalized communities in a privileged context of the center. However, the ultimate goal of decentering the dominant paradigm is to challenge its very dominance and the violence of an epistemology of mastery.

Jo Anne Rey, a Dharug woman,[16] urges that educating "non-Indigenous peoples to become literate in reading, relating with and caring for/as Ngurra is at the heart of sustainable futures" (Rey 2021, 23).[17] A recognition of relationality and interdependence with place is critical for our living together well, and—at this stage—is essential to planetary survival. Rey writes, "With a Country-centric way of being, our ways of knowing are also going to be centred in Ngurra [Country] and involve knowing through *experiential*, contextual learning for the pragmatic purpose of doing-as-caring. Such a praxis involves reciprocity with/as Ngurra" (Rey 2021, 16, emphasis added). The Country-centric way of being and knowing—this place-based onto-epistemology—that Rey describes involves attentive and responsive embodied practices.

Learning from embodied and place-based epistemologies to develop one's own—located—epistemic practices might not be straightforward for folks located in the Western paradigm. Yet it is critical. And it is equally critical that this learning takes place in ways that do not appropriate Indigenous epistemic wealth in an extractivist manner—that those of us located in close proximity to the dominant paradigm of epistemology work continuously to extract ourselves from extractivism.

NOTES

1. All names of research participants are pseudonyms.
2. See, for instance, Simpson (2014) and López López and Coello (2021).
3. I use "dominant" and "dominating" interchangeably to emphasize that the particular epistemology I aim to decenter is dominant because it is dominating. It works to subjugate alternative frameworks such as various Indigenous epistemologies and other epistemologies marginalized through its power.
4. I here use the term "more-than-human" to challenge the anthropocentrism of the binary pair human–nonhuman that, in a way, thinks the nonhuman as that which the human is not. Moreover, I am thinking here of interrelationships of humans not only with other animals but with all that surrounds us.
5. While First Nations people on Turtle Island mostly do not use this term (opting for Indigenous and other names instead), in the Australian context it is widely used by First Nations people—it emphasizes that Aboriginal people where connected to this land "from the beginning."
6. See Boulton and Brannelly (2015) on the connections between care ethics and key Māori values and practices. See also Doucet, Jewell, and Watts in this volume (chapter 7) on resonance and refusal in the exchanges about care between Indigenous and non-Indigenous frameworks. Here, Vanessa Watts (chapter 7) emphasizes the important difference between ecological and ecofeminist approaches to care and an Indigenous-informed one: "Though resonances on the topics of other-than-humans and white heteropatriarchy can and will be found, Indigenous-based relationships with other-than-humans are inscribed with diverse territorial protocols and cosmological, onto-epistemological ideas of care. Further, Indigenous-based relationships with white heteropatriarchy are marked by violent policies of *Care* intended for Indigenous peoples and rationalized as a particular sort of caring *of* Indigenous peoples."
7. See María Puig de la Bellacasa (2017) for an exception.
8. Discussing how songspirals (aka songlines) bring Country into existence, Bawaka Country et al. share how Country is continually created through singing—to this day. Songspirals hold knowledge, but they are more than "knowledge" in the Western sense. The embodied performance of singing is central to knowledge formation and sharing, but not only. Bawaka Country et al. (2022, 3–4) write, "Songspirals are Yolŋu life—they are the doing, being, thinking, understanding of Yolŋu life-worlds. They are a generative ontological manifestation of relationality, of the ongoing emergence of everything in relation with everything else, of the co-becoming of time and place. . . . For us, the land sang itself into existence and it still sings. . . . So, bringing the world into existence is a collective, relational, more-than-human endeavor. It is not just humans who sing. Animals, plants, trees, the wind, all the beings of Country sing. They sing for themselves and they sing to us. . . . We sing the bird and the bird sings us. We sing winds and they sing us."
9. In Aboriginal Australian usage, the word "Country" cannot be translated to land only. Country encompasses culture, nature, landforms, trees, animals, foods, medicines, stories, songs, other cultural practices, law, lore, knowledge, all people (including ancestors and future generations), and more.
10. Welch's use of procedural knowing is different from Habermasian or other Western notions of proceduralism. In the Native paradigm that Welch elaborates a procedural analysis of knowledge and Truth is opposed to a propositional one. Procedural knowing is about a connection to performances and praxes and emphasizes the action-centeredness of this epistemological tradition.
11. "Epistemology of care" here refers to the knowledges and ways of knowing that could emerge from the men's located and embodied practices of care. This is not to be confused with

Dalmiya's (2016) "full-blown" care-based epistemology—an epistemological framework based on care.

12. Andrea Doucet (2006) is a noteworthy exception as she works on men and care and is interested in questions of epistemology.

13. Elsewhere, I have written about the hierarchies of different tasks of social reproductive labor and how "mundane" domestic labor and the more valued work of fathering are interconnected—also through an international division of male reproductive labor (Prattes 2022). Research finds that it is precisely by relying on the work of migrant handymen and domestic cleaners for less valued forms of social reproduction that well-educated men manage to both hold on to their status-giving roles of breadwinners and be involved fathers (see Palenga-Möllenbeck 2016).

14. While I cannot go into this here, it is important to note that complicating my efforts is the fact that "place" and tradition coupled with violence have been used in the very same location I write about here to subjugate, dehumanize, and annihilate "others"—be it as part of imperial endeavors or Nazism. These moves collude with the violent extractivist paradigm that Simpson and others critique.

15. See also Linda Martín Alcoff (2022, 16), who elaborates four corrective epistemic norms to counter extractivist epistemologies: "(i) acknowledging the incompleteness of all knowledge, (ii) developing an approach that recognizes plural epistemologies and seeks productive relationships of inter-epistemology, (iii) practicing relational epistemic humility, and (iv) regularizing the assessment of epistemic relationships in projects of knowing."

16. Dharug Country is located in the western part of Sydney and covers the majority of the city.

17. *Ngurra* is the word for Country in the Dharug language.

REFERENCES

Alcoff, Linda Martín. 2022. "Extractivist Epistemologies." *Tapuya: Latin American Science, Technology and Society* 5 (1). https://doi.org/10.1080/25729861.2022.2127231.

Australian Institute of Aboriginal and Torres Strait Islander Studies (AIATSIS). 2021. "The Marlaloo Songline." https://aiatsis.gov.au/explore/marlaloo-songline?fbclid=IwAR20WL zlD8VVXUlt7po5fVh_MNVZ6JBiouoS5sbBpbNtrnKM37JQnus8WnA.

Bawaka Country including Sandie Suchet-Pearson, Sarah Wright, Kate Lloyd, and Laklak Burarrwanga. 2013. "Caring *as* Country: Towards an Ontology of Co-becoming in Natural Resource Management." *Asia Pacific Viewpoint* 54 (2): 185–197.

Bawaka Country including Laklak Burarrwanga, Ritjilili Ganambarr, Merrkiyawuy Ganambarr-Stubbs, Banbapuy Ganambarr, Djawundil Maymuru, Kate Lloyd, Sarah Wright, Sandie Suchet-Pearson, and Lara Daley. 2022. "Songspirals Bring Country into Existence: Singing More-Than-Human and Relational Creativity." *Qualitative Inquiry* 28 (5): 435–447.

Boulton, Amohia, and Tula Brannelly. 2015. "Care Ethics and Indigenous Values: Political, Tribal and Personal." In *Ethics of Care: Critical Advances in International Perspective*, edited by Marian Barnes, Tula Brannelly, Lizzie Ward, and Nicki Ward, 69–82. Bristol: Policy Press.

Cheney, Jim. 2002. "The Moral Epistemology of First Nations Stories." *Canadian Journal of Environmental Education* 7 (2): 88–100.

Code, Lorraine. 1991. *What Can She Know? Feminist Theory and the Construction of Knowledge.* Ithaca, NY: Cornell University Press.

———. 1993. "Taking Subjectivity into Account." In *Feminist Epistemologies*, edited by Linda Martín Alcoff and Elizabeth Potter, 49–82. New York: Routledge.

———. 2006. *Ecological Thinking: The Politics of Epistemic Location.* New York: Oxford University Press.

Collins, Patricia Hill. 1991. *Black Feminist Thought: Knowledge, Consciousness, and the Politics of Empowerment*. New York: Routledge.

Coulthard, Glen. 2010. "Place Against Empire: Understanding Indigenous Anti-colonialism." *Affinities: A Journal of Radical Theory, Culture, and Action* 4 (2): 79–83.

Dalmiya, Vrinda. 2001. "Knowing People." In *Knowledge, Truth, and Duty: Essays on Epistemic Justification, Responsibility, and Virtue*, edited by Matthias Steup, 221–234. Oxford: Oxford University Press.

———. 2016. *Caring to Know: Comparative Care Ethics, Feminist Epistemology, and the Mahābhārata*. New Delhi: Oxford University Press.

Dalmiya, Vrinda, and Linda Martín Alcoff. 1993. "Are 'Old Wives' Tales' Justified?" In *Feminist Epistemologies*, edited by Linda Martín Alcoff and Elizabeth Potter, 217–244. New York: Routledge.

Davis, Emmalon. 2018. "On Epistemic Appropriation." *Ethics* 128 (3): 702–727.

de la Cadena, Marisol, and Mario Blaser. 2018. *A World of Many Worlds*. Durham, NC: Duke University Press.

Doucet, Andrea. 2006. *Do Men Mother? Fathering, Care, and Domestic Responsibility*. Toronto: University of Toronto Press.

Douglas, Mary. 1996. *Purity and Danger: An Analysis of the Concepts of Pollution and Taboo*. London: Routledge.

Elliott, Karla. 2016. "Caring Masculinities: Theorizing an Emerging Concept." *Men and Masculinities* 19 (3): 240–259.

———. 2019. "Zum Problem von Macht und Dominanz im Konzept Caring Masculinities." In *Caring Masculinities: Männlichkeiten in der Transformation kapitalistischer Wachstumsgesellschaften*, edited by Sylka Scholz and Andreas Heilmann, 201–212. Munich: Oekom Verlag.

———. 2020. *Young Men Navigating Contemporary Masculinities*. Cham: Palgrave Macmillan.

Escobar, Arturo. 2018. *Designs for the Pluriverse: Radical Interdependence, Autonomy, and the Making of Worlds*. Durham, NC: Duke University Press.

FitzGerald, Maggie. 2021. "Precarious Political Ontologies and the Ethics of Care." In *Care Ethics in the Age of Precarity*, edited by Maurice Hamington and Michael Flowers, 191–209. Minneapolis: University of Minnesota Press.

Grosfoguel, Ramón. 2019. "Epistemic Extractivism: A Dialogue with Alberto Acosta, Leanne Betasamosake Simpson, and Silvia Rivera Cusicanqui." In *Knowledges Born in the Struggle: Constructing the Epistemologies of the Global South*, edited by Boaventura de Sousa Santos and Maria Paula Meneses, 203–218. New York: Routledge.

Hamington, Maurice. 2002. "A Father's Touch: Caring Embodiment and a Moral Revolution." In *Revealing Male Bodies*, edited by Nancy Tuana, William Cowling, Maurice Hamington, Greg Johnson, and Terrance MacMullan, 269–285. Bloomington: Indiana University Press.

Hanlon, Niall. 2012. *Masculinities, Care and Equality: Identity and Nurture in Men's Lives*. Basingstoke: Palgrave Macmillan.

Haraway, Donna. 1988. "Situated Knowledges: The Science Question in Feminism and the Privilege of Partial Perspective." *Feminist Studies* 14 (3): 575–599.

Harding, Sandra. 1991. *Whose Science? Whose Knowledge? Thinking from Women's Lives*. Ithaca, NY: Cornell University Press.

———. 1993. "Rethinking Standpoint Epistemology: What Is Strong Objectivity?" In *Feminist Epistemologies*, edited by Linda Alcoff and Elizabeth Potter, 49–82. New York: Routledge.

Jackson, Aaron J. 2021. *Worlds of Care: The Emotional Lives of Fathers Caring for Children with Disabilities*. Oakland: University of California Press.

Klein, Naomi. 2013. "Dancing the World into Being: A Conversation with Idle No More's Leanne Simpson." *YES!*, March 6, 2013. https://www.yesmagazine.org/social-justice/2013/03/06/dancing-the-world-into-being-a-conversation-with-idle-no-more-leanne-simpson.

Kusenbach, Margarethe. 2003. "Street Phenomenology: The Go-Along as Ethnographic Research Tool." *Ethnography* 4 (3): 455–485.
López López, Ligia (Licho), and Gioconda Coello. 2021. *Indigenous Futures and Learnings Taking Place*. Abingdon: Routledge.
Marriott, McKim. 1976. *Hindu Transactions: Diversity without Dualism*. Chicago: University of Chicago Press.
Moreton-Robinson, Aileen. 2013. "Towards an Australian Indigenous Women's Standpoint Theory." *Australian Feminist Studies* 28 (78): 331–347.
Palenga-Möllenbeck, Ewa. 2016. "Unequal Fatherhoods: Citizenship, Gender, and Masculinities in Outsourced 'Male' Domestic Work." In *Paid Migrant Domestic Labour in a Changing Europe*, edited by Berit Gullikstad, Guro Korsnes Kristensen, and Priscilla Ringrose, 217–243. London: Palgrave Macmillan.
Prattes, Riikka. 2017. "Outsourcing Responsibility: Towards a Transformative Politics of Domestic Work." PhD diss., Institute for Social Justice, Australian Catholic University.
———. 2020. "'I Don't Clean Up After Myself': Epistemic Ignorance, Responsibility and the Politics of the Outsourcing of Domestic Cleaning." *Feminist Theory* 21 (1): 25–45.
———. 2022. "Caring Masculinities and Race: On Racialized Workers and 'New Fathers.'" *Men and Masculinities* 25 (5). https://doi.org/10.1177/1097184X211065024.
Puig de la Bellacasa, María. 2017. *Matters of Care: Speculative Ethics in More Than Human Worlds*. Minneapolis: University of Minnesota Press.
Ranson, Gillian 2015. *Fathering, Masculinity and the Embodiment of Care*. Basingstoke: Palgrave Macmillan.
Rey, Jo Anne. 2021. "Changing Places: Weaving City Learnings into Country Futures." In *Indigenous Futures and Learnings Taking Place*, edited by Ligia (Licho) López López and Gioconda Coello, 10–36. Milton: Taylor & Francis.
Shotwell, Alexis. 2011. *Knowing Otherwise: Race, Gender, and Implicit Understanding*. University Park: Pennsylvania State University Press.
———. 2014. "Implicit Knowledge: How It Is Understood and Used in Feminist Theory." *Philosophy Compass* 9 (5): 315–324.
Simpson, Leanne Betasamosake. 2014. "Land as Pedagogy: Nishnaabeg Intelligence and Rebellious Transformation." *Decolonization: Indigeneity, Education & Society* 3 (3): 1–25.
———. 2017. *As We Have Always Done: Indigenous Freedom through Radical Resistance*. Minneapolis: University of Minnesota Press.
———. 2021. *Dancing on Our Turtle's Back: Stories of Nishnaabeg Re-creation, Resurgence and a New Emergence*. Winnipeg: ARP Books.
Smith, Linda Tuhiwai. 2002. *Decolonizing Methodologies: Research and Indigenous Peoples*. New York: Zed Books.
Strathern, Marilyn. 1988. *The Gender of the Gift: Problems with Women and Problems with Society in Melanesia*. Berkeley: University of California Press.
Tronto, Joan C. 1993. *Moral Boundaries: A Political Argument for an Ethic of Care*. New York: Routledge.
———. 2013. *Caring Democracy: Markets, Equality, and Justice*. New York: New York University Press.
Tuck, Eve, and Marcia McKenzie. 2015. "Relational Validity and the 'Where' of Inquiry: Place and Land in Qualitative Research." *Qualitative Inquiry* 21 (7): 633–638.
Vergès, Françoise. 2021. *A Decolonial Feminism*. London: Pluto Press.
Welch, Shay. 2019. *The Phenomenology of a Performative Knowledge System: Dancing with Native American Epistemology*. Cham: Palgrave Macmillan.
Woodly, Deva. 2020. *The Politics of Care*. Edited by the New School. YouTube, June 30, 2020. https://www.youtube.com/watch?v=ih6F6N9pg-A.

5 · DECENTERINGS ELSEWHERE AND THE EPISTEMIC DIMENSIONS OF CARE

VRINDA DALMIYA

The Sanskrit epic *Mahabharata* has a short chapter ("The Book of the Women") that abruptly interrupts the epic's narrative of valor. In the aftermath of the righteous but apocalyptic war between the princely cousins, the Pandavas and the Kauravas, we find Queen Gandhari describing in graphic detail (to none other than Lord Krishna himself) a scene of women grieving the dead on the abandoned battlefield. Gandhari, the Kaurava queen, mourns her own kinsmen killed in the fight, but while doing so she constantly references the distraught Pandava princesses in the *enemy* camp, who are also bemoaning the loss of warriors on *their* side. The following are two excerpts that give us a flavor of the gritty power of her laments.

Gandhari tells Krishna, "[Upon] seeing headless bodies and bodiless heads, the women, unaccustomed to these things, are bewildered. After joining a head to a body, they stare at it blankly, and then they are pained to realize, 'This is not his,' but do not see another one in that place. And these [women] over here, joining arms, thighs, feet, and other pieces cut off by arrows, are overwhelmed by the misery" (Mbh 11.16.51–53; Fitzgerald 2004, 68).[1] She continues in another couplet, "[Oh look] this wife of [the warrior] Yupadhvaja's, her waist no bigger than [what] two hands might measure, having put her husband's arm in her lap, mourns pitiably. That hand of his would undo her belt, rub her full breasts, caress her navel, her thighs, her bottom, and pull off her skirt" (Mbh 11.24.17, 19; Fitzgerald 2004, 68).

The corporeal (dis)membering and (re)membering in these descriptions mark the *body* as a site of violence and sorrow as well as of pleasure and desire. Filtered through the lens of contemporary feminist theory, the brutal encounter with physical vulnerability pictured in the chapter signals subtly different conceptual moves. The scene of the weeping women could well be emphasizing Bonnie Honig's (2013) "mortalist humanism" that shifts the essence of the human from rationality to *being mortal*. Alternatively, the episode could be a gesture toward

Judith Butler's (2004) dissolving of us/them binaries through reconstituting norms of grievability. A third interpretation subsumes these conceptual configurations of physical vulnerability under the normativity of care. I develop this last option. Thus, the laments are read here as the care ethical voice, but in a "different" temporal and cultural context.

In general, attempting care ethical readings of episodes from the epic is significant on two levels.[2] Methodologically, it is an "epistemic disobedience" that grounds theorizing care in an *elsewhere* (a non-Western Sanskrit epic) and an *elsewhen* (in a text from ancient times), thereby dislodging care's conceptual moorings from contemporary Western feminism. On a substantial level, analyzing the *Mahabharata* in this way helps nuance the concept of care itself. "The Book of the Women," for instance, shifts the focus in care ethics from the "inevitable dependencies" of embodiment highlighted by Kittay (1999) to a more capacious fragility, including what can be called "epistemic vulnerability" and "moral vulnerability." Going beyond physical injurability and dependency to notions of uncertainty or not-knowing (epistemic vulnerability) and moral failure (moral vulnerability) radically enriches care ethical agency. Thus, the cross-cultural articulation of care attempted here is both formally and substantively transformative and could be the beginning of imagining feminist futures "in-between" different traditions (Chakrabarti and Weber 2015).

My argument starts by establishing that grief in "The Book of the Women" functions as an epistemic route to alternative moral truths. This dislodges classical tropes in *Indian* moral theories to make room for the relational everyday of caring *in those traditions*. But while paralleling the decentering of rational and autonomous agency in the Western mainstream, the "different voice" in this episode also shows how confronting corporeality can spill over into accepting limits to our knowledge or uncertainty. The next section picks up on another episode in the *Mahabharata* called "The Tale of the Hawk and the Pigeon" to reinforce the connection between embodiment and epistemic vulnerability or uncertainty. But it then segues into emphasizing a notion of moral vulnerability or moral failure. Physical fragility is therefore decentered and care ethical agency opens up to dependencies beyond the corporeal. The last part of the chapter brings the *Mahabharata*'s embrace of vulnerabili*ties*—an intertwined physical, epistemological, and moral precarity—into conversation with Bernard Williams's (1981) notion of moral luck and Lisa Tessman's (2015) work on moral failure. I show that this initiates a further shift of care from an ethics (as traditionally understood) to a politics that can sustain robust political solidarities.

Multiple decenterings are therefore attempted in this chapter. Recovering the differently configured "different voice" from the *Mahabharata*, first and foremost, disrupts the epistemic injustice of routinely ignoring non-Western textual sources in feminist theorizing. This is *methodological* decentering initiated by cross-cultural philosophy. However, turning toward care can often *recenter* an oppressive, albeit a non-Western, patriarchal mainstream.[3] Heteropatriarchy is not disrupted by foregrounding domestic, caring identities in contexts where mothers as goddesses coexist with rampant gender oppression and in cultures that are communitarian (nonindividualistic) to begin with. A "critical transformation" of traditional care concepts (Robinson 2016) is needed to deconstruct oppressive but "Indian" conceptions of moral life or *dharma*. For this we move to the substantive intervention of exploring how physical/corporeal dependencies play out in the cognitive/epistemic domain (as epistemic vulnerability) and in the agentive domain (as moral vulnerability). Finally, rearticulating care agency through such multiple vulnerabilities helps politicize the "ethic" of care by decentering its moral dimensions and enabling robust coalitions across various divides of power and privilege.

MOVING TOWARD CARE AND EPISTEMIC VULNERABILITY

Deconstructing the rational and independent ethical agent is said to open up alternatives to neoliberal agency (Tronto 2017). The relational and affective self of care troubles the vision of solitary individuals maximizing self-interest and market values through privatized notions of responsibility. But theorizing this alternative is squarely centered in the West. When care does step outside its Eurocentric home, it is usually to observe practices of caring in different geographical locations (Raghuram 2016) and explore how the migration of care workers across national borders (Weir 2005) complicates care relations. However, as outlined above, this chapter travels to non-Western *theoretical* locations to see whether and how care decenters the centers of these *other* worlds. The latter move is neither obvious nor straightforward. Note that inevitabilities of sickness, disability, and old age—the starting point of care ethics according to many—are encapsulated in the Buddha's First Noble Truth and in discussions of expiatory suffering underlying the Vedic theory of Karma. Beginning with embodied subjects and physical suffering is therefore not unknown in mainstream South Asian philosophies. Yet the latter remain patriarchal. Such dissonance raises questions like these: *Is* there a voice of "care" in Sanskrit textual sources (like the *Mahabharata*) that can align with *feminist* forms of the embodied and relational agent? And does care have to be configured differently than it has been in order to dismantle the bodied but oppressive moral agent of *Indic* traditions? Reading two episodes from the epic against their grain suggests affirmative answers to both questions. Let us begin with "The Book of the Women."

After the Great War between the princely cousins (the Pandavas and the Kauravas), the king ordered that the women of the court be driven to the abandoned battlefield awash with blood and resounding with screeches of vultures and hyenas picking at the bodies of fallen soldiers. The decree to bring grieving women out into the public space of the battlefield not only is in sharp contrast to Socrates's asking that the crying Xanthippe to be taken back to her private chambers (in the *Apology*) but was unusual even for *Mahabharata* times, when upper-caste women remained in *purdah*. Thus, "The Book of the Women" seems to be swimming against the current and is consciously designed to foreground the women's voice.

That voice, however, takes the form of staging spectacular grief when confronted with battle-scarred physical dismemberment of loved ones. Since Gandhari bemoans the loss experienced by *all* the women across enemy lines, we find here a bipartisan lament bridging "us" and "them" in a *collectivized* female wailing. The grieving is "public" both in the sense of being out in the open as well as in expressing the sorrow of a multitude. But given that standard readings of the epic see the battleground as a metaphor for the "field of morality," the question becomes, what do women *crying together* in that space mean for moral theory?[4]

The laments are multilayered. First, one cannot overlook a clear conservative strand that preserves the status quo and keeps social hierarchies intact. Women wail for their menfolk as "protectors" and cry out to follow them to the "Other World" to remain under their protection. Even though the warriors lie inert, incapable of shielding even themselves, their death is still taken as evidence of valor and a means for rewards in the afterlife. The women's suffering (in spite of their having done no discernible wrong) is accounted for by *their* own misdeeds in *past lives* in accordance with the Law of Karma.

Alternatively, appealing to Sanskrit poetics, some commentators make the case that graphic descriptions of devastation signify the *meaninglessness* of worldly pursuits (Hudson 2013). The weeping women, therefore, are designed to induce an aesthetic tranquility (*shanta rasa*) in the *reader* by underscoring the futility of *dharma* to prevent suffering. This makes the point that freedom from pain is possible only in an otherworldly state, thereby reinforcing *moksha* as the ultimate goal of human life. Such an interpretation also "contains" grief within the structural confines of conventional morality and props up orthodoxy of the times.

My suggestion, however, is that an "excess" in the laments unsettles conceptions of a good life presupposed in the above interpretations. They are thus moments of both questioning received views and discovering a different moral truth. The self-reflexivity of the epic and the constant reversing of its own answers make this reading of the chapter prima facie plausible. Accordingly, grief here is not a helpless response to mortality but an apt emotional response that registers a moral wrong that was missed by the prevailing ethical systems.[5] More specifically, grief of the wailing women becomes an epistemic route for decentering traditional *dharma* and establishing the normativity of care. The following contextualization of the episode is important for this interpretation.

A closer look at Gandhari's laments shows sorrow gradually morphing into rage against Krishna for not having stopped the carnage. She openly blames him—the upholder of *dharma* and hence by implication, *dharma* itself—for the destruction. She is even sarcastic and dismissive about *karmic* explanations that trace her suffering and loss to *her* past actions. But this overt critique is supplemented by a positive message embedded in a peculiar twist later in the narrative.

Note that the protagonists of "The Book of the Women" never really stopped grieving. In a subsequent episode,[6] Gandhari once again launches into a description of how she and the other women—all mentioned by name—remain desolate.[7] This time she is in conversation not with Krishna but with Vyasa, the author of the *Mahabharata*. She demands that he *rewrite* the story so that the grieving women be allowed to "meet" the deceased warriors one last time. Vyasa agrees to the revision. In a miraculous and surreal moment within the narrative world, the dead soldiers come to life: there is a joyous meeting of "father-son, mother-son, husband-wife, brother with brother, and friend with friend" (Mbh 15.33.3).[8]

The step to an argument for care lies here: the change in the narrative script is a change in the moral script initiated by the women. The transformation is facilitated by the fact that grief registers what *matters* through our losing it and thus can well be one of the "alarm bell" emotions of Tessman (2015). The women desire as a balm for their sorrow immersion in particularized togetherness with their fathers, sons, brothers, friends, and lovers. Even a fleeting experience of such intimacy appeases their pain, indicating thereby its *importance*. The literary device of rewinding to the past not just in memory but by reliving what the battle and justice had destroyed—remember that the carnage was caused by a "just" war—records personal relationships as a *value* that was overlooked by conventional morality justifying the war. Consequently, the women grieved not just loss of life but a *betrayal* by extant moral conventions: moral codes meant to prop up life had ended up ignoring our relational bonds of intimacy, the very source of meaning in life.

Interestingly, the later Gilligan (2014) also speaks of a similar betrayal as a distinct form of "moral injury." Analyzing the PTSD of Vietnam War veterans, the trauma of war in Gilligan's analysis is also confined to material destruction, but to conventions that willfully ignore what we all know to be true (that killing innocent children is wrong). Thus, both the epic and Gilligan emphasize loss of trust in mores and philosophical systems that fail to value relational bonds. The weeping women, therefore, "interrupt" the ontology of world transcendence supported by Karma and *moksha*. They celebrate quotidian life—the personal bonds of "father-son, mother-son, husband-wife, brother with brother, and friend with friend." Hence, prioritizing *this-worldly relationships* that embody practices of everyday care could well be their normative message. In this way, "The Book of the Women" aligns with the scholarship of Laugier (2015) and Das (2018), who ground care ethics in face-to-face relationships of "everyday" intimacy.

Now, the violence of war as the route to this moral truth is importantly different from starting with facts of infancy, sickness, disability, and old age that lead theorists like Kittay (1999) to the dependency relationships of care. Gandhari is responding to unexpected and horrific death and *unexpected* annihilation associated with having a body. Such extreme fragility in the face of violence cannot be reversed by dependency relationships: the dead do not come to life through caretaking. Therefore, the *Mahabharata*'s transition from violent *mortality* to dependency and care is bound to be different, if not more complicated.

The inherent ambiguity of the body as a site of violence *and* as a site of desire becomes important now. The porousness of physical bodies to the "outside" can be a source of both violence as well as comfort. Embodiment itself holds the key to the possibility of appeasing bodily pain. Consequently, it is not necessary to leave the body behind (as the *dharmic* order does) in order to respond to suffering. Quests for transcendent states like *moksha* forget to explore the affiliative potential inbuilt in bodied relationships. And by retrieving this possibility, the warrior women bring Indic traditions back to earth—to Veena Das's (2018) "everyday" and Sandra Laugier's (2015) "ordinary." Thus, the voice of care is recovered here as the flip side of violence. This is an important reminder that the relational self is tangled in both disruption and connection and that violence routinely erupts within caring practices.[9] The *Mahabharata*'s robust concept of care hence can check the overly celebratory and romanticized strands of Western care theory.

However, in spite of this advantage, the weeping women's turn to personal relationships must incorporate further critical resources in order to be truly "feminist" care. Without a reworking of the terms of relationships the women would simply be substituting the violence of war with the violence of a *patriarchal* everyday. The desirability of caring relations might be empirically evident, yet an "ethics" needs resources to bridge the gap between how we actually care and the ideal of how we ought to relate to others (Kittay 2019). Without qualitative reconfiguring of intimacies, the voice of the weeping women, like the voice of care generally, cannot be a *liberatory* moral alternative. Are there resources in the laments to justify this further normative move?

The macabre corporeal framing and physical vulnerability that trigger the shift to personal relationships in the first place also transform the texture of those bonds. Note that the *Mahabharata* chapter is grounded in trauma associated with embodiment. In the beginning of the episode, the encounter with sudden death of those deemed indestructible turned the privileged lives of the warrior women upside down. A feminist phenomenology of trauma shows that experiencing such extreme disorientation (Harbin 2016) can be followed by radical conceptual change.

More specifically, Susan Brison's (2002) exposition of what trauma makes us *turn to* and *how we recover* from it motivates a transition to feminist care in the episode. According to Brison, trauma introduces a mathematical "surd"—a nonsensical entry—into a "normal" series. The sense of absurdity experienced after trauma makes it "impossible [for those who have experienced trauma] to carry on with the series" (Brison 2002, 103) that had hitherto constituted normal life. However, Brison is insistent that survivors *do* recover, and what is remarkable is *how* they continue to live. In life after trauma, she claims, commonplace tropes of "coherence of the past," "control over the present," and "predictability of the future" no longer make sense and have to be given up. Thus, survivors abandon *certainties* that had hitherto structured their lives in order to continue living.

Mapping this onto the *Mahabharata* makes the surreal scene of havoc on the battlefield an "absurdity" or "unthinkable" in the worldview of the warrior women.

Yet as survivors of trauma, they carried on with life *without appealing to the sense-making mechanisms* they were used to. Particularly, notions of Karma and *moksha*-inspired visions of the good life were hollowed out by their exposure to violence. Notice that Brison's three tropes that were rendered ineffective in life post-trauma involved "mastery" and "control" over the unexpected. Notice also that the "Law" of Karma is similarly about taking control of and ordering the future in terms of the present. The traumatized wailing women thus are led to abandon these principles as "illusions." Their turn to a relational reality involves giving up a quest for law-like certainties for a deep *lack of control*: life after trauma is a *reorientation* to living with uncertainty or, in our terminology, a living with epistemic vulnerability.

Interestingly, uncertainty was mentioned in Carol Gilligan's early work (1982, 32) as defining the care perspective; but it was not picked up in subsequent literature until very recently. Maggie FitzGerald (see chapter 6) revives this insight by arguing that the successful practice of care as a process *in time* leads to an "epistemic decentering," which, she argues, entails acknowledging the limits to our knowing. "The Book of the Women," however, reaches this conclusion through an encounter with *bodily vulnerability*. The temporal dimension of caring emphasized by FitzGerald comes to the fore, as we shall see, in the episode called "The Tale of the Hawk and the Pigeon." We turn to that next.

FROM EPISTEMIC TO MORAL VULNERABILITY

The protagonists in "The Tale of the Hawk and the Pigeon" are not women but a male king and two birds. It also involves gory, corporeal dismemberment (physical vulnerability) and reinforces acceptance of cognitive limits. But it does so in a different way—one that leads into an embrace of moral failure. Let us look at the story first.

In its attempt to dodge a predatory hawk, a trembling, scared pigeon once alighted on the thigh of King Shibi, giving rise to a classic moral dilemma. The king felt obligated to offer protection to this particular pigeon that had wordlessly and without invitation established a proximate, physical connection with him. Shibi's moral stand was not based on principles of absolute nonviolence or on vegetarianism, for he pointed out the other birds/creatures that the hawk could kill for food while sparing the pigeon. The hawk, however, found the king's intervention in the natural laws of predation unacceptable, arguing that sheltering the pigeon amounted to risking *the hawk's* death by withholding life-giving nutrition from it. This would, in turn, endanger the lives of many others who depended on the hawk's care to stay alive themselves. Thus, the hawk staked its moral claim (on the pigeon) on both deontological and utilitarian grounds. Shibi, however, was not to be moved. As a way out of the deadlock, Shibi offered the hawk a chunk of his own flesh equal to the weight of the pigeon. But no matter how much of his own flesh he put on the scales, the pigeon always weighed in heavier. Ultimately, in desperation, the king was ready to mount his entire body—by this time almost totally dismembered—on to the scales. As in many *Mahabharata* stories, the pigeon and the hawk were gods in disguise. Manifesting their true forms, they halted the proceedings and praised Shibi's moral excellence.

Now, the web of physical relationships between different bodies in the story (the hawk and the pigeon, the pigeon and the king, the king and the hawk) charts a relational and embodied ontology that comes close to the varying ways the *body* figures in care theory.[10] However, the moral of the story, which I argue lies not in what Shibi *does* but in the way the episode *ends*, suggests interesting connections between corporeality and a capacious vulnerability.

First, the episode interrupts King Shibi, who is working with the substitutability of his flesh and the pigeon's. The king's earlier attempts to show that the hawk's hunger could be appeased by killing a host of other creatures also presupposed a material parity or replaceability of the pigeon by other bodies. But in *stopping* Shibi from becoming a stand-in for the pigeon as it were, the story expertly foregrounds the particularity or *unsubstitutability* of moral subjects even as bodied. This is the care ethical point that embodied agents are particulars exceeding corporeal "sameness."[11] A caring response reaches beyond general facts about embodiment to specific precarities constituting a cared-for's specific needs. Spelling out the "material dialectics of dependency work" through a phenomenology of caring for his grandfather, Joel Michael Reynolds speaks of alternating between treating his cared-for as "merely a body," as "an object to be cleaned by my body," as "exchangeable with any other body" (2016, 784), on the one hand, and as a "concern for him as a singular person" and the need to respond to his "infinite, radical alterity," on the other. In the moral tale therefore, Shibi's enthusiasm about the equality/physical parity with others—which is only the first step of the ethical dialectic—needs to be curtailed by a reminder of their inevitable *difference*. This message can ground accepting uncertainty or epistemic vulnerability spoken of in the previous section. Reynolds articulates the second moment of caring in terms of epistemic vulnerability: "I *do not know* how the other might respond to my care; I *do not know* when, where, or why they might respond to this or not to that. I *do not know* the other in any thick sense" (784, emphasis added).

Furthermore, the king's protective response toward the pigeon is a *commitment to the hawk* to barter his own flesh. But this quickly becomes a moving target literally requiring "more" of Shibi than ever imagined. The parable, therefore, models a future-orientedness of *"taking* responsibility" that tangles caregivers like Shibi with the yet unknown, the uncertain, and even the unthought of. There is a temporality in caring—in committing (now) to fulfilling needs in the yet-to-be-realized future. Care agency, therefore, involves open-endedness of the future and all the multiple forces (besides the agent) that bring it into being. Because of this, we can never be sure what a present commitment could require of us. An epistemic vulnerability is thus built into forward-looking responsibility, making it inherently risky. Besides contending with physical frailties, our moral lives need to embrace epistemic limitations arising from being responsible but embodied beings *in time*.[12]

Eva Kittay's (2019) revival of the "reciprocity/receptivity condition" of care in the notion of "completion" of caring takes this risk a step further in a more direct way. She reminds us that successful caring requires "uptake" by the cared-for. Efforts of the caregiver must affect the cared-for positively and actually meet her needs in order to be successful caring—I have not cared for a patient, for instance, unless she is comforted. But since the cared-for is radically different from us, whether this happens or not is beyond the caregiver's control. But Kittay (2019, 213) claims that care is a "success word." Now, if success is indexed to uptake by the other, then care is inevitably linked to moral luck. Luck introduces fragility in the form of *moral vulnerability* because success of an agent's endeavors becomes beyond her control. Reckoning with failure is imminent.

The story reinforces failure when it ends with Shibi not being able to fulfill what he started out to do and still being regarded as exemplary. Shibi, of course, is actively stopped from fulfilling his commitment to the hawk. Though it remains unclear whether sacrificing his entire body would have equaled the weight of the pigeon, it certainly would have *ended* his moral agency. By preventing that, the parable indicates the importance of ongoing effort in the face of epistemic fragility and realization that we often are unable to fulfill what we started out to do. Shibi's embrace of failure, paradoxically, makes him exemplary. For embodied agents, ethical life is inevitably "open to the outside" because of the porousness of the body. Since being bodied is central to an ethics of care in different ways (Kittay 1999; Hamington 2004, 2015; Vaittinen 2015), so is acceptance of moral vulnerability in this sense.

However, besides underscoring the risk of disruption by external forces—whether it be the will/intentions/condition of an Other that scuttles uptake or the "stepmotherly" forces of an indifferent world whose causal order is independent of our intentions—the parable also points to the *inevitability* of moral failure given the imperative to fulfill needs of multiple and different others. The king's responsibility to protect the pigeon conflicted with his obligation not to harm the hawk. The spectacle of carnal substitution was meant to mop up this "moral remainder" that shadowed the choice of saving the pigeon. Even if Shibi had *not* been stopped, sacrificing *himself* would have been a care ethical failure. Shibi thus came up short—the harm to the hawk was, after all, not addressed.[13] He is deemed excellent not just *in spite of* but *because of* accepting unavoidable failure. The next section teases out this puzzling configuration of failure and excellence within the perspective of care ethics.

THE CARE ETHICAL SIGNIFICANCE OF VULNERABILITIES

Theorizing agency in the context of failure can be of significant feminist interest because oppression often comes with a first-person experience of being "impossibly required." Social constructions of race and gender are the moral luck of an "unnatural lottery" (Card 1996), burdening some with unfair demands but fewer resources. However, let us first understand the *Mahabharata*'s own rationale for applauding someone who fails.

In a didactic verse (Mbh 12.329.40) the epic gives a two-tiered articulation of moral life. A commonplace understanding of moral endeavor sees it as a decentering or "renunciation" of selfish interests. Thus, *dharma* begins in *tyaga*—where *tyaga* is "sacrificing" or giving up self-interest and making oneself a transparent conduit for others' interests. But then, in a surprising second move, the epic urges us to "give up," that is, sacrifice or renounce, "that by which we have given up [our self-interest]."[14] Now the step to decenter selfishness and reach out to the interests of others involves acquiring virtues like compassion, hospitality, or "transparency." In this context, the second step calls for *decentering* the *acquiring of these other-regarding virtues* that enabled us to be moral to begin with. This layered analysis of moral life appeals to the uncontroversial insight that "being ethical" lies in *not prioritizing myself*, that is, "my" joys/sorrows over "yours." But then success in this venture can go along with claiming the excellence of "*my* character," "*my* virtues," and "*my* carings." Since centering of the self undermines ethical life, a second-order self-exceptionalism or pride in one's virtuous character would also vitiate the ethical project. Thus, keeping a sense of failure alive and downplaying one's virtuosity even in moments of imminent success blocks vestigial clingings to self and, therefore, is necessary for morality.

We now begin to see why Shibi is exemplary in the epic world. He enacts unselfishness by being *literally* willing to "give himself up" to save the hawk. But stopped in his tracks, he was faced with moral failure. Realizing that his best efforts could not avoid harm, Shibi confronts a vulnerability that diffuses the possibility of moral pride. And in doing so he becomes exemplary.

But surely giving up *all* claims to "mine" or "ours" is overkill for the caring subject. Such self-evacuation can be attractive for the *spiritual* state of egoless subjectivity or *moksha*. But our reading of the contemporary relevance of "The Book of the Women" depended on dislodging that esoteric, traditional goal. Does the parable of Shibi, then, lose the care ethical plot set up by the earlier episode? To see why not, we would need to establish the non-soteriological significance of moral vulnerability. Building on feminist work on moral failure (Tessman 2015) can help show how the *Mahabharata*'s Shibi does not contradict but nuances feminist care agency in a distinct way.

However, there is an obvious problem in pushing for such embrace of failure.[15] Reinforcing failure slides into resigned passivity and into a moral skepticism that dissipates the "I can" in the "I must" and undermines effort itself. Stripped of ideological baggage, the second-order decentering of a virtuous first-order decentering of the self drives a wedge between moral agency on one hand and moral praise on the other. Owning moral failure is to recede from claiming praiseworthiness for oneself. But then since responsibility is typically cashed out in terms of praise- and blameworthiness, receding from entitlement to praise could also undermine effort and evacuate responsibility of all content. A response to this worry is to imagine forms of ethical involvement detached from praise and blame. Contemporary discussions of moral luck (Williams 1981) already speak of *agent-regret* as a kind of ethical involvement not linked to blame. Taking this as a cue, we can conceive accountability in care ethics as consistent with shrugging off praiseworthiness.

When a child darts out in front of a truck moving at the safe speed limit and tragically dies, both the driver and a bystander are saddened, though neither is to blame. However, the driver is *expected* to show what is called agent-regret because she is immersed in the tragedy in a specifically causal way even though *we* do not blame her for what happened. However, for a *bystander* to apologize and show the "recompense" expected of the *driver* is bizarre and inappropriate. The kind of regret in question registers a fine-grained and thinner first-person moral entanglement in such situations that is not, of course, indifference, but neither is it a full-fledged blameworthiness. However, just as bad luck interfered with the truck driver case and led to tragedy, moral successes too depend on *good* luck. This no doubt reinforces the view that we play causal roles in something good happening, but this need not be pinned down to an *entitlement* to praise for the occurrence of the good.

In this way, space for not "owning" success is made between the two extremes of believing that my will is "the" reason something has happened and complete detachment from it. Susan Wolf (2001), in her discussion of moral luck, calls adopting this stance a "nameless virtue." It expresses "recognition that we are *beings who are thoroughly in-the-world*, in interaction with others whose movements and thoughts we cannot fully control." Thus, moral life is interacting with others "whom we affect and are affected by *accidentally* as well as intentionally" (14, emphasis added). The *Mahabharata*'s attempt to curb ethical pride by embracing moral vulnerability could be a reaching out to this "nameless virtue." I am morally expected to mark my involvement *as one force among many others* that results in a good (or something bad) happening. But this "involvement" is being concerned and responsible without full-fledged entitlement to praise or blame.

The importance of such a disposition for care ethical agents should be clear. Remember that caregivers are "thoroughly in-the-world" in Wolf's terms. The relational ontology of care fits in with Wolf's (2001, 10) spelling out the nameless virtue as "living with an expectation and a willingness to be held accountable for what one does." In caring, one does not step back from "what one does" even when the relational matrix deflects it into becoming something unforeseen. To care is a willingness to remain engaged with *how* our actions end up affecting others irrespective of our intentions. For instance, even when efforts to reduce my daughter's pathological anxiety fail through no fault of mine, or when it is caused by events having nothing to do with me, and in fact may have a lot to do with her own neurochemical makeup, I remain committed to her mental health. My feeling remorse (though not guilt) when my actions trigger her is qualitatively different from, say, *your* concern for her. My "taking responsibility" is an involvement with what *happens to her* even due to contingencies beyond my control. The Shibi episode, therefore, points to a virtue that sustains continued engagement with our cared-fors in spite of moral luck and other reasons for likely failures. It is the root of fallibilist *persistence* and an echo of the strength and agency of survivors.

Care ethical agency understood in this way—as involving a triad of corporeal, epistemic, and moral vulnerability—captures the phenomenology of responsibility experienced by frontline responders in COVID-19 times. Consider Mary, a healthcare worker in the early days of the pandemic, who is compelled by a vulnerability-responsive obligation to take care of Sunita. Even while *not knowing* what will actually help, Mary tries and experiments with ways of making Sunita comfortable. Assuming that her efforts are not actively rejected by Sunita, a successful relationship of care is established even though Mary fails to actually reduce Sunita's discomfort. When Sunita dies, Mary is not blamed, and she does not quite "blame" herself either. Yet her regret is qualitatively different from, say, mine. Moreover, even when a few patients do recover, Mary rarely owns them as *her* success. She is aware of the teamwork that took place, and she is mindful of all those not saved or even triaged out because of the attention given to Sunita. What we have here is a deep sense of failure—but one that does not excoriate moral life from being action guiding for first responders. The pandemic highlights not just vulnerability at the physical cellular level but forms of epistemic and moral vulnerability that do not undermine the "I must" in spite of repeated and even inevitable failures to save lives in the absence of knowledge of how to do so.

Such widespread vulnerability opens up robust engagements with power and privilege. Scenarios of vulnerability-infused ethical action drift into political agency in a number of ways. First, we often take ourselves off the moral hook by claiming "not knowing how or what to do." But this is often an exercise in power (Tronto 2013) sustained by various forms of willed ignorance. If uncertainties of forward-looking responsibility make it constitutively failure-accommodating, then, not-knowings, doubts, and unsuccesses can no longer be "excuses" for shaking off a responsibility to act. Retooling responsibility with epistemic vulnerability, therefore, removes one of the central cogs of Joan Tronto's (2013, 59) inequity-producing "irresponsibility machine." The powerful can no longer hide behind ignorance—willful or not—to justify their lack of commitment for change. Of course, the motivation for action in the absence of knowledge will have to be rethought; but that project remains a promissory note here. Suffice it to say that dislodging true belief or knowledge as the spring of action opens up the possibility of exploring alternative emotional states like hope as the ground for political action.

Second, as indicated, "taking responsibility" for another bodied being as an embodied caregiver oneself renders responsibility an interactive performance dependent on how *others* act. But if so, an agent's failing does not necessarily signal *individual* incapacity. It could well register a lack in the *network* within which individual actions are embedded. Attention thus shifts from navel-gazing projects of self-perfection to a mindfulness of the underlying social and institutional structures that can vitiate intentions and lead actions astray. Such sensitivity to "plurality" outside oneself is the heart of politics. Consequently, agency does not remain agent-centric in the typical way: to care, we need to *care with* others, as Tronto has argued so forcefully. Privatized ethical responsibility now moves toward becoming a political notion involving multiple wills in a truly "caring democracy" (Tronto 2013).

Third, vulnerability-accommodating responsibility enables solidarity across social divides and agendas. "Taking responsibility" for racial and colonial oppressions is now a forward-looking stance for change even if we cannot be blamed for the historical rifts in the first place. Such responsibility underlies solidarity. But working together across hierarchies implies fragile and risky coalitions held together not by commonalities in identities or locations but by a vision for a just future. However, those we are in solidarity with could conceive of change differently and in ways unimaginable to us. "Standing with" genuinely different groups therefore also requires openness about the nature of the "joint future" being aimed at. This must accommodate acknowledging not-knowing on our part. Acknowledging epistemic vulnerability now becomes sensitivity to the cognitive significance of power differentials and therefore to giving marginalized others a voice. A capacious care responsibility, therefore, is not undermined by uncertainties, unknowing, and even failures when those at the fringes speak up. Rather, it underwrites the political in forms (or expressions) of solidarity that are resilient and that do not balk when faced with disappointments and failures.

CONCLUSION

Bodies are associated with dependence on the world and on others. This "opening up" to the outside, however, introduces fragility on multiple registers. Our attempt has been to show how acceptance of physical vulnerability leads to the embrace of forms of epistemic and moral fragility as central for moral life. A deep dive into experiences of such failures can push us to be caring in more effective and nonoppressive ways. But recognizing the inevitability of individual missteps points to the importance of rallying *others* to our cause—which is a political will to involve others in constructing safety nets that ensure the sustainability of what is important for us. Preserving everyday relationships of caring therefore morphs from a personal to a political responsibility. Of course, such care ethical agency does not fit into traditional frameworks of consequentialism, deontology, virtue theory, or even the *Mahabharata*'s *dharma*-ethics. Consequently, the privileged position of "ethics" as ordinarily understood is itself decentered. Moral life consists in relinquishing narratives of mastery and hence must ultimately be open to relinquishing its own privilege. However, we must remember that this conceptual journey of gradually embracing more capacious senses of vulnerability began by turning to insights of the *Mahabharata*. Stepping back from power and authority of an exclusively Western intellectual corpus when crafting alternative models of living together might be the most difficult embrace of vulnerability and *tyaga* (sacrifice) of privilege in our story.

ACKNOWLEDGMENTS

I am grateful for the comments of Maggie FitzGerald and Sophie Bourgault. Their persistent engagement helped me clarify the argument. A version of this chapter was presented at the May 2021 CERC Conference "Decentering Ethics: Challenging Privileges, Building Solidarities," where I benefitted from audience responses.

NOTES

1. References to the Sanskrit text are from the Gita Press Edition of the *Mahabharata*. Translations are from Fitzgerald (2004).
2. For further readings along these lines, see Dalmiya (2016).
3. See Kanchana Mahadevan (2014, esp. chap. 1) for a discussion of the complexities of "Indian" femininity.
4. This analogy is made clear in the very first line of the *Bhagavad Gita*, which incidentally is also part of the *Mahabharata*.
5. I use the term "apt" in the sense in which Amia Srinivasan (2017) speaks of anger.
6. Mbh 15.33.
7. The particularism here is pronounced. For instance, when bewailing the lost intimacy between a particular queen, Uttarā, and her young husband, Abhimanyu, the latter is identified not as a generic "warrior" but as having a unique constellation of prowess, beauty, and relationships. He is not only Uttara's husband but the son, nephew, and grandson of various other individuals who are all "named" in turn.
8. It should be noted that after this epiphany of worldly togetherness, the menfolk enter the river and disappear. They are accompanied by some women who choose to drown in the river along with them. Clearly the critiques of patriarchy in the text are quickly papered over, preserving the conservative tone of the epic.
9. For the exclusions and oppressions routinely perpetuated by care, see Narayan (1995) and Malatino (2020).
10. For the different ways in which contemporary care theorists emphasize the *corporeality* of care, see Hamington (2004) and Vaittinen (2015).
11. This is different from Vaittinen's notion of care as a "corporeal relation," which emphasizes the sameness of bodies as "bare life." I am grateful to Maggie FitzGerald for this reference.
12. Once again, this comes close to what Maggie FitzGerald argues in her chapter for this volume (chapter 6).
13. There is a fair amount of ambiguity here of course. Does the end of the story signal a negotiating away of the moral demand of hawk to settle for a pragmatic resolution to the dilemma?
14. Mbh 12.329.40.
15. Maggie FitzGerald (chapter 6), who also speaks of failure, avoids this problem by parsing caring as the constant dynamic between decentering and *recentering* of the self. The solution suggested here is different.

REFERENCES

Brison, Susan. 2002. *Aftermath: Violence and the Remaking of a Self.* Princeton, NJ: Princeton University Press.

Butler, Judith. 2004. *Precarious Life*. London: Verso.
Card, Claudia. 1996. *The Unnatural Lottery: Character and Moral Luck*. Philadelphia: Temple University Press.
Chakrabarti, Arindam, and Ralph Weber, eds. 2015. *Comparative Philosophy without Borders*. New York: Bloomsbury.
Dalmiya, Vrinda. 2016. *Caring to Know: Comparative Care Ethics, Feminist Epistemology, and the Mahabharata*. New Delhi: Oxford University Press.
Das, Veena. 2018. "Ethics, Self-Knowledge, and Life Taken Together as a Whole." *Journal of Ethnographic Theory* 8 (3): 537–549.
Fitzgerald, James L., trans. and ed. 2004. *The Mahābhārata: The Book of the Women and the Book of Peace*. Pt. 1. Chicago: University of Chicago Press.
Gilligan, Carol. 1982. *In a Different Voice: Psychological Theory and Women's Development*. Cambridge, MA: Harvard University Press.
———. 2014. "Moral Injury and Ethic of Care: Reframing the Conversation about Difference." *Journal of Social Philosophy* 45 (1): 89–106.
Hamington, Maurice. 2004. *Embodied Care: Jane Addams, Maurice Merleau-Ponty, and Feminist Ethics*. Champaign: University of Illinois Press.
———. 2015. "Care Ethics and Engaging Intersectional Difference through the Body." *Critical Philosophy of Race* 3 (1): 79–100.
Harbin, Ami. 2016. *Disorientation and Moral Life*. New York: Oxford University Press.
Honig, Bonnie. 2013. *Antigone, Interrupted*. Cambridge: Cambridge University Press.
Howard, Veena Rani. 2018. "Lessons from 'The Hawk and the Dove': Reflections on the Mahabharata's Animal Parables and Ethical Predicaments." *Sophia* 57:119–131.
Hudson, Emily T. 2013. *Disorienting Dharma: Ethic and Aesthetics of Suffering in the Mahabharata*. New York: Oxford University Press.
Kittay, Eva F. 1999. *Love's Labor: Essays on Women, Equality, and Dependence*. New York: Routledge.
———. 2019. *Learning from My Daughter: The Value and Care of Disabled Minds*. New York: Oxford University Press.
Laugier, Sandra. 2015. "Ethics of Care as a Politics of the Ordinary." *New Literary History* 46:217–240.
Mahābhārata. n.d. Translated by Sahityācāra Pandit Ramnarayandutta Shashtri Pandey "Ram." Gorakhpur: Gita Press.
Mahadevan, Kanchana. 2014. *Between Femininity and Feminism: Colonial and Postcolonial Perspectives on Care*. New Delhi: ICPR and D. K. Printworld.
Malatino, Hil. 2020. *Trans Care*. Minneapolis: University of Minnesota Press.
Narayan, Uma. 1995. "Colonialism and Its Others: Considerations on Rights and Care Discourse." *Hypatia* 10 (2): 133–140.
Raghuram, Parvati. 2016. "Locating Care Ethics beyond the Global North." *ACME: An International Journal for Critical Geographies* 15 (3): 511–533.
Reynolds, Joel Michael. 2016. "Infinite Responsibility in the Bedpan: Response Ethics, Care Ethics and the Phenomenology of Dependency Work." *Hypatia* 31 (4): 779–794.
Robinson, Fiona. 2016. "Paternalistic Care and Transformative Recognition in International Politics." In *Recognition and Global Politics: Critical Encounters between State and World*, edited by Patrick Hayden and Kate Schick Manchester, 159–174. Manchester: Manchester University Press.
Srinivasan, Amia. 2017. "The Aptness of Anger." *Journal of Political Philosophy* 26 (2): 123–144.
Tessman, Lisa. 2015. *Moral Failure: On the Impossible Demands of Morality*. Oxford: Oxford University Press.

Tronto, Joan C. 2013. *Caring Democracy: Markets, Equality, and Justice.* New York: New York University Press.

———. 2017. "There *Is* an Alternative: *Hominus Curens* and the Limits of Neoliberalism." *International Journal of Care and Caring* 1 (1): 27–43.

Vaittinen, Tiina. 2015. "The Power of the Vulnerable Body: A New Political Understanding of Care." *International Feminist Journal of Politics* 17 (1): 100–118.

Weir, Allison. 2005. "The Global Universal Care Giver: Imagining Women's Liberation in the New Millennium." *Constellations* 12 (3): 308–330.

Williams, Bernard. 1981. *Moral Luck.* Cambridge: Cambridge University Press.

Wolf, Susan. 2001. "The Moral of Moral Luck." *Philosophic Exchange* 31 (1): 5–19.

6 · THE COMMITMENT TO CARE
An Unwavering Epistemic Decentering
MAGGIE FITZGERALD

"Decenter" means to pull from the center, to displace from a central location. This chapter argues that the ethics of care—and the commitment to care that such an ethics demands—involves an unwavering epistemic decentering, operating across several registers and epistemic resources at once. Epistemology "addresses both *what we know* and *how we know*" (Hamington 2004, 44, emphasis original). The epistemic decentering that I speak of here involves both of these (interconnected) questions: my argument is that because the ethics of care conceives of "how we know" as an ongoing and iterative process of decentering the self to know the other, it necessarily and continually results in a decentering of "what we know," including what we know care itself to be.

The impetus for this argument is to consider and engage with the question, what is "care" from a care ethical standpoint? This is a tricky question, and it has increasingly haunted the care ethics literature. On the one hand, the idea that there is some universal definition of care, or cohesive set of care practices or values, risks obfuscating differences in and across sociopolitical groups and culturally specific meanings and practices of care (which come from various forms of life). Far too often, such universal definitions smuggle in notions of care as universal truths based on hierarchies of power and epistemic privilege, which works to delegitimize or render invisible care knowing and care practices of oppressed groups. The scholarship of care theorists like Parvati Raghuram (2016, 2019), for example, has highlighted that care literature (broadly defined) sometimes focuses on white, bourgeois care practices from the Global North, presenting them as the whole of care and thereby marginalizing practices and relations of care from elsewhere. On the other hand, however, if care is evacuated of all content and claims, it would seem that care ethics offers us very little in terms of an ethical trajectory that can help us with moral contemplation and deed. Given these concerns, how can we understand "care" from an ethics of care perspective?

This chapter argues that the framing of this issue as one of defining care misses fundamentally the epistemic dimensions of care ethics. I contend that a key part of care, as an ethical theory, is that it demands an unwavering epistemic commitment to decentering ourselves, our knowledge claims, and therefore our specific notions and practices of care. In other words, "what we know" care to be must always be decentered by the "how we know" of care ethics. From a care ethical epistemological standpoint, an understanding of care is asserted or enacted, and then it must be decentered—we engage with others, we decenter ourselves and center the other in that engagement, and we try to listen attentively so as to consider, in a serious manner, competing versions of care. In so doing, we come to revise our own notions of care and enlarge the possible ways in which we conceive of care as both a practice and a value. This unwavering commitment to decentering what we know care (as practice and value) to be is difficult work: knowledge is co-constitutive of "forms of life," which makes it both "true" (part of the bedrock of a particular way of being) and also revisable (as forms of life themselves are mutable, although change can be slow) (Walker 2007). Tracing this decentering, discussing the resources that help us in this task—most notably, our bodies, our imagination, and epistemic humility—and demonstrating how this decentering is an essential part of the epistemic dimensions of an ethics of care (a part that allows us to decenter continually our very understandings of care) is the central aim of this chapter.

DECENTERING I: SELF

To understand the care ethical epistemology, it is useful to begin with a discussion of the ontology of care ethics. The ethics of care conceives of subjects as deeply relational beings who emerge in and through their relations with one another, broader social-political systems, and our natural world. Selves are thus infinitely unique, as they are constituted by unique sets of relations (Hekman 1995). It is also in and through these sets of relations (and the practices that sustain these relations) that the self comes to know: knowledge, from a care ethical perspective, arises from practices and relations that constitute a form of life. Given the complex webs of relations we find ourselves in, knowledge (and the forms of life knowledge comes from) will be multiple and unique too. We cannot a priori know which of these knowledges are "better" than others—the best we can do is engage with people, who may be very different from ourselves, and commit to the slow and difficult process of trying to understand various epistemic claims and the good to be found therein.

Starting with this relational social ontology leads us, then, to the first epistemic decentering that is key to a care ethical epistemology: the ethics of care involves a decentering of the self so as to attempt to know the other. That is, on the one hand, our interdependencies commit us to the other: we are dependent and vulnerable beings, embedded in relations that alternatively sustain and harm us, and we thus enact such relations ourselves. An ethics of care, and its relational social ontology, orients us to the ethical consequences of this relationality. We must be attentive and respond as well as is reasonably possible to the other. This commitment to care, then, inherently requires knowledge: as Vrinda Dalmiya (2016, 7, emphasis original) writes, "*Carers* always need to know." In order to care for another, we must commit ourselves to knowing their hopes, desires, wishes, interests, needs, and concerns as clearly as possible. On the other hand, however, as unique selves, this attempt to be attentive, to know and understand the other, is also always limited. We cannot project ourselves into the other; we cannot know the other fully. The radical alterity implied by the relational ontology I describe here (i.e., the radically different selves that emerge from complex sets of relations) means that there will be irreconcilable gaps between/across subjects. In this way, the relational self of the ethics of care also *limits* knowing: the singularity of relational selves means that we are—each and every one of us—somewhat unknowable to the other. Because each subject is in/of a different lived experience, context, and web of relationships, their knowing is specific to them. And while there are, surely, many overlaps between experiences, contexts, and relationships—these overlaps form the collective epistemic terrain that we find ourselves in—there are often excesses characterizing this terrain (see, for example, FitzGerald 2022), and not everyone can traverse it equally (or even parts of it at all). For the ethics of care, our relational being thereby presents an epistemological tension: relations constitute both the possibility of knowing *and* the limits of our knowing in complicated ways.

Navigating this tension, I contend, involves an unwavering struggle to decenter oneself: "We struggle toward the reality of the other" (Noddings 2003, 14), a reality that we cannot ever really or fully comprehend, as we are always pulled back to ourselves (i.e., we cannot eschew our context and the relations that constitute us). Or as Nel Noddings (2003, 16) writes, while "caring is always characterized by a move away from self," as we must strive to receive, communicate, and work with the other (31), this is not equivalent to "emptying" oneself of all of one's own contents (Noddings 2015, 78). Certainly, as relational beings, this is not possible. Instead, an ethics of care, by foregrounding our relational being and the responsibilities that our relations demand of us (and that we demand of others), asks that we put aside our "own projects for the moment and allow the expressed needs of [the other] to take precedence" (Noddings 2015, 78). But understanding others' needs, even when "expressed," is difficult business. Attempting to hold space for other knowledges (when we ourselves are constituted by ways of knowing particular to our form of life) is hard. Further, as knowledges are grounded in specific contexts and sets of relations—contexts that we may not be a part of—it may be impossible to access that knowledge in a fulsome way. But certainly, these limits to knowing cannot absolve us from our care responsibilities; the commitment to caring implicit in an ethics of care holds us accountable for knowing (albeit a humble knowing), even in such cases. Indeed, "care ethics and care epistemology are thus joined at the hip" (Dalmiya 2016, 3): the ethical commitment to care requires us to engage continually in an epistemological process of decentering the self to know the other.

We are fortunate to have many epistemological resources to help us with this messy and challenging work—resources that the ethics of care values and foregrounds as holding great moral and epistemological merit. Perhaps most significant of these resources is an ability to be attentive, to practice what Sophie Bourgault (2016) calls "attentive listening." It is through active, engaged, and sustained listening to those we are in relation with that we come to know them and their needs (even if only ever tentatively). Attentive listening engages a variety of skills and resources—although, as I discuss now, these skills and resources often involve their own decenterings.

Embodiment

First, as care ethicists like Bourgault (2016) and Maurice Hamington (2004) show, attentive listening is possible in large part because of our bodies. Attentive listening "requires physical presence" (Bourgault 2016, 317), and "much of what is communicated between people is found in the subtleties of facial expressions, hand gestures, posture, inflection, and eye contact. When one is actively attending to someone else face to face, these subtleties can be absorbed consciously and subconsciously through the body" (Hamington 2004, 109). Listening in an attentive way demands that our senses—our corporeal resources—receive the other's words, affects, and emotions. Yet attentive listening requires the body's resources (which are therefore epistemological resources) in other ways too: the listeners' bodily movements, stances, energies, and affects also foster the conditions necessary for receiving the other. As Bourgault (2016, 319, emphasis original) writes, "A competent listener will know that the way *her own body* is looked at *by the speaker* greatly matters." Bodies can enact response in an ongoing way without interrupting a speaker. Hamington (2004, 47) writes that perception—the ability to see/hear/understand something through the senses—is "the 'silent conversation' our body has with the world around it" and the people with whom we are in relation.[1] Bodies can, and often do, articulate that listening is happening without requiring that listening to stop.

At the same time, however, our bodies, and the habits they hold (Hamington 2004), will sometimes serve as an obstacle to our listening. Bodies become tired, our senses can be overwhelmed, and there are limits to our ability to listen continually (Bourgault 2016, 316; see also Bourgault this volume [chapter 2]) and with patience. The ways in which caring responsibilities are unequally distributed, and the ways in which many are held accountable for listening while others do not have to listen effectively (Robinson 2011b), shape a body's capacity to engage in sustained listening. Furthermore, as Bourgault (2016, 320) brilliantly illustrates, the epistemic resources of the body and its ability to perceive might at times repel us from listening: "Reading, in the comfort of one's bed, a novel about the life of an alcoholic homeless man who reeks of vomit is quite different from actually listening to his story, standing two feet away from him on a street, in a cold winter night. In all likelihood, the smell of vomit (and the cold) will impede our listening and affect our moral judgement." In cases like this, we must decenter, as opposed to draw upon, our bodies' sensory-perceptive epistemological resources. We must stick with the suffering we are sensing, the unease we feel, and strive to sustain our listening. Similarly, sometimes our bodily responses and habits that demonstrate our listening will need to be decentered to respond appropriately to the speaking other. For instance, people with various neurodivergences may find eye contact—a commonsensical bodily habit of listening for many—to be disruptive and uncaring. In such cases, sustained eye contact would not convey the listening we mean it to, and this habit would need to be decentered to account for the needs of the speaker.

From a care ethics perspective, then, the body as an epistemological resource is necessarily caught in an unwavering decentering. The body is an extremely important site for knowing: the body, its senses, its perceptive capacities, its corporal proximity, and its habits are the very means by which attentive listening can unfold. The body, in many ways, positions us (provides a center) for listening. At the same time, however, these very tools can lead us astray. Certain utterances, statements, feelings, or sensory experiences are difficult to hear; when it comes to listening attentively to suffering, this is often the case. Our bodies might signal that we should turn away from listening in such moments. Our bodies might also enact habits of attentive listening that are inappropriate to a given speaker. In these instances, the epistemological resource that is the body must be decentered. We must struggle against such turning away and be cognizant of revising our embodied listening practices so that they do in fact listen attentively, and convey attentive listening, to the speaker, in all their uniqueness.

Imagination

Our imagination is yet another key epistemological resource for decentering ourselves so as to know the other—one that I believe is exceptionally important when there is a limit to knowing the other that cannot be overcome.[2] My previous work (FitzGerald 2022) has grappled with this question in the context of the pluriverse. The pluriverse is a concept that challenges the idea of a single world with different belief systems, paradigms, or cultures by postulating a world of many worlds. In the pluriversal context, there will be limits to what subjects from one world can know of another world. For example, subjects from a world premised upon sharp subject-object distinctions (such as the modern Western world) cannot truly know the types of deep relations that constitute other worlds, like the worlds of Māori or Quechua people. More simply, I suggest that where difference is most deep and pervasive, there may be times when attentive listening simply cannot overcome the epistemological gaps between different social-political groups (see also Koggel this volume [chapter 1]). We cannot "presume that there can be symmetry. Such perfect identification with the other's position is impossible" (Bourgault 2016, 327). It is here that imagination, as an epistemological resource, can play a crucial role.

Imagination allows us to draw upon our own knowledge and epistemic resources to gain "a glimmer of understanding" (Hamington 2004, 74). It allows us to extend care and concern to situations and particularities that are unknown to us, albeit not in a way that directly translates these particularities (Hamington 2004, 69)—to be sure, such one-to-one translation is often impossible. Imagination, as an epistemological resource for an ethics of care, is not about overcoming limits; it is about acknowledging the impossibility of knowing the other fully while still attempting to move toward the other so as to comprehend what they need and desire. This epistemological process must therefore be a creative one, "a practice of creatively overcoming disconnects between the interests of the self and the other" (Confortini and Ruane 2013, 73; see also van Dijke, Bos, and Duyndam 2020), between different visions of care, and across forms of moral life.

Imagination is also a component of "concrete" thinking, which is key to a care ethical epistemology. "Concreteness is opposed to 'abstraction'—a cluster of interrelated dispositions to simplify, generalize, and sharply define. To look and then speak concretely is to relish complexity, to tolerate ambiguity, to multiply options rather than accepting the terms of the problem" (Ruddick 1989, 93). Abstract thinking, which generalizes and eschews particularity, is not conducive to attentive listening. Attentive listening demands looking closely at the issue and the context in and through which it emerged, inventing options, refusing closure, and valuing ways of conversing that "ask about the circumstances in which a person comes to believe and the consequences of that belief in her life.... Patient, sympathetic listening to the complexities and uncertainties of another's experience" (Ruddick 1989, 96)—especially when that experience is outside of our onto-epistemic framework, and consequently somewhat unknowable to us—is imaginative and creative work.

At the same time, while our imagination is indispensable as we try to navigate "gaps" in/across epistemological claims and resources, our imaginations must also be continually decentered. We cannot assume that we are imagining "correctly" or "accurately," nor can we assume that our imaginations will "overcome" the epistemic distance that might exist between people or across forms of life. We also have to be careful that we do not "extract" epistemological claims and resources from other ways of knowing/being (see Prattes this volume [chapter 4]); for instance, as scholars like Sarah Hunt (2014) and Vanessa Watts (2013; see also Doucet, Jewell, and Watts this volume [chapter 7]) make clear, different Indigenous knowledges that are tied to unique practices and ways of life are easily emptied of the embodied and real content when employed in/by non-Indigenous scholars or groups. A care epistemology must resist extracting other knowledges (as if they could be abstracted from place and transported directly elsewhere in the first place) or projecting fully one's own knowledge into other contexts. Care knowing "leaves open the possibility of imaginative identification being wrong" (Dalmiya 2016, 251), and it does not try to overcome difference. It "lets otherness be" (Ruddick 1989, 122). Attentive listening requires imagination to help creatively reframe problems and develop connections that allow us to understand the other (particularly when there are ontological and epistemological differences at play) without letting these imaginative solutions ossify into firm claims that obfuscate the fact of the difference. The best measure to protect against such ossification is to decenter our imaginative constructions through ongoing practices of engaging with others in embodied and embedded ways (Dalmiya 2016, 280).[3]

Humility

Finally, humility, and a deep acknowledgment of the vulnerability of all knowledge claims (including, or perhaps even principally, one's own), is essential to the type of attentive listening prioritized in care ethical knowing. As Dalmiya (2016, 259) writes, "An active listening is possible only when a prior disposition to question our own convictions *and* an inclination to believe that the [other] has something new and important to say are set in place." This "prior disposition" is an epistemic humility, which comes from an understanding that all "judgement is unsafe" (Hutchings 2013, 26). We are fallible, and knowledge claims are not transcendentally true but emerge from actual relations and practices and find their meaning only in and through these relations and practices (Hekman 1995; Hutchings 2013; Ruddick 1989).

Because all knowledge emerges from specific forms of life (which, while concrete, do not stand on some transcendental ground but arise in and through changeable relations and practices), we must foreground continually the vulnerability of our knowledge claims and humbly commit to revising these claims when confronted with other knowledges, which themselves are not universally "true" or even "more true," but again find meaning and correctness only in and from other forms of life (Hekman 1995). Epistemic humility thus involves a "prior motivational openness of self-ascribing ignorance and other-ascribing epistemic authority" (Dalmiya 2016, 25). Self-ascribing ignorance allows us to foreground the riskiness and vulnerability of our own claims and helps us commit to self-reflection, while other-ascribing authority orients us continually toward hearing and learning from other knowledges and other knowers. Moreover, it is through such an ongoing and iterative process of asserting, testing, and assessing our own claims, in conjunction with listening to, testing, and assessing other claims, that we can come to revise knowledge claims more generally; in this way, foregrounding the riskiness of judgment reveals knowledge itself to be fully social and political. We collectively work together to agonize over which knowledges we want to guide our care practices and care ethical decision making, that is, which knowledges we want to live in and with (FitzGerald 2022; Ruddick 1989; Walker 2007). We also must be attuned to the ways in which power permeates this collective process of mutual correction, often in ways that "stack the odds" against the knowledge claims of those already marginalized and oppressed by relations of power. "Moral relations are thick with unequal levels of power, voice, influence, and independence" (Robinson 2011b, 851), and this shapes fundamentally which knowledge claims circulate, gain currency, and occupy positions of authority. Without acknowledging the vulnerability of our judgment, we cannot undertake this important epistemic work.

At the same time, while this epistemic humility is a crucially important resource for a care ethics epistemology, this humility, I suggest, must also sometimes be decentered—via a recentering of the self—for two reasons. First, we cannot "allow the acknowledgement of vulnerability to let [our]selves off the hook of judgement" (Hutchings 2013, 26). Our humility cannot prevent us from making claims, nor can it prevent us from acting. Over-agonizing our knowledge to the point of "freezing" will not be conducive to a care ethical life. Sometimes we will have to act, based on what we know, although this too can be part of an ongoing process (see the next two sections below for more on the temporality of care knowing). Second, our humility, I believe, also cannot lead us to abdication. Sara Ruddick (1989, 111–112) describes the dangers of abdication when discussing maternal thinking:

> Under the gaze of others, mothers punish behaviour they would otherwise gently correct or accept blame for "failures" that, in private, they would not recognize as such. Relinquishing authority to others, they lose confidence in their own values and in the perception of their children's needs. . . . I call this particular kind of self-loss the "abdication" of maternal authority. . . . The abdication I speak of exists when a mother hides from her child her real feelings and the realities of the power situation as she sees them. The abdicating mother talks as if the authorities are legitimate, as if their will should be obeyed.[4]

While speaking specifically of the relation between mothers and children, this point is, I believe, crucially important in all contexts. Because we are enmeshed in relations of power, we sometimes relinquish authority to others and "second-guess" our knowledge claims—we lose our voice. While the collective endeavor of knowledge (re)production demands that we take seriously the knowledge claims of others, the riskiness and vulnerability of this process can be scary. We might fear the judgment we will meet in asserting our own claims and responding to the claims of others. This, as Ruddick (1989, 111) demonstrates so well in her discussion of mothers, is even more probable when the listener is less powerful than the speaker or when the listener (who might be more powerful than another speaker) is under the gaze of others who are more powerful than herself (this is often the case for young mothers in patriarchal societies where "experts" and masculinist norms and sources of authority "conspire to undermine the confidence" [Ruddick 1989, 112] a mother might have). The fear of the judgment of others or the "fear of the gaze of others can be expressed intellectually as 'inauthenticity,' a repudiation of one's own perceptions and values" (Ruddick 1989, 112). While epistemic humility is invaluable, power relations can easily warp this humility into a fearful lack of confidence, resulting in a repression of one's own epistemic authority that is, in fact, a harmful loss of oneself (as opposed to a generative decentering of self, as is key to the care ethical epistemology described here). Such humility does not correct power imbalances; it reinforces them.

Given this, it is important to emphasize that the degree to which different listeners might need to practice epistemic humility should be judged with serious consideration for the relations of power in which they find themselves: the riskiness of foregrounding one's vulnerability (including the vulnerability of one's knowledge claims) is not equally distributed. Those who occupy privileged positions, and whose knowledge claims are never questioned (even by themselves), must learn to orient themselves toward epistemic humility in fuller ways. Those whose voice and authority have already been diminished by existing power relations might sometimes need to decenter their humility—assert themselves, their voice, and their knowledge more fully—so as not to undermine their own knowledges and values, so as not to self-renounce in harmful ways. "Degenerative humility or passivity" (Ruddick 1989, 72) cannot guide our epistemological processes.

Countering such degenerative humility requires a recentering of the self. A care epistemology, as a result, involves decenterings all the way down: it is an endless process of decentering the self to try and know the other and then decentering the other to return to one's voice. Just as decentering oneself is difficult, recentering one's voice is demanding work because, first and foremost, a relational self inherently must (re)consider their thoughts, feelings, aims, desires, wishes, and so on, through and within their ongoing relations with others: one's voice, to be certain, is a product of the relations that constitute the self, and returning to one's voice does not mean eschewing the complexities of these relations, even if it does mean foregrounding one's voice over the voice of the other. And, of course, this recentering can be even harder for those who have been encouraged (through socialization, because of various norms and relations of power, as a result of trauma, etc.) to forgo their own voice so as to preserve relations with others. Carol Gilligan's (1993) work has long been instructive on this point: women frequently lose their voice as they have been positioned in patriarchy to preserve relationships with others, even at extraordinary personal costs. As Gilligan has shown, recentering the self for women (given patriarchal power relations) is often difficult. While genuine epistemic humility is necessary for the "slow, often puzzling, and sometimes painful and costly tasks of mutual correction" (Walker 2007, 257), this humility must also be continually decentered, in part via critical reflection on the ways in which power relations position and shape the speaker, the listener, and those who may be witnessing the dialogue.

The messy and difficult task of attempting to decenter oneself (never fully possible) so as to learn attentively about other forms of life and other selves (again, never fully possible), and then again recentering oneself so as not to lose one's voice, is, I suggest, the key epistemological process ("how we come to know, how we know we know") from an ethics of care perspective (FitzGerald 2022, 218). It is through this process of decentering and recentering that we assert, assess, test, and revise our knowledge claims; it is through this decentering that we listen attentively, consider, and accept or reject other knowledge claims; and it is through this process that we collectively come to enlarge the "possibilities and the goods of [our] shared lives" (Walker 2007, 258). Decentering and recentering the self depend on many other epistemological resources, although these, as I have argued above, must be decentered too. Our bodies, our imaginations, and an ongoing orientation toward humility are both our resources for knowing better as well as potential hindrances as we strive toward mutual correction. Without doubt, the unwavering commitment to these interconnected decenterings is "hard, uncertain, [and] exhausting" (Ruddick 1989, 123); the epistemology underpinning an ethics of care demands much of us insofar as it is a "practice of living with dissonance" (Confortini and Ruane 2013, 73), of striving toward the impossible task of holding both self and other at the fore.

DECENTERING II: TIME AND SUCCESS

There are two additional decenterings related to a care ethical epistemology that I wish to highlight, where I am again focusing on the "how we know" register of epistemology as opposed to the "what we know" register. A care epistemology, I argue, decenters dominant understandings of time and success in relation to the ways in which we come to know. More precisely, this slow process of coming to know through a decentering of self in relation with the other means that the process of knowing is not a linear one that unfolds through time toward a "successful" conclusion. Instead, care ethics conceives of knowledge as emerging through "messy feedback loops" (Tronto 2015, 264) in which claims are asserted, assessed, and justified based "on their effects on the practices and relationships to which they give rise" (Robinson 2014, 103). These effects, it is important to note, include both intended and surprising effects: "Care does not leave unintended consequences outside of its own process" (Tronto 2015, 264). From this perspective, knowledge does not accumulate or even necessarily become more precise through linear time (although perhaps it might), and success is not measured by a simple assessment of cause and effect. Rather, the expansion and finessing of knowledge unfold in complex ways as we attempt to know what to do in the here and now, while also holding sustained concern for the future.

For instance, care knowing, as Catia Confortini and Abigail Ruane (2013, 73) argue, is oriented toward "bridging practical goals for surviving the present with more idealistic goals for 'best practices' in the future." Here, the present and the future are decentered from a linear relation, in which we deal with the present "now" and consider the future "later." Knowing how to care demands that we attempt to weave back and forth between a concern for both the now and future and that we account for how the past has shaped / will shape both. In this way, care involves a more layered notion of time, in which the past, present, and future are all bound up, shaping caring needs, and the ways in which needs are or are not addressed. Care knowing must consider these different temporalities all at once: we cannot effectively tend to our caring needs without thinking through past harms, contemplating current unmet needs and suffering, and (at least) considering the unknowable and uncertain futures that are yet to come. Care thus evades linear temporality and requires the care knower to decenter any particular concern for the past, present, or future by instead moving back and forth across all three of these temporal planes at once. We must constantly decenter our concern with the present by turning toward a concern for the future; we must decenter our concern for the future by addressing the present; and doing both of these things will require taking the time necessary to understand how the past has both limited and opened possibilities for the here and now, as well as for moving forward. Attempting to address the harms of the present while also "transforming the conditions that make caring difficult or impossible" (Noddings 2003, xxii) involves focusing on the present, examining the past, and considering the future all at once.

This weaving across temporalities and listening attentively to the needs of others (and how they themselves make sense across past, present, and future) is time-consuming: it takes time to hold the past-present-future (i.e., to decenter continually our thinking from the past to the present to the future, and back again) at the front of our concern and to understand how others do the same. As Bourgault (2016, 316, emphasis original) notes, attentive listening, as is characteristic of a care ethics epistemology, unfolds slowly and is time-intensive; it means we need *"to stop and to wait."* This can be an extremely difficult task, especially when we want to know how to respond to others. Often, our desire "to take care" urges us to act and respond (not to mention the ways in which "rushing" is increasingly valued in Western societies that promote efficiency at all costs). However, coming to know "how to care" requires time. Care knowing implores us to slow down thinking and listen patiently. At the same time, this slowing down must also sometimes be decentered, as at some point we must respond to the needs of the other. Our urge to act must be decentered by the crucially important task of listening, which takes time. But there are times when our patient listening must be disrupted so that we respond.

Relatedly, a care ethical epistemology decenters dominant notions of "successful" knowing, in which we employ our knowledge to address an issue which is then resolved. In contrast, the knowing that emerges from a care ethical lens understands that "humanly ordinary failure" (Ruddick 1989, 104) will very often be the norm. Because knowledges are multiple and contextually specific, and because we can never completely know the other, the "accumulation" of knowledge does not lead to a universal knowing in and through which we can always "get it right." As Bourgault (2014) again reminds us, there will necessarily be failures, and we ought to begin with this fact. More acutely, beginning with this fact decenters the very notion of success in the first place. While of course we might say that a certain type of knowledge is more successful in terms of how it helps us address a need, the real measurement of success, I assert, will come from our commitment to responding to the other in a continual and ongoing way. That is, while we might know incorrectly in a given circumstance, we may still be successful in our care knowing if we listen to the other, learn from their response to our care knowing, and revise what we believe(d) to be correct in light of that. The response of the other is key here: the knower "explicitly gets *confirmation* on whether the assessments" (Dalmiya 2016, 251, emphasis original) they have made are effective from the response of the other. Success, from this vantage point, is not simply about whether what we know is right; it is much more related to our sustained attempt to center the other, to listen, to receive, to respond, and then to listen again as the other responds to our response. When our care knowing does not yield successful outcomes, or when it brings about unintended negative consequences, our epistemological processes can still be considered a success if we humbly listen to the other, revise our knowledge accordingly, and "make amends and start again" (Ruddick 1989, 109). I believe that so often, because of the sheer difficulty in attempting to decenter the self/center the other, the success of our care knowing can only ever be measured by our ongoing commitment to know better. While we may fail many times before we understand the other well enough to care for them, the fact of our perseverance toward such understanding is a success of its own.

DECENTERING III: CARE

Having illustrated how the question of "how we know" is answered from a care ethical perspective via a plethora of decenterings, I return to the question that prompted this investigation: What, then, is care from a care ethics perspective? My closing argument is that this question is, in many ways, beside the point—at least as a question that could ever be answered definitively. Because the ethics of care conceives of "how we know" as an ongoing and iterative process of decentering and recentering self and other, it necessarily and continually results in a decentering of what we know, including what we know care, itself, to be. Care, like all knowledges and practices, emerges from sets of relations and forms of life. Given the multiplicity of our relations, care practices and values will be multiple and unique, and they will change as we together partake in the process of mutually assessing and correcting knowledge claims about care.

Importantly, when I speak of defining care, I mean in terms of both practices of care as well as values related to caring. The practices of care and our values of care must both, from a care ethical perspective, decenter one another. Through attentive listening, learning from others, and critically examining our care practices, we can see if the ways in which we organize and live our lives align with our stated values, and we can reflect on whether our practices and morals make sense to all those involved (Robinson 2011a, 26). The effects of our caring practices and knowledges, and the response from those with whom we are in caring relation, are significant not only because the outcome of care practices matter (which, assuredly, they do) but also because it is through assessing the outcomes of practices of responsibility and care that knowledge and deed are tested, evaluated, and revised.

Last, it is worth emphasizing again that this constant decentering—of self, of practice, of value—is tough work. The attentive listening, reflection, and humility that underpin the epistemology described here (that guide the processes by which we come to know) are a constant struggle, and we must commit to this struggle without fail from a care ethics perspective. C. Thi Nguyen (2020, 142) explains that an "epistemic bubble is a social epistemic structure in which some relevant voices have been excluded from omission," while an echo chamber "is a social epistemic structure in which other relevant voices have been actively discredited." Bubbles are relatively fragile; "it is possible to pop an epistemic bubble by exposing a member to relevant information or arguments that they have missed. Echo chambers, on the other hand, are significantly more robust" (Nguyen 2020, 145), as voices that might decenter the epistemological claims of the chamber are actively discredited. Without negating the important political problem of chambers, I think it is crucial to foreground that most epistemic claims are rooted in neither bubbles nor chambers: most epistemic claims are "rooted in [the knower's] social, historical, linguistic, and cultural situation" (Hekman 1995, 129–130), in their form of life. In this way, simple exposure to "new" knowledge or "new" voices does not instantly or easily change the claims that constitute a form of life (à la epistemic bubbles); neither are these new knowledges and voices necessarily and expressly discredited and dismissed (à la echo chambers).[5] Instead, we must commit to the hard work of decentering our epistemological claims (which both constitute our forms of life and yet can be changed) in an unwavering way. We must struggle to hear different knowers meaningfully without always abdicating to those different knowledges and therein losing our voice. We must grapple with the task of making sense of gaps in epistemic resources without thinking we have fully overcome them. We must strive continually to be open and attentive to the other, a struggle that will be "sometimes brief, sometimes long and agonizing" (Noddings 2003, 53). Furthermore, we must understand that in/through this patient struggle, we may encounter one another in ways that transform us and our knowing—this is, in so many ways, the point. Indeed, when particular notions and practices of care come to be presented as the whole of care (as argued by Raghuram and her critique of the dominance of white/Western understandings of care in the existing care ethics literature, for example), and when others draw our attention to this fact (when others respond to this ossification of certain conceptualizations of care), we can see that we are failing in our commitment to care and the epistemological decenterings this commitment demands. We are failing to enact the decentering that, from a care ethical lens, is the very mechanism by which we come to know, the very process in and through which ourselves and our knowledge can be transformed in ways that together move us toward more caring relations and forms of life.

The commitment to care, from this vantage point, takes "courage" (Noddings 2003, 39): the constant decenterings discussed here are never resolved, never finalized. The best we can do is commit to "liv[ing] with the conflict" (Noddings 2003, 13) that such decenterings generate (and I use generate here purposively, as these struggles are frequently productive). It is only by moving back and forth—between self and other, between practices and values, between past-present-future, failure and success—that we can consciously assess practices, decisions, and claims in light of the values we hold, and in turn assess those values, and whether or not they are reflected in practices, or generate relations, with which we want to live.

ACKNOWLEDGMENTS

I wish to thank Marion Paradis Noppen, without whom this chapter would not exist. Marion, I am so grateful to be able to experience the challenges and joys of decentering with you.

NOTES

1. This quote cites David Abram's (1996, 52) work on Maurice Merleau-Ponty.
2. I struggled with making "Embodiment" and "Imagination" two distinct subsections here, as I am well aware of the ways in which this separation mirrors the mind/body dualism characteristic of dominant Western epistemologies that devalue emotions, corporeality, and vulnerability. I wish to be clear that I see embodiment and imagination as inextricably intertwined. Our imaginative capacities literally are the result of various biological processes, and they are nurtured and informed by our embodied, lived experience. Further, how we think (our imaginations, our cognitions) has clear and direct impacts and consequences on our bodies, the ways we treat our bodies, and the ways we regard other bodies. However, I have maintained this separation for organizational and clarity purposes here. See Hamington (2004, 64) for more on this point.
3. One exception here would be cases where others do not want to engage with us—when social groups, for instance, ask to be left alone (often for very legitimate reasons). This is a specific problem that merits further attention but, due to scope, cannot be tended to here.
4. For Ruddick (1989, 40) a mother is defined as "a person who takes on responsibility for children's lives and for whom providing childcare is a significant part of her or his [or their] working life."
5. Clearly, so many forms of life are structured by relations of power that do implicitly discredit specific voices, often along lines of various axes of oppression, like race, class, and gender. Miranda Fricker (2007) calls this "testimonial injustice," and I do not mean to gloss over the pervasiveness of this phenomenon (see Bourgault in this volume [chapter 2]). However, my point here is that this implicit bias is not quite the same as that which upholds echo chambers, whereby certain voices are actively and explicitly dismissed by members of the epistemological group (as is the case with "anti-vaxxers" for example). Forms of life are both changeable and yet very sticky—they exceed both bubbles and chambers—and they are our most primary epistemic

terrain. (In fact, I would assert that bubbles and chambers both always emerge in and from forms of life and refer to particular epistemic spaces within given forms of life.)

REFERENCES

Abram, David. 1996. *The Spell of the Sensuous*. New York: Vintage.
Bourgault, Sophie. 2014. "Beyond the Saint and the Red Virgin: Simone Weil as Feminist Theorist of Care." *Frontiers: A Journal of Women Studies* 35 (2): 1–27.
———. 2016. "Attentive Listening and Care in a Neoliberal Era: Weillian Insights for Hurried Times." *Etica & Politica* 18 (3): 311–337.
Confortini, Catia C., and Abigail E. Ruane. 2013. "Sara Ruddick's *Maternal Thinking* as Weaving Epistemology for *Justpeace*." *Journal of International Political Theory* 10 (1): 70–93.
Dalmiya, Vrinda. 2016. *Caring to Know*. Oxford: Oxford University Press.
FitzGerald, Maggie. 2022. *Care and the Pluriverse*. Bristol: Bristol University Press.
Fricker, Miranda. 2007. *Epistemic Injustice*. Oxford: Oxford University Press.
Gilligan, Carol. 1993. *In a Different Voice*. Cambridge, MA: Harvard University Press.
Hamington, Maurice. 2004. *Embodied Care*. Urbana: University of Illinois Press.
Hekman, Susan. 1995. *Moral Voices, Moral Selves*. University Park: Pennsylvania State University Press.
Hunt, Sarah. 2014. "Ontologies of Indigeneity: The Politics of Embodying a Concept." *Cultural Geographies* 21 (1): 27–32.
Hutchings, Kimberly. 2013. "A Place of Greater Safety? Securing Judgements in International Ethics." In *The Vulnerable Subject*, edited by Amanda R. Beattie and Kate Schick, 25–42. Basingstoke: Palgrave Macmillan.
Nguyen, C. Thi. 2020. "Echo Chambers and Epistemic Bubbles." *Episteme* 17 (2): 141–161.
Noddings, Nel. 2003. *Caring*. Berkeley: University of California Press.
———. 2015. "Care Ethics and 'Caring' Organizations." In *Care Ethics and Political Theory*, edited by Daniel Engster and Maurice Hamington, 72–84. Oxford: Oxford University Press.
Raghuram, Parvati. 2016. "Locating Care Ethics beyond the Global North." *ACME: An International Journal for Critical Geographies* 15 (3): 511–533.
———. 2019. "Race and Feminist Care Ethics: Intersectionality as Method." *Gender, Place & Culture* 26 (5): 613–637.
Robinson, Fiona. 2011a. *The Ethics of Care*. Philadelphia: Temple University Press.
———. 2011b. "Stop Talking and Listen: Discourse Ethics and Feminist Care Ethics in International Political Theory." *Millennium: Journal of International Studies* 39 (3): 845–860.
———. 2014. "Discourses of Motherhood and Women's Health: Maternal Thinking as Feminist Politics." *Journal of International Political Theory* 10 (1): 94–108.
Ruddick, Sara. 1989. *Maternal Thinking*. Boston: Beacon.
Tronto, Joan. 2015. "Theories of Care as a Challenge to Weberian Paradigms in Social Science." In *Care Ethics and Political Theory*, edited by Daniel Engster and Maurice Hamington, 252–271. Oxford: Oxford University Press.
van Dijke, Jolanda, Inge van Nistelrooij Pien Bos, and Joachim Duyndam. 2020. "Towards a Relational Conceptualization of Empathy." *Nursing Philosophy* 21:e12297.
Walker, Margaret Urban. 2007. *Moral Understandings*. 2nd ed. New York: Routledge.
Watts, Vanessa. 2013. "Indigenous Place-Thought and Agency amongst Humans and Non-humans (First Woman and Sky Woman Go on a European World Tour!)." *Decolonization: Indigeneity, Education & Society* 2 (1): 20–34.

7 · INDIGENOUS AND FEMINIST ECOLOGICAL REFLECTIONS ON FEMINIST CARE ETHICS

Encounters of Care, Absence, Punctures, and Offerings

ANDREA DOUCET, EVA JEWELL, AND VANESSA WATTS

This chapter is a story about three researchers coming together from distinct sociocultural and onto-epistemological locations to explore histories and concepts of care and feminist care ethics. It was shared research projects and some resonances in our critiques of Euro-Western and colonial onto-epistemologies that brought us together. Our initial aim was to think through potential connections between Indigenous and feminist ecological epistemologies. We thus began by noting that the different epistemological terrains we stand on—Indigenous (specifically Anishinaabe and Haudenosaunee) for Eva and Vanessa and feminist ecological for Andrea—have moved along parallel and occasionally intraconnected pathways. Indigenous and feminist ecological scholarship have both critiqued, albeit it in different ways, the ethicopolitical legacies of the "gaze of Western imperialism and Western science" (Tuhiwai Smith 2012, 41), the "Euro-Western epistemology-ontology divide" (Watts 2013, 32), and "epistemologies of mastery" (Code 2006, 4). There are, however, critical differences between Indigenous and feminist approaches to knowledge making and the status of these fields in the academy. For example, although feminist epistemologies still occupy a marginalized position in the epistemological canon (Rooney 2012), Indigenous epistemologies have more brutal histories of exclusion.

These uneven degrees of exclusion and marginalization became even more obvious in our preparatory conversations for this chapter. We knew that our differences across intellectual training, different generations of scholarly thought, and geopolitical histories of care would guide the chapter. Yet we were not fully prepared for how vast these differences would be. Cross-disciplinary writing on care and feminist care ethics has developed with little acknowledgment of Indigenous lives or Indigenous teachings and writing about profound relationalities within and across stories, theories, and onto-epistemologies. Our discussions—which were both generative and challenging—solidified our view that our collaborative writing about care had to start with acknowledging distinct care histories, notably the palpable ongoing impacts of settler colonialism on caregiving and care receiving for Indigenous parents and children. This chapter is thus also a story about making space for abandoned and invisible worlds of care; for acknowledging absences, constructive rage, and relational autonomy within feminist care ethics; and for unfolding articulations of Indigenous care concepts.

From our first meeting, we made the decision to recognize our distinct positionalities by writing the chapter in multiple voices. This decision contrasts with recent writing about Euro-Western and Indigenous collaborations that seek to braid, mesh, or integrate Indigenous and feminist approaches (i.e., Elm et al. 2016). We draw from Tuck and Yang's (2014, 238) "refusal," not as a "prohibitive stance, but as a generative orientation"; from Jewell's (2018, 87) critique of the reconciliatory urge for settler researchers to work "benevolently, non-critically even, with Indigenous knowledges" in their application of two-eyed seeing, which gives insufficient attention to the epistemic violence that Western knowledges invoke through this method; and we connect these to a less well-known tenet of feminist care ethics, "relational autonomy" (Friedman 1997, 2013).

This chapter is organized in two parts. Guided partly by several key principles from feminist care ethics—relationships and relationalities, responsiveness and contextualities, and responsibilities—we begin by positioning ourselves in relation to care ethics, concepts, and histories. The second part of the chapter reflects some of our conversation about feminist care ethics. Andrea maps her current diffractive engagement with feminist care ethics, and Eva and Vanessa respond to each point with offerings and punctures.

FEMINIST CARE ETHICS: WHERE ARE WE EACH SPEAKING AND WRITING FROM?

Feminist Care Ethics, Relational Methods, Feminist Ecological Ethico-onto-epistemologies: *Andrea*

My journey with care concepts and the field of feminist care ethics began about thirty years ago, when I had the opportunity to work closely with Carol Gilligan while I was a doctoral student at Cambridge University. As a visiting professor at Cambridge for two years, she created a research group centered on a relational narrative method of data analysis, the Listening Guide (e.g., Brown and Gilligan 1992). For seventeen months, I was part of a small group of students who met biweekly with Gilligan to engage in collaborative data analysis and writing (see Mauthner and Doucet 2003).

Gilligan's impacts on my research and writing were utterly profound—theoretically, methodologically, epistemologically, and personally. Her writing, along with that of Sara Ruddick, Selma Sevenhuijsen, and Joan Tronto, provided me with ways of thinking beyond the dominant paradigms of separations and binaries in the burgeoning field of "gender divisions of household work and care." Those early years seeded my ever-growing approach to care work in terms of relational connections between care and justice; intradependence, interdependence, and independence; relationships and relational autonomy; rights and responsibilities; and a recognition of both the generative and dark sides of care.

In the years since then, I have engaged in a long-term project of remaking the Listening Guide, connecting it to broader fields of feminist methodologies and epistemologies. Notably, my diffractive engagement with Lorraine Code's *Ecological Thinking* (2006), with its focus on ecological social imaginaries of knowledge making, ethico-onto-epistemological entanglements, and her epistemological case study of the American ecological thinker Rachel Carson instigated a transformative shift in my thinking on care and epistemologies. Two moments stand out at this stage of my journey.

The first moment came from my engagement with Carson; rereading her books and analyses of her writing by Code and ecological thinkers led me to see and feel deep lines of connection between ecological thought and feminist care ethics. Although neither Carson nor Code use the words "relational ontologies" in their writing, it is there in their explications of how all living things—what they *are*, where they come from, and what they *become*—coexist in and through deep intra-affective relations of constant flow, change, growth, decay, and regrowth. I read relational ontologies in Carson's scientific, journalistic, and poetic observations of seashells and shores, birds, fish, and insects, in her view of synergistic human-earth relationalities, how all life is intraconnected, how "nothing exists alone," and where humans are not separate from but "part of nature" (Carson 1962, 4, 188). In short, central dimensions of feminist care ethics (i.e., relationalities, responsiveness, and responsibilities) are deepened in ecological thought and in feminist ecological ethico-onto-epistemologies.

The second moment happened when, deeply immersed in ecological thinking, I attended the 2016 Truth and Reconciliation Conference, which was held in Winnipeg, one year after the tabling of the "Truth and Reconciliation Report" (Truth and Reconciliation Commission of Canada 2015). Incredulously, it was there that I truly heard, saw, and read some expressions of centuries-old Indigenous relational thought, philosophies, teachings, and onto-epistemologies. My encounter with Aimée Craft, an Anishinaabe writer and legal scholar, and her book (*Breathing Life into the Stone Fort Treaty: An Anishinaabe Understanding of Treaty One*; Craft 2013) opened up a new world of reading and writing for me. I began to incorporate Indigenous work, including Vanessa Watts's (2013) seminal piece on Anishinaabe and Haudenosaunee place-thought onto-epistemologies, in my graduate teaching. When I began to collaborate with Eva, I read in her work (Jewell 2018) and observed in her research approach some resonances with the feminist ecological ethico-onto-epistemological frame I was developing.

These encounters also left me with a sense of loss. I wondered, *how could I have missed all of this?* The question of how to move forward, as a descendent of white settlers and as someone who acknowledges that Indigenous relational approaches have been with us all along—unseen, undervalued, and, in some instances, subtly or blatantly exploited by white settler researchers—partly motivated my desire to write this chapter with Eva and Vanessa. I found one good model of respectful acknowledgment in the best-selling book *Finding the Mother Tree: Discovering the Wisdom of the Forest* by Canadian ecologist Suzanne Simard. She writes about how she had to unlearn "the rigid lens of western science," through which she had been taught "to take apart the ecosystem, to reduce it into its parts, to study the trees and plants and soils in isolation" (Simard 2021, 302). She also acknowledges that her paradigm shift—to one emphasizing diversity and relationality, where "everything in the universe is connected—between the forests and prairies, the land and the water, the sky and the soil, the spirits and the living, the people and all other creatures," owes a great deal to the Indigenous elders she worked with and to Indigenous teachings and scholarship. She writes that she could finally see the "deeper socio-ecological linkages that are fundamental to the Indigenous ways of life" and how she was fully aware that "I wasn't the first person to figure this out, that this was also the ancient wisdom of many Aboriginal people."

Care and Colonial Entanglement: *Eva*

I was introduced to feminist care ethics when I worked with Andrea in 2018 on a postdoctoral fellowship specializing in Indigenous methodologies. This was a topic I was thinking and writing about at that time, as I had produced my thesis research in partnership with (and as a loving offer to) my community: Chippewas of the Thames First Nation. With Andrea, I was immersed in the field of gender, work, and care and learned to use and apply the Listening Guide to the research we were conducting with an urban Indigenous community. This methodological tool—particularly the readings of cultural contexts and social structures—gave definition to a practice I had experienced and witnessed in my own life as an Anishinaabe person and scholar: critical, anticolonial perspectives of social and political structures that a mainstream Canadian public seems to consider an unquestioned norm. This layer of reading was one that I was increasingly interested in, taking the opportunity to read for the implicitness of settler colonialism and the tensions that arise when Indigenous peoples navigate these structures without the advantage of intergenerational epistemic and social capital (Jewell et al. 2020).

Andrea continually encouraged me to think about how to be in conversation with feminist care ethics literature. Admittedly, it took me some time to really consider how this literature applied to my evolving work. I was concerned with supporting my community through original governance resurgence and language reclamation and helping my colleagues to build the Indigenous-led spaces I wanted to work in (e.g., Yellowhead Institute). How did feminist care ethics relate, particularly when there wasn't much by way of Indigenous perspectives in this field? I couldn't yet see it. It wasn't until I encountered care ethics' discussion of the social, political, and economic reproduction of the very systems I was critiquing that I finally clued in (see Luxton and Bezanson 2006). Suddenly, care ethics made sense, at least theoretically, for thinking through my practical concern of how to repopulate and reclaim the Anishinaabe governance systems that I've been so passionate about. Once I started reading for this, I developed an appreciation of feminist care ethics as well as many critiques.

As an Anishinaabe scholar (with paternal Haudenosaunee lineage) from a family and communities deeply impacted by Canada's residential schools, my reading of care ethics is contextualized by the violence that Cree scholar Megan Scribe refers to as colonial care (2020). Colonial care, the actual clutches on children that remove them from the care of their original families, works in tandem with settler bureaucracy to enact colonial violence in the lives of Indigenous peoples. Although feminist care ethics examine care subjects of any age, the colonial care that Indigenous children have been subjected to for the entirety of the Canadian settler state's existence is the context of my life and my entry into this discussion. In Western societies, children were subjected to violence as a necessary means to their maturation, and in a settler-colonial framework, Europeans politically constructed Indigenous peoples as "the degraded, not fully human, child" (Rollo 2016, 61). The care for and civilizational progress of Indigenous peoples became a moral duty for the settler state. For me, care is "killing the Indian in the child"; it is the "dark side of care" enacted on several generations of Indigenous children. This genocide is the heavy burden of colonial care.

And yet care is at home in Anishinaabe worldviews and is arguably a vital concept in our onto-epistemologies. Zaagidowin (love) is our first knowledge from which we strive to make our choices. Our philosophies of the good life are centered in being good, responsible relative to all life (notably to life beyond human embodiments), and our principles of noninterference are acts of care and respect of the pathways to which all life has a right. Some of these ideas are similar to what care ethics literature, in some way or another, starts to articulate, albeit in a different trajectory than the land-based, relationship-based worldviews that characterize many Indigenous knowledges.

As a result, I found, time and again in our briefly mentioned difficult discussions, that my affect was resentment. Resentment for the absence upon which Vanessa and I enter this discussion, for my personal and familial struggle to embody original care practices (compromised entirely by the settler-colonial violence of residential schools), and for the general absence, in the field, of what care has meant for Indigenous peoples, both in original worldviews and as subjugated to colonial care's violence. Care, in its many definitions, is the loving actions of our ancestors, the protection they tried to secure for us, the worldviews that gave rise to principles of noninterference, temporal consent, and relationship-based societies. But on the other hand, colonial care also attempted to end and erase Indigenous worlds. And in many ways, the social reproduction of settler-colonial worlds through means of care is the immiseration of Indigenous life.

Entering upon Absence: *Vanessa*

In higher education (and since the release of the Truth and Reconciliation Commission's final report in 2015), the interest in "Indigenous ideas" and not just "Indigenous problems" has taken off, an entanglement of ideas and philosophies across disciplines that can be fruitful. Indigenous studies, a discipline in its own right, has been building theory and methodology for decades. In many fields of study, wherein Indigenous peoples have been present, we have been overwhelmingly defined by our social problems (see also Tuck 2016). Certainly, criticism of the state and state policy has also been present in these problem-oriented framings, but Indigenous-informed theorizing has largely been absent in the ascertaining of who we are as Indigenous peoples, beyond the scope of problemed peoples. As such, in these more contemporary entanglement of ideas, Indigenous scholars might find themselves entering upon absence, despite a presence of ingrained ideas about who we are.

My fields of study are Indigenous studies and sociology. When entering my doctoral program in sociology, I had developed a strong sense of the intellectual scape from my previous training in Indigenous studies. Arriving into social theory, during the first year of my doctorate, I found the closest alignment with ecofeminist literature that we were introduced to, namely Donna Haraway's work. I became more drawn to ecofeminist and ecological literatures during this time, finding parallels but also tensions when holding them alongside Indigenous epistemologies. At times, I was frustrated that intellectual interventions about nonhuman relations and feminist discourse were considered "new" and "novel" ideas, without much attention paid to contributions of Indigenous thinkers, other than small gestures (usually in the form of generalizations) about Indigenous peoples.

With respect to care ethics, it is difficult to not associate the word *care* to the structural and more politicized area of *Care* that Indigenous peoples in Canada have been and are subject to. While the field of feminist care ethics strives to attend to injustices, particularly those enlivened by sexist and patriarchal norms, I feel particularly attuned to very material, racialized, gendered, and colonial forms of *Care* that produce material, racialized, gendered, and colonial forms of injustice for Indigenous peoples. When we consider Indigenous forms of knowledge making in already-established disciplines where Indigenous perspectives have been absent or show up only in the form of social problems, knowledge making often has to start as an unmaking. Even the term "Indigenous" does a disservice to the complexity and diversity of knowledge systems across the territories we are part of. Conversations around epistemologies and ontologies often rely on abstract concepts and processes, whereas material places and other-than-human beings as forms of care relations are fundamental to Indigenous philosophies and societies (see also Llavaneras Blanco in this volume [chapter 10]).

I met Andrea during a panel we were presenting on for the 2018 International Sociological Association meeting in Toronto. Her paper, "Feminist Sociologies: Diffractive Readings of Histories, Contributions, Futures," journeyed through contributions of Canadian feminist sociology, drawing on Haraway's work to map out urgent questions for care and inequality, including Indigenous peoples. Her analysis was critical and commanding. As a junior scholar feeling somewhat outside and new to the discipline, I immediately felt drawn to Andrea's work and hearing her speak sparked a sense of synchronicity. It was through this relationship that I would later meet Eva, someone whom I heard so much of through friends and colleagues. I was first introduced to her work through the Yellowhead Institute, in the "Calls to Action Accountability" report, a project that gained national attention (Jewell and Mosby 2021). The report accounted for those government bodies, institutions, and organizations that had responded to ninety-four *calls* (and those many, many *calls* left unanswered).[1] Through these relationships, we have copresented, published chapters in the same edited volumes, and have now arrived here, to engage with each other. I am grateful for these new friendships sparked by deep intellectual regard.

As a person who navigates the academy as a Mohawk and Anishinaabe woman, I notice more and more attempts to eradicate seemingly irreconcilable differences between properly "non-Indigenous" and "Indigenous" thought motivated by reconciliatory discourse. Indeed, feminist theory has experienced (and continues to grapple with) bringing to bear on established ideas of how knowledge is made, who can hold knowledge, and how it should be disseminated. Important interventions on the ethics of care that Andrea points to also resonate here, as Indigenous ideas about care contain distinctive differences. It is my hope that this chapter, in a dialogical form, will consider ideas, resonances, and punctures that challenge conventions of knowledge *about* Indigenous peoples and center ideas *from* Indigenous peoples.

FEMINIST CARE ETHICS: DIFFRACTIVE MAPPING, OFFERINGS, AND PUNCTURES

In this chapter section we write in two and sometimes three voices (Andrea, and Eva and Vanessa's shared and separate voices). Andrea begins by mapping selective and diffractive readings of some key enduring features of feminist care ethics. Diffractive readings, rooted in Haraway's concept of diffraction, is about "heterogeneous history, not about originals" (Haraway 1997, 273) and reflects key qualities of feminist care ethics, including relationalities, responsiveness, and responsibility. To "read diffractively is to *read through not against*; it means reading texts intra-actively through one another, enacting new patterns of engagement" (Barad 2007, 29, emphasis added). Eva and Vanessa then consider these features with offerings and punctures from Indigenous perspectives.

Care as Relationalities, as Relationship, as Relational Ontologies: *Andrea*

Relationalities, relationships, and relational ontologies are at the heart of feminist care ethics. This is clear from the field's long-held view of human subjectivities as relational and interdependent. The concept of a relational self challenges the dominant presumption in Euro-Western liberal theories that human subjectivity is characterized by individuality, independence, autonomy, and rationality (see critiques by Gilligan 1982; Held 2006) and embraces interconnectedness, interdependencies, vulnerabilities, and embodiment. Relational ontologies have been mainly articulated in terms of relational subjectivities—that is, a "different starting point" where "individuals are conceived as being in relationships" (Tronto 2013, 49). Yet relationalities and relational ontologies are much wider than relational views of human subjectivities. As articulated in new materialist, posthumanist, and feminist ecological ethico-onto-epistemologies, relational ontologies also encompass the deep relationalities of all living things as well as of our knowledge-making practices. This signifies a profoundly radical move from inter-*action*, where two objects come together as separate parts joining, to *intra*-action, which "entails the very disruption of the metaphysics of individualism" while also challenging the "inherent boundary between observer and observed, knower and known" (Barad 2007, 154).

Feminist care ethics *does* lend itself to this kind of thinking because of its deeply relational orientation, but there is still a need for stronger articulations, or diffractive readings that can find nascent ideas in earlier care writing about relational ontologies. This would mean, for example, recognizing relationalities within and between objects and beings of all kinds and how what they *are*, what they *do*, and their processes of becoming are made and remade within, and as part of, a wide array of constantly changing constitutive contexts and habitats. There would also be more attention to the relational human and more-than-human intra-actions (see also Bozalek's work in this volume [chapter 9]; Puig de la Bellacasa 2017; Tsing 2015) and more robust connections between feminist care ethics and relational epistemologies (Dalmiya 2002; Hekman 1995; Robinson 2020) and ethico-onto-epistemologies (see Dionne 2021; Doucet 2018). These gaps in the field also reflect a sustained lack of engagement with Indigenous work (but see Jewell 2024).

How We Care, How We Are Careless: *Vanessa*

Many Indigenous cosmologies contain what might be considered an ethic of care, many forms of which extend beyond the bounds of human to human relations or individuals within social institutions. Relationality in Indigenous societies (in which relations are communicative and agential) is present in human to human relations, other-than-human to human, and other-than-human to other-than-human relations. These constellations of relations are both interconnected and distinct and, perhaps most significantly, *real*. In an earlier work I described the necessity of taking Indigenous cosmologies seriously, not simply as parable or mythical moralistic stories (though these exist too). I impress, rather, that the presence of our cosmologies contain historical, real, and material lineages to our multiplicity of interspecies relations. Mohawk scholar Susan Hill (2017, 3) describes perhaps the most foundational relationship Haudenosaunee have: the one with land. Hill writes, "Yethi'nihstenha Onhwentsya is the Kenyen'keha (Mohawk) name for the earth. 'She-to-us-mother provides-[for our]-needs' describes the relationship between Onkwehonwe (humans) and the earth." In this orientation, humans are viewed as being *of* the earth—specifically, they are made of clay. This is not a symbolic gesture in a mythical story; it is rather a historical account that carries within it the roles and responsibilities with a material being (i.e., "She-to-us-mother provides-[for our]-needs"). When humans are conceived as being materially related to other-than-human beings (such as land), the epistemological is crucially indivisible from the ontological (Watts 2013). We, as humans, are the stuff of the earth, inheriting how we come to know. As such, our epistemological views of the world are reliant on the ontological commitments embedded in our diverse and multiple foundings across Indigenous territories.

Anishinaabe legal scholar John Borrows (1996) describes interspecies relations in his case study: "Crow, Owl, Deer et al. versus the Anishinaabe." In this story, the deer, caribou, and moose leave the territory of the Anishinaabeg and are captured by crows. A battle between the Anishinaabeg and the crows took place when the Anishinaabeg discovered that the deer were being kept in confinement by the crows. Neither side won the battle, and each agreed to a truce. However, the deer were perceived to look at this outcome with indifference. As such, the Anishinabek met with the crow and deer in council, seeking answers: "The Anishinabe asked: 'Why are you so apathetic about our efforts to rescue you from your imprisonment? We have suffered great affliction and hazarded death to save you all on your behalf. It seems as though you could not care less.' The Chief Deer replied: 'You are mistaken if you have imagined that we are here against our wishes. We have chosen to stay with the crows. We are not sad but very happy. The crows have treated us better than you ever did when we shared the same country with you'" (Borrows 1996, 651). The Deer Nation and Anishinaabeg had formerly been parties to an agreement about how deer would be hunted, and Anishinaabeg had violated this agreement. Anishinaabe scholar Hayden King (2017) reads this story as depicting a "rules-based world" that is "not anarchic," in that the terms of permissibility are limited by a mutually agreed-upon treaty. The ability to conduct interspecies communication was thus not only possible but an expectation. From such a perspective, peace and balance are maintained through community-based governance, wherein all peoples and non-peoples were responsible. Care, in this sense, extends beyond human-centered notions of society and relations and, further, beyond what "ecological" might capture. Rather, it centers active and agential care relations across species, where reciprocity is profoundly connected to material practices of care.

In the story, care is positioned as a form of sacrifice and salvation by the Anishinaabe—ultimately decried by the Deer. Rather, care is expressed by the Deer in forms of respect, independence, and boundaries. In feminist care ethics, the implosion of boundaries enforced by patriarchal notions of care is central in addressing injustices. In this story, however, it is the establishment of boundaries that articulates care. For Indigenous communities, land is a central orientation to knowledge making, and just as territorial markers highlight particularities around waters, trees, vegetation, rock, and animal life, so too persist particularities associated with how we come to care and what constitutes carelessness.

Care as Practices: *Andrea*

For more than four decades, care scholars have focused on care as practices and as moral qualities or dispositions that are part of those practices. As well described by British care scholar Hilary Graham forty years ago, "What it means to care for someone and what it entails are closely related" (Graham 1983, 13; see also Ruddick 1995). Tronto is perhaps best known for clearly articulating this line of thought in her continual refinement of how she refers to caring practices and labor as complex processes that includes stages, steps, or phases of care. First developed with Bernice Fisher in the early 1990s (Fisher and Tronto 1990), these include an initial four steps that Tronto (2013) then widened to five; Tronto also added to these what she calls "moral qualities" and "dispositions" (Tronto 1993, 35, 19). Taken together, these steps and their related moral elements are (1) *caring about* someone's unmet needs (*attentiveness*); (2) *caring for* these needs (*responsibility*); (3) *caregiving* and making sure the work is done (*competence*); (4) *care receiving* and assessing the effectiveness of these care acts (*responsiveness*); and (5) *caring with*—which is about collective responsibilities for care (*plurality, communication, trust and respect*) (Tronto 2013, 23, 35).

More recently, Tronto (2020) has given more expression to how feminist care ethics has not given enough attention to ecological and more-than-human matters; and she extends her long-standing views on the politics and dark sides of care: that "care cannot be separated from its deeply political place" (2020, 43) and that "care is often bad care" (Tronto 2020, 50). In response to a series of letters from a new generation of diverse scholars (Karjevsky, Talevi, and Bailer 2020), Tronto (2020, 82) is more explicit and reflective about how white settlers need to address "white silence" and to think about care responsibilities differently and "to begin to take responsibility for what they have, consciously or unconsciously, done."

Despite these developments, there have been three notable absences in the study of care practices. First, the specificity and contexts of Indigenous care practices, as articulated in Indigenous families, communities, and nations, have received little attention (but see Jewell 2024). Second, care has been taken up mainly as practices and theories and in relation to policies and sociopolitical life, but much less so in relation to our research practices and our ethical, ontological, and epistemological responsibilities as knowers and knowledge makers (but see Brannelly 2018; Code 2015; Puig de la Bellacasa 2012). Third, except for ecofeminist work and some research on the care of animals (e.g., Donovan and Adams 2007), care practices as related to the intra-active care of land and nonhuman life have been largely ignored (but see Doucet 2023; Karjevsky et al. 2020; Puig de la Bellacasa 2017).

Relational Care Practice: *Eva*

For many Indigenous nations, original land-based and relationship-based onto-epistemologies frame care and its attendant practices. Watts (2013) contends that for Anishinaabe and Haudenosaunee peoples (and Indigenous peoples' worldviews more broadly), the world we live in and the human knowledge we receive/produce from it are inseparable. *Place-thought*, as Watts explains, is "the premise that land is alive and thinking and that humans and non-humans derive agency through the extensions of these thoughts" (21). Similarly, in her formative text *How It Is,* Jicarilla Apache philosopher V. F. Cordova (2007) writes, "The issues of 'consciousness' that so bedevils the Western philosopher is not a great issue among Native Americans. Consciousness, awareness, is assumed to be a characteristic of the universe" (146–147). The presupposition that humans are not unique in possessing agency and consciousness is at the heart of Anishinaabe and Haudenosaunee care ethics and practices.

In Anishinaabe and Haudenosaunee worlds, care extends to and is received from not only the nonhuman world but worlds beyond the physical plane. From this understanding, Indigenous peoples developed technologies and practices that serve to fulfill our relational obligations with our worlds, a necessity that Watts (2013) expands on: "If, as Indigenous peoples, we are extensions of the very land we walk upon, then we have an obligation to maintain communication with it. A familiar warning is echoed through many communities, that if we do not care for the land we run the risk of losing who we are as Indigenous peoples" (23). For Indigenous peoples, the providers and subjects of care are not confined to human embodiment; our identity and very existence depend on our relational abilities with our nonhuman kin. Scobie, Finau, and Hallenbeck (2024) retrieve social reproduction theory from the Marxist critiques of state biopower to apply in an Indigenous context to state that "[Indigenous] social reproduction cannot be separated from the land" (4). To culturally regenerate and socially reproduce subsequent populations of people who deeply understand that the world around them is not only alive but a relative with whom we can (and indeed must) consult to create knowledge and solve problems requires a completely divergent relational ethos from what is currently practiced in a Euro-Western settler-colonial world.

Eli Baxter's memoir *Aki-wayn-zih* (2021) suggests that this relational ethos is, in fact, the life purpose of Anishinaabeg: to harness the complex knowledge of nonhuman relations in what Kim Anderson (2011) has described as a "mastery of relatedness" (127). While the titular Anishinaabemowin term of Baxter's Aki-waynzih is often translated as elder, it is an honorific given to someone who, with age and over time, achieves advanced knowledge in relation with the land: "'Aki-wayn-zih' means 'a person who is as worthy as the earth'" (Baxter 2021, 11). Baxter's (2021) narrative demonstrates that for Anishinaabe, the most advanced aspiration of our human embodiment is to be in total relational alignment with nonhuman society.

Indigenous relational obligations involve *reciprocal* practices of care, meaning that care is not solely practiced by humans for our worlds around us. Indeed, our worlds care for us as well. In many ways the genealogy of what we know about being human and how to socially reproduce our worlds as Indigenous peoples come from our nonhuman relatives. For example, the Anishinaabeg doodem system, the governing structure by which kin, identity, belonging, and social responsibilities are determined was received from the governing practice of our animal kin (Dumont 2016; Deleary 2016; see also Benton-Banai 1979). Much of the concern of human life, of *mno-bmaadziwin* (the good life), is in being a good relative in the context of our worlds around us.

One can imagine, perhaps, the grounds for our punctures to feminist care ethics and ecological feminist work that theorizes the interconnectedness of human life and land in sociopolitical contexts where settler colonialism has sought to erase Indigenous place thought through violence and genocide. Moreover, the particular violence that Indigenous peoples in settler-colonial contexts (and beyond) endure is under the twisted auspices of care for our well-being. Canada's Indian residential school system was founded under the presumption that Indigenous peoples' existence was permissible only if they assimilated to the lower rungs of Euro-Western society. Settler states and churches forcibly removed Indigenous children from the care of their parents, lands, languages, cultures, and nations. What resulted was a near total devastation of Indigenous worlds; as Billy-Ray Belcourt (2018) describes it, "The past-present-future of settler colonialism is ridden with scenes and technologies of abandonment" (11). It is in the absence of Indigenous peoples, our care, laws, languages, embodiments, and relationships, that some white feminist scholars even developed groundbreaking philosophies about their novel relationship to stolen lands and environments.

Care as Contextuality and Specificity Rather Than Universalistic Principles: *Andrea*

Gilligan (1982, 19) argued that the ethics of care is partly a "mode of thinking that is contextual and narrative rather than formal and abstract." The field's attention to context and specificity, to the concrete, and to differences grew partly out of critiques of Enlightenment thought, liberal political theories, malestream development theories, and logical positivism, which all deal in universal ethical and abstract principles. Feminist care ethics has also provided sustained critiques of Cartesian, Euro-Western, and modernist dualisms and normative hierarchies of subject/object, reason/emotion, nature/culture, mind/body, and public/private binaries (Hekman 1995; Robinson 2020).

Although it has continued to deepen and widen in response to changing historical, socioeconomic, and political contexts, the field has paid less attention to care and colonization. Notably, almost three decades ago, Uma Narayan (1995) argued that while the field "correctly insists on acknowledging human needs and relationships," it failed to address the "very different accounts" of colonization by the "colonizers and the colonized" (133–134). She thus argued that feminist care ethics should focus more on analyzing how "a *colonialist* care discourse" has much resonance with "contemporary strands of the ethic of care" (133–134).

Care to Stop Us from Vanishing? *Vanessa*

In extending the work of Narayan (1995), a colonialist care discourse would seek to understand the very real and material systemic inequities ongoingly produced by racist law and politics against Indigenous peoples while also seeking to further break down binaries between colonizer and colonized; that is, the "colonized" announces a codependency, one in which the colonized is centrally defined by the overpowering machinations of the colonizer.

In her work on situated knowledges, Haraway (1988) aptly describes how feminists of the time involved in debates of science and technology were akin to Reagan-era "special interest groups" (575). In a similar vein, how will Indigenous knowledges enter upon an established field of ethics of care, without first being universalized? In Canada, for example, the "Indian," a special interest group of the colonizer state, was (and is still) universalized as an impediment to the progress of Canada. In this universalizing of hundreds of diverse nations, onto-epistemologies, and sociopolitical systems, the "Indian" is consistently viewed in academia and by the state as a universalized category, stripped of any nuance or active practice of independent ideas that are not beholden to a history of bigger ideas. In academia, universalizing ideas about so-called special interest groups almost always require members of so-called special interest groups who show up to the proverbial ivory tower to fight against these conventions of knowledge. And thus getting to any sort of particularity or nuance about multiple Indigenous contexts must often be an undoing, an unstitching of a blanket of Indigenousness.

Feminist care ethics has provided sustained critiques of dangerous dualisms, binaries, and hierarchies. And yet the formation of these binaries, dualisms, and hierarchies themselves require an obfuscation of specificity about numerous Indigenous contexts into universalized categories under the law. In particular, when it comes to care and Indigenous peoples under the law (the Indian residential school system, child welfare laws as they apply on reserves), universalized categories of Indigenous peoples serve(d) a broader pursuit of the colonial state: saving the Indian. Salvation of Indigenous peoples through white, colonial systems was (and continues to be) delivered through statist arms of care. Given this dynamic, specific contexts of Indigenous forms of care outside of universalized, statist definitions of Indigenous peoples are crucial to understanding care ethics in their many contexts.

Care as "Social Death" Against Indigenous Worlds: *Eva*

"Care" is a fraught term for Indigenous peoples. In 1990, Fisher and Tronto wrote that care is a "species activity that includes everything that we do to maintain, continue, and repair our 'world' so that we can live in it as well as possible. That world includes our bodies, our selves, and our environment, all of which we seek to interweave in a complex, life-sustaining web" (40).

In this quote from early definitive works on feminist care ethics, the complexities of what's described as "our world" and how these worlds are made possible are absent. We entered this discussion to address this absence and to articulate the perspectives of those dispossessed of their care responsibilities and of their worlds, to make way for settler-colonial worlds. Those same settler-colonial worlds would ultimately contain feminist theorizing care atop worlds eroded by that very same practice. In particular, the parts of the "world" Fisher and Tronto describe—the bodies, selves, and environment—are all subjects of care made ontologically possible through the social death of others. Social death, conceptualized by Orlando Patterson and later described by Billy-Ray Belcourt (2018), is "the arrangement of modes of abandonment that empty some populations of moral purchase" (1). Social death is the result of colonial forces "caring" for Indigenous peoples. Social death is, in this telling, the inability to socially reproduce Indigenous worlds to even a portion of their original capacity without the interlopers of settler colonialism, neoliberalism, and late-stage capitalism. Social reproduction of our worlds, the worlds of Indigenous peoples, is marked by ongoing structural violence despite state promises to do better (Jewell and Mosby 2021).

CONCLUSION: SO WHAT—AND NOW WHAT?

Relational Autonomy and Refusal: *Andrea*

This collaboration with Eva and Vanessa has brought me back to concepts and practices of "relational autonomy." First coined by Marilyn Friedman in 1993 to capture her views that "conceptions of autonomy can combine relational and individualistic aspects" (Friedman 2014, 42), relational autonomy suggests that "persons can be independent in some ways while being (more) dependent in other ways" (59) and that there are "reasons why members of subordinated or dominated groups might want to retain independence as an aim of action" (43).

Relational autonomy has been central to how we have thought about our collaboration. Eva and Vanessa's offerings and punctures and feminist care ethics also brought us back to Eve Tuck and Wayne Yang's (2014) writing on refusal—not a wholesale rejection or separation but one that is "always grounded in historical analysis and present conditions" (243). Seeing refusal as "desire" that "refuses the teleos of colonial future" and "expands possible futures" (243) is also one way of thinking about *relational autonomy* between the field of feminist care ethics and Indigenous engagements with, and contestations of, care concepts, practices, and approaches.

My own thinking on feminist care ethics has been centered on a few key Rs, including relationalities, responsiveness, and responsibilities. Writing this chapter has been an act of care in that it has invoked those Rs, while also deepening my sense of what relationalities are, the politics and precarity of responsiveness, and the urgency and complexities of what it means to be a responsible knowledge maker and care scholar.

Care Vanishing: *Vanessa*

What would vanishment look like in this context? A vanishment of colonization-as-care, a vanishment of the poor and feral Indian from discourse. A vanishment of tropes about Indigenous peoples that augment the legacy of practices of *Care* of Indigenous peoples by Canadian social and public institutions. This sort of depoliticized imagining is tempting but ultimately disconnected from justice. Indigenous ideas about care are not designed to be removed from their political scapes. They include intimate acts of care between families and children, peoples and land, and other-than-human beings. Whether it is taking place when fighting for the rights of our territories to survive and thrive, fighting for the rights of our children to access safe and kinship-based homes, expanding our own notions of care ethics, Indigenous ideas about care continue to proceed and adapt. As such, our care practices are big enough to accommodate the messes colonial care has ordained. But more than that, they preexisted colonial messes and exist in their own right. As conversations continue to emerge in feminist care ethics, it will be important to distinguish between ecological and ecofeminist discourse about care and Indigenous-informed ones. Though resonances on the topics of other-than-humans and white heteropatriarchy can and will be found, Indigenous-based relationships with other-than-humans are inscribed with diverse territorial protocols and cosmological, onto-epistemological ideas of care. Further, Indigenous-based relationships with white heteropatriarchy are marked by violent policies of *Care* intended for Indigenous peoples and rationalized as a particular sort of caring *of* Indigenous peoples.

Challenging hegemonic conventions of knowledge and hegemonic tropes of who Indigenous peoples are and what we mean to state interests mean that Indigenous ideas should not simply be a lens to gain insight about something else already articulated and understood. Our philosophies, stories, and cosmologies are place-formed; they are not intended to exist in the abstract as a mechanistic theorem to peer through. Although reconciliation as a national and political imperative has opened doors to important conversations between institutions, peoples, and disciplines, care work is most productive when the seemingly intimate and discreet is taken seriously.

Reclaiming Indigenous Worlds of Care: *Eva*

We approached this conversation with offerings and punctures while keeping in mind the contemporary prevalence of reconciliation (particularly in Canada), which is arguably cause for the increase in the mainstream scholarly appetite for Indigenous knowledge collaboration, however gratingly generalizing that may be. Instead, I look to the kind of reconciliation that is, for Anishinaabe, Haudenosaunee, and Indigenous peoples more broadly, about reclaiming, repairing, and reproducing the care practices anchored in our onto-epistemologies (Lindberg 2017; MacDonald 2019). Our work in reconciliation need not be in holding space for state apologies or forgiving colonial violence but instead might be in reconciling with ourselves, re-creating full relationships with our laws, languages, cultures, lands, and past/future generations. Let this refusal to forgive, as Flowers (2015) puts it, be understood as not only a negation but an affirmation to culturally regenerate and socially reproduce our land-based worlds, in Flowers's case, "my hwulmuhw teachings as a Leey'qsun woman" (42). Let the space of refusal be a resolution to our care practices and an offering to non-Indigenous care scholars to support, listen to, and make way for Indigenous social reproduction as an act of conciliation, the starting place of relationality.

ACKNOWLEDGMENTS

This chapter is equally authored; our names are listed alphabetically. We thank Jessica Falk for research assistance and for facilitating our online writing sessions and the editors of this volume (Sophie Bourgault, Maggie FitzGerald, and Fiona Robinson) for their excellent feedback. This collaboration was partly supported by funding from a SSHRC Partnership grant (no. 895-2020-1011).

NOTE

1. The 94 Calls to Action published in 2015 by the Truth and Reconciliation Commission of Canada can be found at https://nctr.ca/records/reports/#trc-reports.

REFERENCES

Anderson, Kim. 2011. *Life Stages and Native Women: Memory, Teachings, and Story Medicine.* Winnipeg: University of Manitoba Press.

Barad, Karen. 2007. *Meeting the Universe Halfway: Quantum Physics and the Entanglement of Matter and Meaning.* Durham, NC: Duke University Press.

Baxter, Eli. 2021. *Aki-wayn-zih: A Person as Worthy as the Earth.* Edited by Matthew Ryan Smith. Montreal: McGill-Queen's University Press.

Belcourt, Billy-Ray. 2018. "Meditations on Reserve Life, Biosociality, and the Taste of Nonsovereignty." *Settler Colonial Studies* 8 (1): 1–15.

Benton-Banai, Eddie. 1979. *The Mishomis Book: The Voice of the Ojibway.* St. Paul, MN: Indian Country Press.

Borrows, John. 1996. "With or Without You: First Nations Law (in Canada)." *McGill Law Journal* 41 (3): 629–665. https://canlii.ca/t/2bhb.

Brannelly, Tula. 2018. "An Ethics of Care Research Manifesto." *International Journal of Care and Caring* 2 (3): 367–378.

Brown, Lyn Mikel, and Carol Gilligan. 1992. *Meeting at the Crossroads: Women's Psychology and Girls' Development*. Cambridge, MA: Harvard University Press.

Carson, Rachel. 1962. *Silent Spring*. Boston: Houghton Mifflin Harcourt.

Code, Lorraine. 2006. *Ecological Thinking: The Politics of Epistemic Location*. New York: Oxford University Press.

———. 2015. "Care, Concern, and Advocacy: Is There a Place for Epistemic Responsibility?" *Feminist Philosophy Quarterly* 1 (1): 1–20.

Cordova, Viola Faye. 2007. *How It Is: The Native American Philosophy of V. F. Cordova*. Tucson: University of Arizona Press.

Craft, Aimée. 2013. *Breathing Life into the Stone Fort Treaty: An Anishinaabe Understanding of Treaty One*. Saskatoon, Saskatchewan: Purich.

Dalmiya, Vrinda. 2002. "Why Should a Knower Care?" *Hypatia* 17 (1): 34–52.

Deleary, Mary E. 2016. "Dodem Teachings at the 2016 Clan Gathering." Recorded lecture, Chippewas of the Thames First Nation, Ontario, October 29, 2016.

Dionne, Emilie. 2021. "Knowledge Practices as Matters of Care: A Diffractive Dialogue between Lorraine Code's Ecological Thinking and Karen Barad's Agential Realism." In *Thinking Ecologically, Thinking Responsibly: The Legacies of Lorraine Code*, edited by Nancy McHugh and Andrea Doucet, 175–192. New York: State University of New York Press.

Donovan, Josephine, and Carol␣J. Adams. 2007. *The Feminist Care Tradition in Animal Ethics: A Reader*. New York: Columbia University Press.

Doucet, Andrea. 2018. "Feminist Epistemologies and Ethics: Ecological Thinking, Situated Knowledges, Epistemic Responsibilities." In *The Sage Handbook of Qualitative Research Ethics*, edited by Ron Iphofen and Martin Tolich, 73–88. London: Sage.

———. 2023. "Care Is Not a Tally Sheet: Rethinking the Field of Gender Divisions of Domestic Labour with Care-centric Conceptual Narratives." *Families, Relationships and Societies* 12 (1): 10–30.

Dumont, Onaubinasay Jim. 2016. "Dodem Teachings at the 2016 Clan Gathering." Recorded lecture, Chippewas of the Thames First Nation, Ontario, October 29, 2016.

Elm, Jessica H. L., Jordan P. Lewis, Karina L. Walters, and Jen M. Self. 2016. "'I'm in This World for a Reason': Resilience and Recovery among American Indian and Alaska Native Two-Spirit Women." *Journal of Lesbian Studies* 20 (3–4): 352–371.

Fisher, Bernice, and Joan Tronto. 1990. "Towards a Feminist Theory of Caring." In *Circles of Care: Work and Identity in Women's Lives*, edited by Emily K. Abel and Margaret K. Nelson, 35–62. New York: State University of New York Press.

Flowers, Rachel. 2015. "Refusal to Forgive: Indigenous Women's Love and Rage." *Decolonization: Indigeneity, Education & Society* 4 (2): 32–49.

Friedman, Marilyn. 1993. "Beyond Caring: The Demoralization of Gender." In *An Ethic of Care: Feminist and Interdisciplinary Perspectives*, edited by Mary Jeanne Larrabee, 258–274. London: Routledge.

———. 1997. "Autonomy and Social Relationships: Rethinking the Feminist Critique." In *Feminists Rethink the Self*, edited by Diana Tietjens Meyers, 40–61. Boulder, CO: Westview.

———. 2013. "Independence, Dependence, and the Liberal Subject." In *Reading Onora O'Neill*, edited by David Archard, Monique Deveaux, Neil Manson, and Daniel Weinstock, 111–129. Abingdon: Routledge.

———. 2014. "Relational Autonomy and Independence." In *Autonomy, Oppression, and Gender*, edited by Andrea Veltman and Mark Piper, 42–60. New York: Oxford University Press.

Gilligan, Carol. 1982. *In a Different Voice: Psychological Theory and Women's Development*. Cambridge, MA: Harvard University Press.

Graham, Hilary. 1983. "Caring: A Labour of Love." In *A Labour of Love: Women, Work and Caring*, edited by Janet Finch and Dulcie Groves, 13–30. London: Routledge and Kegan Paul.

Haraway, Donna. 1988. "Situated Knowledges: The Science Question in Feminism and the Privilege of Partial Perspective." *Feminist Studies* 14 (3): 575–599.

———. 1997. *Modest_Witness@Second_Millennium. FemaleMan_Meets_OncoMouse: Feminism and Technoscience*. New York: Routledge.

Hekman, Susan J. 1995. *Moral Voices, Moral Selves: Carol Gilligan and Feminist Moral Theory*. Cambridge: Polity.

Held, Virginia. 2006. *The Ethics of Care: Personal, Political, and Global*. New York: Oxford University Press.

Hill, Susan M. 2017. *The Clay We Are Made Of: Haudenosaunee Land Tenure on the Grand River*. Winnipeg: University of Manitoba Press.

Jewell, Eva M. 2018. "Gimaadaasamin, We Are Accounting for the People: Support for Customary Governance in Deshkan Ziibiing." PhD diss., Royal Roads University.

———. 2024. "Towards an Anti-Colonial Feminist Care Ethic." In *Making Space for Indigenous Feminism*, 3rd ed., edited by Gina Starblanket, 168–192. Halifax: Fernwood Publishing.

Jewell, Eva M., Andrea Doucet, Jessica Falk, and Sue Fyke. 2020. "Social Knowing, Mental Health, and the Importance of Indigenous Resources: A Case Study of Indigenous Employment Engagement in Southwestern Ontario." *Canadian Review of Social Policy* 80:1–25.

Jewell, Eva M., and Ian Mosby. 2021. "Calls to Action Accountability: A 2021 Status Update on Reconciliation." Yellowhead Institute. https://yellowheadinstitute.org/trc/.

Karjevsky, Gilly, Roasario Talevi, and Sascia Bailer, eds. 2020. "Letters to Joan." New Alphabet School. https://newalphabetschool.hkw.de/wp-content/uploads/2020/06/Letters-to-Joan-CARING-edited-by_BAILER-KARJEVSKY-TALEVI.pdf.

King, Hayden. 2017. "The Erasure of Indigenous Thought in Foreign Policy." Open Canada. https://opencanada.org/erasure-indigenous-thought-foreign-policy/.

Lindberg, Tracy. 2017. "Reconciliation Before Reconciliation with Dr. Tracey Lindberg." Interview by Paul Kennedy. *Ideas with Paul Kennedy*, June 21, 2017. CBC Radio.

Luxton, Meg, and Kate Bezanson. 2006. *Social Reproduction: Feminist Political Economy Challenges Neo-liberalism*. Montreal: McGill-Queen's University Press.

MacDonald, David B. 2019. *The Sleeping Giant Awakens: Genocide, Indian Residential Schools, and the Challenge of Conciliation*. Toronto: University of Toronto Press.

Mauthner, Natasha, and Andrea Doucet. 2003. "Reflexive Accounts and Accounts of Reflexivity in Qualitative Data Analysis." *Sociology* 37 (3): 413–431.

Narayan, Uma. 1995. "Colonialism and Its Others: Considerations on Rights and Care Discourses." *Hypatia* 10 (2): 133–140.

Puig de la Bellacasa, María. 2012. "'Nothing Comes without Its World': Thinking with Care." *The Sociological Review* 60 (2): 197–216.

———. 2017. *Matters of Care: Speculative Ethics in More Than Human Worlds*. Minneapolis: University of Minnesota Press.

Robinson, Fiona. 2020. "Resisting Hierarchies through Relationality in the Ethics of Care." *International Journal of Care and Caring* 4 (1): 11–23.

Rollo, Toby. 2016. "Feral Children: Settler Colonialism, Progress, and the Figure of the Child." *Settler Colonial Studies* 8 (1): 60–79.

Rooney, Phyllis. 2012. "The Marginalization of Feminist Epistemology and What That Reveals about Epistemology 'Proper.'" In *Feminist Epistemology and Philosophy of Science: Power in Knowledge*, edited by Heidi E. Grasswick, 3–24. London: Springer.

Ruddick, Sara. 1995. *Maternal Thinking: Towards a Politics of Peace*. Boston: Beacon.

Scobie, Matthew, Glenn Finau, and Jessica Hallenbeck. 2024. "Land, Land Banks and Land Back: Accounting, Social Reproduction and Indigenous Resurgence." *Environment and Planning A: Economy and Space* 56 (1): 235–252.

Scribe, Megan. 2020. "Indigenous Girlhood: Narratives of Colonial Care in Law and Literature." PhD diss., University of Toronto.

Simard, Suzanne. 2021. *Finding the Mother Tree: Discovering the Wisdom and of the Forest*. London: Allen Lane.

Tronto, Joan C. 1993. *Moral Boundaries: A Political Argument for an Ethic of Care*. New York: Routledge.

———. 2013. *Caring Democracy: Markets, Equality, and Justice*. New York: New York University Press.

———. 2020. "Dear Yayra." In *Caring: Letters to Joan*, edited by Gilly Karjevsky, Rosario Talevi, and Sascia Bailer, 50–51. New Alphabet School. https://newalphabetschool.hkw.de/wp-content/uploads/2020/06/Letters-to-Joan-CARING-edited-by_BAILER-KARJEVSKY-TALEVI.pdf.

Truth and Reconciliation Commission of Canada. 2015. "The Survivors Speak: A Report of the Truth and Reconciliation Commission of Canada." Winnipeg, Manitoba: Truth and Reconciliation Commission of Canada.

Tsing, Anna Lowenhaupt. 2015. *The Mushroom at the End of the World: On the Possibility of Life in Capitalist Ruins*. Princeton, NJ: Princeton University Press.

Tuck, Eve. 2016. "Suspending Damage: A Letter to Communities." *Harvard Educational Review* 79 (3): 409–427.

Tuck, Eve, and Wayne K. Yang. 2014. "R-Words: Refusing Research." In *Humanizing Research: Decolonizing Qualitative Inquiry with Youth and Communities*, edited by Django Paris and Maisha T. Winn, 223–248. Thousand Oaks, CA: Sage.

Tuhiwai Smith, Linda, ed. 2012. *Decolonizing Methodologies: Research and Indigenous Peoples*. London: Zed Books.

Watts, Vanessa. 2013. "Indigenous Place-Thought and Agency amongst Humans and Non-humans (First Woman and Sky Woman Go on a European World Tour!)." *Decolonization: Indigeneity, Education & Society* 2 (1): 20–34.

8 · CRAFTING A NEW CORPO-REALITY IN CARE ETHICS

Contributions from Feminist New Materialisms and Posthumanist Ethics

ÉMILIE DIONNE

In her work on moral developmental psychology, Carol Gilligan, a pivotal figure in care ethics, aimed to foster new ways of listening and caring. With her *listening guide*, addressed to psychologists and qualitative researchers, she helps them develop "sensible skills," such as attentiveness and empathy, to become good listeners (or good witnesses) (Gilligan and Eddy 2017, 2021; also Doucet, Jewell, and Watts this volume [chapter 7]). This idea echoes the work of feminist philosopher Lorraine Code, who, in *Ecological Thinking* (2006), recognizes the inherently political and ethical dimensions of epistemology, given that knowing is always and only a "situated" practice, that is, that knowledge emerges only from somewhere, such as from a person or from a community of knowers, with social, cultural, political, and gendered histories and stories (Code 2006; also Code 1991). For Code, would-be knowers are endowed with the responsibility of making themselves *sensibly available* to others, specifically to those whose voices are and have been systematically and systemically marginalized and silenced and whose epistemic capacity is systemically thwarted (e.g., women, people of color, Indigenous and 2Q+LBGT people). Yet because of their situation (including their positionality in systems of power), would-be knowers often cannot hear/receive the voices/testimonies of marginalized others; they cannot understand their truths as epistemic positions in their own right. Their own epistemic capacity is "captured" (i.e., framed) by the dominant/normative regime of thought, akin to Michel Foucault's (1966) notions of *episteme* and regime of thought, which inform what one can and cannot know or think. To correct this, Code argues that would-be knowers, because of their position, have the ethical duty to be/come *epistemic advocates* who, while they may have yet to hear/receive/understand the testimonies of marginalized others, can however act as champions, allies, and advocates and help those voices to be voiced and heard. With time and generosity, new sensibilities will be created, thereby enabling them to be heard and understood (Code 2006).

Both thinkers recognize the important and inherent role the sensible plays in knowing. It is with and through our senses that we can experience and engage with the world and its inhabitants. They argue that it is possible to adopt a more ethical and *caring* approach when a person engages in activities like caring or knowing. Such is the goal of the listening guide and Code's work on advocacy epistemology. Elsewhere, I have coined the term "corpo-real configuration" to encompass this sensible reality and possibility (Dionne 2019, 2020). Equipped with contributions from feminist new materialists (FNM) and posthumanist ethicists (PE) regarding matter as dynamic, open, agentic, and ontologically relational, it is possible to understand better *and transform* one's sensible corpo-reality and work toward ensuring that one's practices are caring well ethically (i.e., enacting social justice).

Care ethics aims to contribute to the improvement of our living conditions by positioning care at the core of human practices, including knowledge practices and justice. In their now well-known definition of care, Fisher and Tronto (1990) state that care is "a species activity that includes everything that we do to maintain, continue and repair our world so that we can live in it as well as possible. This world includes our bodies, ourselves and our environment, all of which we seek to interweave in a complex, life-sustaining web'" (Fisher and Tronto 1990, 40). For Tronto, care is also not quite *something*, a given or even a disposition, but dynamic, a process and a practice always renewed, (re)made, and improved (Tronto 2020a, 103; cf. Bozalek this volume [chapter 9]).

As others have pointed out however (see notably Bozalek this volume [chapter 9]; Flower and Hamington 2022; Tronto 2020a, 2020b), although there is an undeniable recognition of the planet and of nonhumans in the canonical definition of care presented above, it remains undeniably a human-centered definition. The focus remains on humans as a species. Yet, as feminist PE argue, in order to *care well* even for humans, we need to challenge many of our categories of thought and further care ethics' relational conception of ontology. Various disciplines of knowledge (which are always and only ontological practices and practices of care) need to (further) decenter themselves because nonhumans are much more present and active than is known and recognized by these humanist approaches, including in many "human" activities, such as politics, care, sciences, and so on.[1] They act, affect, influence, and are also affected, in ways that are material and irreversible; that is, they bear traces and these traces are ongoing and "mattering"/ lively marks of enactments. Care practices are an example of such enactments with material/"mattering" effects. Consider, as an example, this case reckoned by Jane Bennett (2010, 90):

> In *Pandora's Hope*, Latour tells a story about Amazonian rather than English worms, and ... we see that worms play a more important part in the history of (that part of) the world than most persons would at first suppose. The story begins with the puzzling presence, about ten meters into the rainforest, of trees typical only of the savanna. The soil under these trees is "more clayey than the savanna but less so than the forest." How was the border between savanna and forest breached? Did "the forest cast its own soil before it to create conditions favorable to its expansion," or is the savanna "degrading the woodland humus as it prepares to invade the forest"? This question presumes a kind of vegetal agency in a natural system understood not as a mechanical order of fixed laws but as the scene of not-fully-predicable encounters between multiple kinds of actants. Savanna vegetation, forest trees, soil, soil microorganisms, and humans native and exotic to the rainforest are all responding, in real time and without predetermined outcome, to each other and to the collective force of the shifting configurations that form.

There are numerous concepts and categories that "we" (scholars or not) use to make sense of the worlds and our engagements with it. These require urgent rethinking, reimagining, and decentering. Examples of such categories include that of the "human." With novel scientific developments, it is now known that the human body is host to many life-forms that interact in complex ways to enable our existence, affects, and thoughts. In light of their engagements with the sciences, FNM and PE put forth a more profound understanding of (and a commitment to) the inherently relational, dynamic, and porous conception of ontology, whereby different "things" do not exist prior to or outside of relationships. They emerge from them.

Yet how can care ethicists (among other scholars) consider "better" (i.e., more strongly, ethically, and in committed ways) nonhumans? In this contribution, I argue that a better understanding of matter is needed, including the affective capacity of the human body, to this effect. This means working at our corporeal/sensible configuration (our senses), which is what allows connections, engagements in and with the world, and knowledge, in an ontology that is fundamentally relational. Alongside others, I argue that our current sensible configuration is affected by an *ontology of precarity*, which I discuss further in this chapter and elsewhere (Dionne 2020, 2021). Echoing the work of FNM, these corpo-real configurations are *ontology-making projects*; that is, they always participate actively to how the world and what inhabits it and is possible within it "matter," that is, as discursive-material and open entanglements. In the context of an ontology of precarity, what "matters" and how it does do so by creating *more* precarity. Here sentient beings' ability to sense, care, and practice care participates in making the world *matter precariously*.

This chapter is organized as follows. First, I define more fully the concepts introduced in this introduction (i.e., corpo-reality, matter as dynamic/open, the ontology of precarity). Then, I draw from the work of FNM Elizabeth Wilson, who develops the approach of *organic empathy* to explore how "damaged organic matter" can be engaged in positive and healing ways to work toward more positive reconfigurings from which knowledge and care practices that are ethical and positive can take place. Finally, I provide examples of engagements and experiments in scientific practices with nonhumans that participate in the reconfiguration of one's sensible configuration, thus making new ways of knowing and new knowledges possible.

CORPOREAL CONFIGURATION AND DISPOSITION: A FEW WORDS ON EMBODIMENT

Body Talks and the Sensible: Configuring the Human Body to Sense Otherwise

Sociologists and anthropologists of the sciences and technology, feminist scholars, and French phenomenologists have contributed significantly to the recognition of the diverse roles played by the human body, and specifically the senses, in knowledge practices. Inherently, given embodiment and the "situatedness" of any embodiment (geographical, socially, politically, historically, and so forth), all knowledge comes from somewhere (cf. Haraway 1991) and from multiple bodies in relation *and intra-action* (defined further below). Embodiment cannot be abstracted or subtracted from the operation of knowledge. It is from it, *with it*, that knowledge exists. This means not that knowledge is not possible but that knowledge can be only a partial view, from somewhere, a situation. Building communities of knowers becomes important because other knowers will have other situations and other views. Through connection, knowledge can be enriched, but a single person can never hope to achieve a totalizing view.[2]

In the introduction, referring to Gilligan's and Code's respective works, I mentioned their insistence that *good and ethical*—responsive—knowers must work on "themselves," as sensible and sentient selves, to receive well the stories or testimonies of the person they listen to. In "How to Talk about the Body?," science and technologies studies scholar Bruno Latour (2004a) provides a good illustration of the work involved in crafting embodiment to know specific things in specific ways. Latour uses the example of the connoisseur (wine expert) and explains how the person can develop, through rigorous and attentive training, skills and capacities to distinguish odors and flavors in the wine that others, who have not trained intensively, cannot. Through this rigorous and dedicated work, new abilities/skills (i.e., senses) can become available. However, in the process, choices are made regarding the sensible configuration of the body, meaning that not all possibilities will remain. Some will cease to be (i.e., they "virtualize"). The time spent at acquiring *these* abilities is also not spent acquiring *other* abilities (e.g., to become a physicist or marathon runner). But, in choosing, options *do* become available. Put otherwise, without such choices, none would. Our bodies are thus inherently the key to knowing.

Matter as Agentic and Relational: Barad's Contribution of a Relational Ontology

With her work in physics, Barad brings us a radically novel conception of physics/matter that eschews the conventional view of matter as stable and permanent, immutable throughout time and space. Rather, reality is always in the process of being made, affecting and affected, dynamic and fluid. "Things" (configurations) do emerge when they are stabilized, but only in *and with* context, such as through a scientific experiment and in social-cultural-historical location. And even then, their emergence is inherently and irrevocably "situated," that is, located within a larger condition of *inseparability, indeterminacy,* and *connectivity*. Finally, this configuration remains temporary, for reality is not fixed or even given but always in motion, in the process of *being-made* (and therefore *unmade*).

This process whereby "things" acquire a configuration, Barad describes it as an *intra-action* as opposed to an *interaction*. This is the case because things do not have a fixed essence or identity. "Intra-action" is the concept Barad uses to identify and describe the meeting between matter and meaning as yet indeterminate. There is nothing ("no thing") that preexists/precedes *relata*. Hence, the "identity," contextually bound, is achieved relationally (including the context). The identity includes all the other relationships (e.g., bonds, ties) with *other "things,"*[3] be they concepts/ideas, theories of knowledge, agencies of observation—*and including* things that are not necessarily "actual" (e.g., the past). "Other" things, actual or virtual, are tantamount (i.e., as important and for consideration) to truly "know" the thing (i.e., develop accurate knowledge about it). "Things" (i.e., their "identity") are created (configured) through the enactment that is an encounter and can be a scientific experiment or theory of knowledge. Barad explains that an *agential cut*, or separation, is enact*ing*, within the larger "instances of wholeness" (Barad 2008, 119), where "wholeness" does not have a transcendent status. The cut "cuts" multiply at once (more than one thing), which Barad calls *together-apart*.

One more important contribution of Barad is her description of matter as *performative,* here inspired by Judith Butler's concept (2006). She explains that the practices (e.g., knowledge practices) that aim to develop knowledge have to engage with the "fabric" of matter, meaning that practices do not leave matter untouched, unchanged. Knowledge practices are *interventions* that must engage directly, tangibly (materially), *and* irreversibly with matter, to "know" it (i.e., to develop knowledge).[4] These necessarily "material" engagements thus have material (and *mattering*) consequences. They leave marks that cannot be erased or removed. These remain and inform the future configurations that matter can take (in being opened, dynamic, future oriented). Here, it is helpful to think of "matter" as akin to plastic: it can take other/new forms, is not congealed, can become otherwise in the future. Yet erasure is not possible, only inheritance (and transformation).

The Sensible Is Relational

Building on these accounts of Latour and Barad, I now move to the contribution of French Philosopher Jacques Rancière who makes the case for the ontological contribution of the arts and artists given their different (read: sensible/sensibly available) way of being, that is, appreciating, engaging, and existing in the world, and whereby, given this different mode of being, they participate in the ongoing and changing distribution of the "sensible," that is, the world (in-the-making), including how it is / makes itself accessible to us, through our embodiment/senses: "The first possible meaning of the notion of a 'factory of the sensible' is the formation of a shared sensible world, a common habitat, by the weaving together of a plurality of human activities.... The idea of a 'distribution of the sensible' implies something more. A 'common' world is never simply an *ethos*, a shared abode, that results from the sedimentation of a certain number of intertwined acts. It is always a polemical distribution of modes of beings and 'occupations' in a space of possibilities" (Rancière 2000, 43). The sensible, for Rancière, is the real, our physical reality. Accessing it, empirically, requires our senses, and "sensible/sensual" disposition. Plus, the real itself *is* sensible, that is, the world must be engaged in particular and different ways to become available, sensibly, to us, and allow actions in the world (i.e., becoming). The engagements of artists are such unique/different practices.

The sensible configuration of the world (i.e., how it is sensibly available and accessible) "matters" because in some sensible configurations some *things* (e.g., the voices and epistemic capacity of those who are systemically marginalized) cannot be "sensed" (i.e., perceived, heard, etc.). Because of their sensible, sensorial, and aesthetical *tuning*, unique to their praxis and ways of being/inhabiting/dwelling in the world, artists redistribute this sensibility whereby what was previously unseen/unsensed can now be. This recalls Code's idea of knowers as epistemic advocates rather than always knowers themselves. They allow a redistribution of the sensible whereby, subsequently, certain things *can* be sensed (seen, heard, felt) by those who do not have the artists' sensible configuration. This is why artists play a critical social and political role in Rancière's view. Because of their particular way(s) of being in the world, artists "understand" (i.e., experience and engage) it differently and therefore give rise to new affective capacities in the world. As seen with Barad, the world itself "matters" differently in these contacts/encounters, making other possibilities possible and actual. Artists' "renderings" (i.e., artistic productions) offer (or provoke) new sensorial experiences, who will subsequently see, sense, and engage the world in new ways and participate differently in its ongoing "mattering."

Good examples are provided by French philosopher Maurice Merleau-Ponty in his work on visual artists (painters) and phenomenology in "Eye and Mind" ([1964] 2003). He gives the example of the sketches of women drawn by an artist that initially provoked laughter and were denigrated: viewers could see no resemblance to women's bodies. Yet after exposure to the sketches, viewers' senses started to change, often imperceptibly and without any intention on their part. Not only did the viewers come to see the drawings as "speaking" of women (e.g., capturing motion); eventually, they also started to look differently at bodies, through the renderings of the artists.

CORPOREAL INDISPOSITION

With Rancière, we have seen the social, political, ontological—and aesthetic—contribution of artists in redistributing the "sensible." In this section I discuss what I mean by an "ontology of precarity" to explain the importance of a better understanding of materiality and agential matter for care ethics.

The Case of Precarious Ontology

The concepts of *precarity* and *precariousness* have been at the center of preoccupations of various scholars in feminist and cultural studies. For example, in what is now largely recognized as a key intervention on this topic, Butler has proposed the two concepts of *precariousness* and *precarity* to describe how the lives of some people and groups can be made precarious socially. *Precariousness* speaks of the biological, the organic, and the social "entities" that humans are, therefore making us fragile/vulnerable to threats (of various kinds) as well as "ontologically placed" in a constant and diverse situation of (multiple) (inter)dependencies for selfcare and survival. (This echoes Fisher and Tronto's definition of care.) The *order of precarity* is the social and political response and organization whereby precariousness is addressed (viewed) and responded to through social provisions (e.g., health care, social benefits, education, child care). This "ordering," however, is political, normative, and ideological in that not *all forms* of precariousness are seen, recognized or responded to—and therefore, made to "matter" in a discursive-material entanglement. This means that the lives (and conditions, situations) of some are made *precarious*: their precarity is viewed as the result of their individual situation, fault, and responsibility (rather than the result of social, political, normative, environmental, historical situations and forces). This ordering can even further exacerbate precarity; in denying precariousness, the ordering makes some people the target of criticisms, violence, and marginalization by the "normalized" (i.e., privileged). (See also Butler [2016] on "ungrievable lives.")

Scholars suggest that this situation further intensifies and expands itself in the context of late/advanced capitalism and neoliberalism, and that a new ontology (immanent/dynamic) is constituted, in which "things" *matter* (as material-discursive entanglements) *through* precarity. This is what can be called an *ontology of precarity* (cf. Butler 2004, 2012, 2016; Puar 2012; Hamington and Flowers 2021). In it, we can speak of the subject as *precarious*, or her condition as precarious, that is, a situation whereby the person (or a social/cultural group) no longer envisions a future for themselves and lives in a permanent (at times latent, but often active) situation of uncertainty and unknowability. In the neoliberal era, there is less and less support provided to individuals and groups that are ontologically precarious and significantly more barriers to recognizing the social and political ordering of precarity. The burden of responsibility for an increasingly growing number of needs (e.g., education, care, health care, economic, social) is "downloaded" onto the shoulders of individual people (or marginalized groups and communities). Care itself can actually be and contribute to *uncare*, as discussed by Doucet, Jewell, and Watts in this volume (chapter 7).

Vulnerability

Elsewhere, I have argued that the ontology of precarity creates a corpo-reality where people shy away from sensibility and therefore their senses and ability to sense (i.e., be available to the otherwise, such as the testimonies and voices of marginalized people and groups). In our current *precarious* ontology, individuals fear / come to apprehend their ontological sensibility (that makes them vulnerable to threats, or even the target of them). This has material consequences, following Barad's conception of matter (and Wilson's, which I discuss below). Attempts are recurrently made to make oneself *less* vulnerable (and *more* insensible). Yet in actuality, it is this sensibility / vulnerability / capacity for vulnerability that enables humans to know, to care, as sentient beings (cf. Dionne 2019, 2020).

In order to correct/transform this "sensible situation" (configuration) and revalue vulnerability, FNM and PE insist on the need to attend to one's sensible capacities, to notice anew. Only this way can they know well (ethically) and consequently *care well*, for both humans and nonhumans (or both as inherently entangled).

THINKING AND DOING WITH THE NONHUMAN: CONTRIBUTIONS FROM FNM, POSTHUMANIST ETHICS, AND ECOMATERIALISM

For care ethics to consider well/better the nonhuman, I argue that a better (more accurate and ethical) conception of (material) matter is needed, as well as more sensible attention and engagement with nonhumans in an environmental and ecological perspective. But first, it is important to attend to our *current* corpo-real configuration. From an ontology of precarity where we *matter* precariously and relying on Barad's conception of matter as dynamic, open, and performative, in this section I introduce the work of FNM Elizabeth Wilson, whose work on organic matter that has been hurt/damaged in the context of living with a mental health issue or engaging with narrow pharmaceutical treatments gives us a helpful tool—that of *organic empathy*—to initiate our work toward a new sensible corpo-reality.

In her work on biology and the human gut, Wilson (2015) uses emerging findings in biology and the context of developing pharmaceutical treatments to address various mental health issues such as depression and food disorders to show how biological (i.e., organic) matters are more lively, affective, and agentic than previous biological approaches (or feminist scholars) have recognized. In light of this, Wilson proposes the approach of *organic empathy*, inspired by psychotherapy, as a way to adopt a more caring and respectful approach to organic matter (i.e., various organs and organic processes), one that recognizes but also capitalizes on the agential capacity and role of nonhumans. Wilson argues that this approach can be particularly helpful in some specific health contexts where organic matter has experienced trauma and is therefore marked negatively by these experiences. She argues that in such cases, the organic processes or *viscera* may require particular forms of attention and care to resolve the health concern. Current practices, she maintains, continue to have a too narrow or indifferent attention toward other organs, that are not considered the main "site" of a mental health issue (e.g., depression). In such practices, the brain remains the sole interest of the pharmaceutical developments and treatments.

Like other new materialists, Wilson argues that organic matter, approached otherwise, that is, caringly, could contribute in more helpful, productive, and interesting ways to care practices and treatment—and it may have a lot to contribute. Additionally, she argues that because current biomedical practices tend to engage the body *atomistically* (individual organs, not "defined" by their relationality or network-like configuration), they miss out on the role and agency played by organs-as-network (organic processes, or *viscera*). Pharmaceutical developments approach the body as a set of distinct organs with relationships, and not the body *as* relational, a complex and processual network in the first place, where *relata* would precede organs. In their "insensibility," they also can further affect negatively the person and the body, with effects that leave marks that may be engaged differently in the future but cannot be removed.

When pharmaceutical drugs are developed (e.g., to address a mental health issue such as depression), the focus is primarily and often exclusively on the brain; to bring the drug to the brain and circulate through the other organs (e.g., the gut) and organic processes (e.g., metabolism); but because they are not the "main sites," these engagements remain minimal, accessory. Wilson's work however shows that a mental health condition can nonetheless have effects *throughout* the body, spread differentially. The treatment, too, will affect organs and organic processes differently. Here, it is useful to think of such experiences as leaving *bodily memories* throughout the body and specific to each organic process and entanglement. The body's ability to respond in the future (e.g., to treatment) is informed and influenced by traces.[5]

Organic matters are approached as mere things, from an objectified and heteronomous perspective (i.e., without agential role or capacity). However, Wilson argues that they can be/come powerful allies in treatment—as well as knowing *endeavors*, or partners, caringly. In fact, they do; see, for example, Bennett's/Latour's account of worms presented above. Wilson's suggestion is that pharmaceutical scientists take inspiration from psychotherapy, which emphasizes the importance and roles of relationships and relationality as key mechanisms to entice behavioral changes. Psychotherapy understands people, when they have issues, as having created *coping* relationships/pathways with others, ideas, and so on; these are "helpful," in the short term, but ultimately damaging, or preventing the person from achieving other goals, more durable, positive, sustainable in the long run. Through relationality and new relationships, psychotherapy will attempt to create new pathways, more positive and emancipatory ones, to help the person leave these damaging ones behind, and truly resolve or live well with her mental health. *Organic empathy* is akin to a psychotherapy with organs and organic processes that, too, can have been hurt and have experienced trauma. This approach proposes that particular attention and care for *these* organic processes be paid to their stories and histories, the specific traces of past enactments on them, and how they now respond / can respond. This is needed to heal, to entice new responses. Importantly here, the past cannot be erased, but it can be engaged differently, inheriting differently, cared for, so that it can "matter" (discursively and materiality) differently.[6]

HOW TO CRAFT *CORPOREAL DISPOSITION*: THE *ARTS OF NOTICING* WITH MATERIAL ECOCRITICISM, AND MULTISPECIES ETH(N)OLOGY

In this final section, I draw from works in environmental ethics and material ecocriticism to help care ethicists work toward the (re)configuration of our (and others') *sensible corpo-reality*. The goal here is to see how one can work—*and also be sensibly available*—in new ways to the "otherwise," that is, to nonhumans as well as to people, including those that are no longer or yet to become "actual." In other words, how can we acquire new sensibilities to connect, all the while addressing and redressing the *precarious corpo-reality* we inherited?

The scholars I discuss here are proposing that knowers and scholars across disciplines, and care ethicists and care practitioners in particular, work actively at mastering the *arts of noticing*. Noticing well is yet to be done adequately by humans, but likely, by other entities "that sense" as well. A precarious ontology, I argue, renders one scarred, vulnerable in a negative way; additionally, one likely does not know that they are insensible and unavailable, or how to become otherwise. Noticing well requires making oneself vulnerable in a positive way; accepting and welcoming this vulnerability, notably through experiences and experimentations and through sensory engagements that often put aside rational/cognitive processes. The "method" favored by these scholars is that of storytelling, that is, of creating, telling, writing stories—and *new ones*, too—as well as new *forms* of stories, for example, unexpected narrative forms such as a poem mixing multiple languages or drawings, colors, and so on. Haraway, in particular, has taught us that "storying" is what the sciences and knowledge practices do to create and develop knowledge. Storying is actually a way of being in the world for humans (and likely for other entities, too; see the works of Eduardo Kohn [2013], Thom van Dooren et al. [2017], van Dooren and Deborah Bird Rose [2012, 2016], Eben Kirksey [2014], for examples). It is a way of rendering the world meaningful and creating relationships through which we can become and act. Humans create stories, but storying is not limited to humans (much like caring or knowledge practices, argue these scholars). In Haraway's words, "It matters what stories we tell to tell other stories with; it matters what concept we think to think other concepts with.... My stories are suggestive string figures at best, they long for a fuller weave that still keeps the patterns open, with ramifying attachment sites for storytellers yet to come.... String figures are like stories; they propose and enact patterns for participants to inhabit, somehow, on a vulnerable and wounded earth. My multispecies storytelling is about recuperation in complex histories that are full of dying" (Haraway 2016, 10–12).

"Storying" has thus been further used as an approach by scholars to help in imagining differently, and from there, participating to the "different mattering" of the world (in constant motion and transformation). To this effect, Haraway proposes *SF*, initials that stand for either science fiction, science fantasy, speculative fiction, speculative fantasy, and so forth (Haraway 2018) to know the world otherwise. Such scholars argue that *all scholars*, knowers, who always create stories, need to be more intentional, forceful, ethical, and responsive in creating their own "storying practices," *but also*, in doing so *with* nonhumans, who are always and already participating, influencing, and being affected.[7] These scholars also embrace the idea that stories/storying affect/inform our corporeal/sensible configuration, much like Rancière's argument that artists/arts participate in the redistribution of the sensible.

In their work in environmental ethics and on the Anthropocene, scholars such as Anna L. Tsing (Tsing et al. 2017), Rose and van Dooren (2017; van Dooren and Rose 2012, 2016) thus propose new methodologies and approaches to cultivate what they call the *arts of noticing*, akin to my concept of corpo-reality. These arts will enable new knowledges and new knowledge approaches. Below are some examples of their experiments that can inspire care ethicists to work toward the (re)configuration of their current corpo-reality to decenter care ethics and participate in an ethico-ontology.

Environmental anthropologists van Dooren, Rose, and Kirksey use storying to create new stories *with* nonhumans, a method they call *multispecies eth(n)ologies*, which enable them to develop new knowledges of environmental matters (van Dooren and Rose 2012, 2016; Rose and van Dooren 2017; Kirksey 2014). In their words,

> Noticing Attunes Us to Worlds Otherwise. When nineteenth-century Japanese polymath Minakata Kumagusu campaigned to maintain the local shrines that the Meiji government planned to raze, he did so both as a scientist and as a participant in local forms of knowledge. Local shrines were sites of remnant old forest, and

Minakata hoped to preserve their biodiversity, including the slime molds and fungi that were subjects of his research. At the same time, he felt that folk knowledge, including stories of strange beings and eerie shadow biologies, was key to his ability to learn about nature. Rather than dismissing folk knowledge, he incorporated approaches from it into his scientific work. Indeed, while generally unacknowledged, vernacular—and even "spooky"—insights have informed some of the most important science all over the world. This is a reason to learn from ghosts, however unfamiliar their forms.... In the midst of disaster, stones bring a gift of hope: of fortune, of insight, of the possibility of living-with. In the Anthropocene, multiple conversations with stones are necessary. After all, the Anthropocene is a geological epoch proposed by geologists, climate chemists, and stratigraphers—scientists used to studying stones, rocks, sediments, and chemical cycles. In the Anthropocene, they suggest, humans have become a geological force. Modern industry is laying down indelible strata on the earth that will remain even after we have vanished from the surface of the planet.... To learn the stories of stones, geologists might use the insights of ethnographers and poets. In her poem "Marrow," writer Ursula K. Le Guin urges us to listen to stones without forcing our will on them. Might such listening be necessary to know the Anthropocene? (Tsing et al. 2017, 10–11)

Another example comes from the work of material ecocritics Serpil Oppermann and Serenella Iovino, who engage in "storying with matter" to produce new meanings and new ways to sense and engage the world. Material ecocriticism is itself a philosophy/scholarship that considers "stories," "storying," and "narratives" as powerful tools to develop ethical (or rather *onto*-ethical) knowledge:

Material ecocriticism has emerged from the new materialist paradigm, co-opting its fundamental conceptualization of matter and agency, and more generally, its intellectual horizon. But, reformulating the concept of agentic matter in terms of its expressive potential, material ecocriticism has developed its own interpretive practice, which takes into account agentic matter as a narrative agency producing its own stories, as well as the representations of agentic matter's expressive power in literary, cultural, and visual texts. As the most obvious and the most self-evident narrative sites, literary texts, for example, open up the vitality inherent in matter and extend it over time, endlessly producing a performative mirror that does not just reflect the world, but creates worlds. Like the stories of matter, literary stories shed light on the intra-action of human creativity and the creative expressions of material agencies. (Oppermann 2019, 108)

A last example comes from the work of environmental anthropologist and dancer Natasha Myers, who in the past decade has significantly refined her own *affective methodologies* whereby she engages her astute and multidisciplinary knowledge of the body (embodiment) and different artistic practices to engage in knowledge practices. Of late, she has engaged plants—and specifically their epistemic, aesthetic, and sensible capacities—as ways to inspire and transform our imagination (i.e., what we think our body can do) and from there create new practices, new embodiment:

> [McClintock] recounted to her biographer, Evelyn Fox Keller, "I start with the seedling, and I don't want to leave it. I don't feel I really know the story if I don't watch the plant all the way along. So I know every plant in the field. I know them intimately, and I find it a great pleasure to know them" (Keller 1983: 198). [A]s she worked closely with the plants, [McClintock] cultivated new modes of sensory perception and attention. It was only by gearing her attentions and labours to the temporalities of her plants that she was able to cultivate her celebrated "feeling for the organism" (Keller 1983). Eventually she saw past the static forms we normally register and recognized plants as active agents.... In the process of their careful work, plant scientists learn to pay attention to what it is that plants pay attention to: from the subtlest shift in the gradient of nutrients in the soil; to the most minute changes in the chemical bouquet of their surrounding atmosphere; to reconfigurations in the webs of relation that they catalyze with microbes, fungi, pollinators, herbivores, and other plants. To do their work well, scientists must give themselves over to their inquiry. They must get entrained to plant behaviours, rhythms and temporalities, and they must learn to elicit and observe a range of phenomena that many others will never behold. (Myers 2015, 40–41)

CONCLUSION

As I reach my conclusion, I want to draw from a recent article by Anna Krzywoszynska (2019), who provides a critical account of the focus on attention and attentiveness in care ethics. In the context of her fieldwork with farmers and agriculture in the United Kingdom, specifically their relationship with soil, Krzywoszynska highlights some of the limits and potential dangers of attention and attentiveness when inappropriately supported (i.e., embedded in a strong "strings" of relationships). She presents how attention and attentiveness can become a deterrent (i.e., a limit, a hindrance) to ethical transformation, such as working toward more (onto-)ethical "worldlings," notably in the larger context of late capitalism, neoliberalism, and the ontology of precarity I discussed. Her fieldwork reveals that, with *this* context, the capacity of (individual*ized*) people or like-minded small groups, the embrace of new values and the attempt to live by them (i.e., attentiveness to nonhumans and to a relational ontology) can be thwarted by the larger, inhospitable, and unfavorable context of neoliberalism/capitalism, a context that consistently puts the burden of responsibility on individual shoulders, further individualizing people and social groups as well as denying the many forms of interdependency that enable each of our lives (and deaths). Trying to embrace the values of attentiveness and care, in such contexts, can drag on and exhaust "individualized" people, "small" communities, as well as socially underrepresented, marginalized, people, who are likely to feel overwhelmed, alone, and paralyzed by the vastness and greatness of what is needed, thus leading to adverse effects for attentiveness (cf. Bourgault this volume [chapter 2]).

For care ethics, this insistence on attention and attentiveness as a means to care as an (onto-)ethics raises important questions and considerations. First, one has to achieve an appropriate *ethico-sensible* attention, toward both humans and nonhumans, specifically regarding how "humans" are always and already composed and enabled through multiple (nonhuman) others. These new practices of noticing will help increase attention and attentiveness in ways that are ultimately about being and becoming *response-able* (i.e., able to respond and to participate in ways that cultivate the diversity of forms and abilities for others to respond, engage, and inhabit the world).[8] Yet, it is important that this is done by also understanding and inheriting *well* the larger context, which can be inhospitable. This can be done by creating supporting and "caring" niches from which those who work to achieve more caring/attentive "corpo-configurations" (that include humans and nonhumans) will be supported to do so in safe and nurturing ways. For environmental ethics, this starts with becoming aware of the multiple ways in which nonhumans already care, provide care, and support us. This can also help us feel less alone, cognizant that we are part of a relational ontology (cf. Doucet, Jewell, and Watts this volume [chapter 7]). Being corpo-really available is also about the following: attending to what we, as vulnerable and relational "beings," plug ourselves onto and allow ourselves to be plugged onto, so "we" can *intra-act*, and become a new "we" (i.e., a sensible configuration/corpo-reality). This humility is borne of the recognition that we are always embodied, situated, partial; that we cannot be or know everything and are always ignorant of something (i.e., not sensible to it) and, therefore, dependent on communities that may take us many years to become "sensitive" to.

The world *is* complex and thick. This thickness *matters*, as a discursive-material dynamic entanglement, and those advocating for the arts of noticing push for stronger and better consideration for this thickness, which requires more than words; it requires active bodily work. Such work, however, is not without danger and risk, notably because it recognizes and taps into the ontological vulnerability, that is the condition of organic beings. We have to embrace our vulnerability, and we will be transformed through this work; "we" will change. "We" will become a new "we." These are ethico-epistem-ontological projects, participating in configuring of corpo-realities (i.e., our capacity to sense, to be available, how we are, and so forth).

In relata only, "we" become and inherit. We thus must work at bettering how we inherit, too, our relations with the past, our past, and the futures we can create.

NOTES

1. See Puig de la Bellacasa (2011, 2017) and Latour (2004b).
2. There can never be a total view even with the accumulation of partial perspectives because the world is not given, fixed, but always in the process of changing, of being made and unmade. A totalizing view would not make sense in this ontology.
3. Things include people, concepts, objects of observation that are scientific objects, agencies of observation that are former subjects of knowledge but now include theories as well as instruments of knowledge such as measurements.
4. This is called, by various feminist / new materialists, the tradition of "representationalism" in science whereby sciences aim to create a copy of reality. For more on this, see Barad (1996, 2008) and Thrift (2008).
5. On how memories are embodied and can inscribe themselves corporeally to inform future responses, see the work of N. Katherine Hayles (1999) and Dionne (2010, 2013).
6. See also Puig de la Bellacasa (2011, 2017) on "matters of care."
7. An important contribution pertains to considering the politics and policing of what stands and can stand as a story. See Dionne (2013).
8. On the concept of response-ability, see Barad (2008) and Haraway (2016).

REFERENCES

Barad, Karen. 1996. "Meeting the Universe Halfway: Realism and Social Constructivism without Contradiction." In *Feminism, Science, and the Philosophy of Science*, edited by L. H. Nelson & J. Nelson, 161–194. Springer: Netherlands.
———. 2008. *Meeting the Universe Halfway*. Durham, NC: Duke University Press.
Bennett, Jane. 2010. *Vibrant Matter: A Political Ecology of Things*. Durham, NC: Duke University Press.
Butler, Judith. 2004. *Precarious Life*. New York: Verso.
———. 2006. *Gender Trouble*. New York: Routledge.
———. 2011. *Bodies That Matter: On the Discursive Limits of "Sex."* New York: Routledge.
———. 2012. "Precarious Life, Vulnerability, and the Ethics of Cohabitation." *Journal of Speculative Philosophy* 26 (2): 134–151.
———. 2016. *Frames of War: When Is Life Grievable?* New York: Verso.
Code, Lorraine. 1991. *What Can She Know? : Feminist Theory and the Construction of Knowledge*. Cornell: Cornell University Press.
———. 2006. *Ecological Thinking: The Politics of Epistemic Location*. Oxford: Oxford University Press.
Dionne, Émilie. 2010. "The Deconstruction of Dolls: How Carnal Assemblages Can Disrupt the Law from Within in Ghost in the Shell: Innocence." *Rhizomes* 21 (1). http://www.rhizomes.net/issue21/dionne/index.html.
———. 2013. "Thinking the Pluri-Person through Ironic Practices of Storytelling." PhD diss., York University.
———. 2019. "The Pluri-Person: A Feminist New Materialism Figure for a Precarious World." *Symposium* 23 (2): 94–112.
———. 2020. "Slowing Down with Non-human Matter: The Contribution of Feminist New Materialism to Slow Scholarship." In *Posthuman and Political Care Ethics for Reconfiguring Higher Education Pedagogies*, edited by Vivienne Bozalek, Michalinos Zembylas, and Joan Tronto, 99–106. New York: Routledge.
———. 2021. "Resisting Neoliberalism: A Feminist New Materialist Ethics of Care to Respond to Precarious World(s)." In *Care Ethics in the Age of Precarity*, edited by Maurice Hamington and Michael Flower, 229–259. Minneapolis: University of Minnesota Press.

Fisher, Berenice, and Joan Tronto. 1990. "Toward a Feminist Theory of Caring." In *Circles of Care: Work and Identity in Women's Lives*, edited by Emily K. Abel and Margaret K. Nelson, 35–62. Albany: State University of New York Press.

Flower, Michael, and Maurice Hamington. 2022. "Care Ethics, Bruno Latour, and the Anthropocene." *Philosophies* 7 (2): 1–31.

Foucault, Michel. 1966. *Les Mots et les choses. Une archéologie des sciences humaines*. Paris: Gallimard.

Gilligan, Carol, and Jessica Eddy. 2017. "Listening as a Path to Psychological Discovery: An Introduction to the Listening Guide." *Perspectives on Medical Education* 6 (2): 76–81.

———. 2021. "The Listening Guide: Replacing Judgment with Curiosity." *Qualitative Psychology* 8 (2): 141–151.

Hamington, Maurice, and Michael Flower. 2021. *Care Ethics in the Age of Precarity*. Minneapolis: University of Minnesota Press.

Haraway, Donna. 1991. *Simians, Cyborgs, and Women*. London: Free Association Books.

———. 2016. *Staying with the Trouble*. Durham, NC: Duke University Press.

———. 2018. *Modest_Witness@Second_Millennium. FemaleMan_Meets_OncoMouse: Feminism and Technoscience*. New York: Routledge.

Hayles, N. Katherine. 1999. *How We Became Posthuman: Virtual Bodies in Cybernetics, Literature, and Informatics*. Chicago: University of Chicago Press.

Iovino, Serenella. 2010. "Ecocriticism, Ecology of Mind, and Narrative Ethics: A Theoretical Ground for Ecocriticism as Educational Practice." *Interdisciplinary Studies in Literature and Environment* 17 (4): 759–762.

Iovino, Serenella, and Serpil Oppermann. 2012a. "Material Ecocriticism: Materiality, Agency, and Models of Narrativity." *Ecozon@: European Journal of Literature, Culture and Environment* 3 (1). https://doi.org/10.37536/ECOZONA.2012.3.1.452.

———. 2012b. "Theorizing Material Ecocriticism: A Diptych." *Interdisciplinary Studies in Literature and Environment* 19 (3): 448–475.

Kirksey, Eben, ed. 2014. *The Multispecies Salon*. Durham, NC: Duke University Press.

Kohn, Eduardo. 2013. *How Forests Think: Toward an Anthropology beyond the Human*. Oakland: University of California Press.

Krzywoszynska, Anna. 2019. "Caring for Soil Life in the Anthropocene: The Role of Attentiveness in More-Than-Human Ethics." *Transactions of the Institute of British Geographers* 44 (4): 661–675.

Latour, Bruno. 2004a. "How to Talk about the Body? The Normative Dimension of Science Studies." *Body & Society* 10 (2): 205–229.

———. 2004b. "Why Has Critique Run Out of Steam? From Matters of Fact to Matters of Concern." *Critical Inquiry* 30 (2): 225–248.

Merleau-Ponty, Maurice. (1964) 2003. "Eye and Mind." In *The Primacy of Perception*, edited by James E. Edie, translated by Carleton Dallery, 159–190. Evanston, IL: Northwestern University Press.

Myers, Natasha. 2015. *Rendering Life Molecular: Models, Modelers, and Excitable Matter*. Durham, NC: Duke University Press.

———. 2017. "From the Anthropocene to the Planthroposcene: Designing Gardens for Plant/People Involution." *History and Anthropology* 28 (3): 297–301.

Oppermann, Serpil. 2008. "Seeking Environmental Awareness in Postmodern Fictions." *Critique* 49 (3): 243–253.

———. 2012. "Bodily Natures Science, Environment, and the Material Self." *Environmental Ethics* 34 (1): 103–106.

———. 2016. "From Posthumanism to Posthuman Ecocriticism." *Relations* 4 (1): 23–37.

———. 2017. "Nature's Narrative Agencies as Compound Individuals." *Neohelicon: Acta Comparationis Litterarum Universarum* 44 (2): 283–295.

---. 2019. "Storied Seas and Living Metaphors in the Blue Humanities." *Configurations* 27 (4): 443–461.
Puar, Jasbir, ed. 2012. "Precarity Talk: A Virtual Roundtable with Lauren Berlant, Judith Butler, Bojana Cvejić, Isabell Lorey, Jasbir Puar, and Ana Vujanović." *TDR: The Drama Review* 56 (4): 163–177.
Puig de la Bellacasa, María. 2011. "Matters of Care in Technoscience: Assembling Neglected Things." *Social Studies of Science* 41 (1): 85–106.
---. 2017. *Matters of Care: Speculative Ethics in More than Human Worlds*. Minneapolis: University of Minnesota Press.
Rancière, Jacques. 2000. *La partage du sensible: Esthétique et politique*. La Fabrique Éditions.
Rose, Deborah Bird, and Thom van Dooren. 2017. "Encountering a More-Than-Human World: Ethos and the Arts of Witness." In *The Routledge Companion to the Environmental Humanities*, edited by Ursula K. Heise, Jon Christensen, and Michelle Niemann, 136–144. New York: Routledge.
Strathern, Marilyn. 2004. *Partial Connections*. Lanham, MD: AltaMira Press.
Thrift, Nigel. 2008. *Non-Representational Theory: Space, Politics, Affect*. New York: Routledge.
Tronto, Joan. 2020a. *Moral Boundaries: A Political Argument for an Ethic of Care*. New York: Routledge.
---. 2020b. "Afterwords: Response-Ability and Responsibility: Using FNMs and Care Ethics to Cope with Impatience in Higher Education." In *Posthuman and Political Care Ethics for Reconfiguring Higher Education Pedagogies*, edited by Vivienne Bozalek, Michalinos Zembylas, and Joan Tronto, 153–160. New York: Routledge.
Tsing, Anna Lowenhaupt, Nils Bubandt, Elaine Gan, and Heather Anne Swanson. 2017. *Arts of Living on a Damaged Planet: Ghosts and Monsters of the Anthropocene*. Minneapolis: University of Minnesota Press.
van Dooren, Thom, Deborah B. Rose, and Matthew Chrulew, eds. 2017. *Extinction studies: Stories of time, death, and generations*. New York: Columbia University Press.
van Dooren, Thom, and Deborah Bird Rose. 2012. "Storied-Places in a Multispecies City." *Humanimalia* 3 (2): 1–27.
---. 2016. "Lively Ethography: Storying Animist Worlds." *Environmental Humanities* 8 (1): 77–94.
Wilson, Elizabeth. 2015. *Gut Feminism*. Durham, NC: Duke University Press.

9 · DIFFRACTING CARE AND POSTHUMAN ETHICS

Responsibility, Response-ability, and Privileged Irresponsibility

VIVIENNE BOZALEK

This chapter considers how diffracting care ethics through posthuman ethics may potentially evoke new insights for thinking about responsibility, response-ability, and privileged ir/responsibility.[1] While issues of race, indigeneity, class, and gender are crucial to consider in relation to privilege, responsibility, and response-ability, it is important also to pay heed to decentering the human by incorporating the nonhuman and more-than-human. This is so particularly in the face of what has variously been called the Anthropocene, Capitalocene, or Plantationocene (Haraway 2015, 2016). Care ethics theorists have hitherto not paid enough attention to the privilege of human exceptionalism and the damage that humans have wrought on our planet, with a few exceptions (see, e.g., Boulet 2021; Dionne 2020; Fraser and Taylor 2021; Puig de la Bellacasa 2017; Rogowska-Stangret 2020; Schrader 2015). We need to consider issues of privileged irresponsibility from a wider lens, beyond human exceptionalism. One way to do this is to put care ethics in conversation with posthuman ethics in relation to "think-with" notions of responsibility, responsiveness or response-ability, and privileged irresponsibility (Haraway 2016, 7). This chapter considers how diffracting care and posthuman ethics might bring new imaginaries for engaging differently in our collective non-innocence and implicatedness for our damaged planet, which can never be erased. The chapter thinks-with notions like "hauntology" (Derrida 1994; Barad 2010), "grievable lives" (Butler 2004, 2020), "shadow places" (Plumwood 2008), "non-innocence," (Haraway 2008, 2016), entangled empathy (Gruen 2015), and "transcorporeal culpability" (Alaimo 2016) in relation to privileged irresponsibility.

DIFFRACTION—WHAT IS IT?

The notion of a diffractive methodology was suggested by Donna Haraway (1992) as an alternative to reflection and reflexivity and taken forward by Karen Barad (2007). Both diffraction and reflection are optical phenomena, but Haraway and Barad maintain that reflection and reflexivity are problematic as pervasive tropes for thinking and knowing. Reflection and reflexivity require that the human subject assume a distance from the object of reflection, whereas in diffraction subject and object do not precede process or relation but contingently come into being through process and relation. Similarly, individuals or entities do not preexist relations or processes but come into being through them. Reflection and reflexivity are also seen to be grounded in a representational logic and concerned more with epistemological rather than ontological aspects of research. Thus, for Haraway (1992) and Barad (2007) diffraction provides a useful counterpoint to reflection. This is because reflection is caught up in mirroring and sameness and diffraction is about difference or more precisely patterns of difference that matter. A diffractive methodology is respectful of entanglement of ideas and other materials in the way other reflective methodologies aren't according to Barad (2007). Diffraction "enables genealogical analyses of how boundaries are produced" (Barad 2007, 30) rather than starting from the assumption of existing binaries.[2]

Barad (2007) actually refers to diffraction as a *physical phenomenon* that is part of wave behavior—which pertains to light, water, or sound waves. Diffraction is where waves "combine when they overlap and the apparent bending and spreading out of waves when they encounter an obstruction" (Barad 2007, 28), such as an obstacle or a slit in an apparatus. These waves bend and spread out in the area beyond the barrier or slit producing a new pattern. In combining, waves can be amplified by being superimposed upon one another.

Barad uses this physical process of diffraction as a methodology that engages affirmatively with difference. In a diffractive methodology the details of one theory or philosophical position (in this case the political ethics of care) are read attentively and with care through another (feminist posthumanism or feminist new materialism) in order to come to more creative insights about a certain issue. Barad proposes a diffractive methodology rather than critique, which she regards as a potentially epistemologically damaging process of distancing, othering, and putting another theoretical or philosophical position down. Critique thus requires a viewing of the work of others from a distance, assuming a position of superiority and exteriority, knowing better and feeling entitled to interrogate the work of others. Diffraction is also a matter of doing justice to the fine details of texts. For such justice entails "acknowledgment, recognition, and loving attention, is not a state that can be achieved once and for all" (Barad 2007, x). A diffractive methodology is not setting up one approach/theory/oeuvre *against* another but rather a detailed, attentive, and care-full reading of the ideas of one *through* another, leading to generative ideas that come from the possibility of multiple transdisciplinary approaches to viewing responsibility, response-ability, and privileged irresponsibility.

Diffraction can be both temporal or spatial. A given particle can be in a superposition—which means it can be in two or more *places* at one time. Less well known, however, is that it can also be in multiple *times* simultaneously. Temporal diffraction refers to the proposition that the past is not something that can ever be left behind but exists in the present and in the future—where temporalities are entangled and thickly threaded through one another. Temporal and spatial diffraction are crucial to understand when considering privileged irresponsibility (see, e.g., Bozalek et al. 2021). Temporal diffraction allows us to understand how the past is never done with and how it exists inside the present and future, and spatial diffraction allows us to understand that even if we are separated from something in terms of space, we are still entangled with it. Both Barad (2017, 2018) and Derrida (1994) have used the notion of hauntology to refer to how the ghosts of the past continue to haunt the present and the future. As Barad (2010, 264) notes, "Only by facing the ghosts . . . and acknowledging injustice without the empty promise of complete repair (of making amends finally) can we come close to [hearing the silent speaking, the speaking silence of the ghosts]. The past is never closed, never finished once and for all, but there is no taking it back, setting time aright, putting the world back on its axis. There is no erasure finally. . . . The trace of all reconfigurings are written into . . . what was/is/to-come." Privileged irresponsibility and hauntology have been considered in relation to social work in South Africa, where Bozalek and Hölscher (2022) explore how the effects of South Africa's colonial and apartheid past continue to reverberate into the present and future. The profession of social work in South Africa has not engaged sufficiently with the reality of how Indigenous populations, their kin as men, women, children, their land, houses, and animals were expropriated and exploited by the settlers who colonized the country, forms of which continue to date. Although promoting itself as a profession that is defined by social justice, social work has been slow to recognize its complicity in the forms of violence to which this past has given rise. Hoosain and Bozalek's (2021) chapter in *Post-Anthropocentric Social Work* also shows how the violences of apartheid and colonial legacies, such as slavery and forced removals, continue to affect present-day circumstances. The chapter explains how in/determinacy and dis/continuity can help understand how intergenerational trauma in South Africa was manifested through colonialism and the institutionalized racism of apartheid.

Bozalek and Hölscher (2021) also think about the inherited ghosts of the past in relation to higher education in a diffraction writing piece during coronatime. In this chapter, we think-with hauntology and the rupturing of time, which the coronavirus brought, and where higher education was an opportunity to reassess obsessions with progress and success in its realization that human lives are seriously under threat—and with this sensibility, the opportunity for an accountability and response-ability toward all human and non/more-than-human lives.

RELATIONAL ONTOLOGIES

Tronto's (1993, 2013) political ethic of care, Haraway's speculative fabulation, science fiction, fin de siècle, or "staying with the trouble" (2016), Despret's cosmopolitics/cosmoecology (Despret and Meuret 2016) and Barad's (2007) agential realism are all predicated on a relational ontology, which starts from the premise that entities do not preexist their relationships but rather come into being through relationships. From this perspective, individuals or entities are not separate with neat discrete boundaries, but rather individuals or entities *intra-act* and are entangled with each other across space and time as phenomena. We are all part of the world, entangled with the world's becoming and both discourse and matter are entangled as material-discursive phenomena, "entanglements of spacetimemattering" (Barad 2012, 32). It is through agential cuts (cutting together/apart at the same time), differentiating and entangling in one move (rather than Cartesian cuts, which assume a separation between subject and object) that entities come into being. "Agential cuts necessarily exclude some aspects and include others. The agential cut creates exteriority-within phenomena: inside/outside are undone. What exists outside the cut is still entangled with what is being focused on" (Bozalek and Fullagar 2022, 30). From an agential realist perspective, the world is indeterminate as it is always in a process of coming into being. Indeterminacy is ontological and eschews the idea of individually existing determinate entities, but proposes instead phenomena-in-their-becoming, and a radically open relating of the world. Agential cuts creating subject and object, wave and particle are therefore temporary and contingent separations (and which are still entangled), and are made through material conditions, not necessarily by intentional humans. This might entail part of the world making itself intelligible to another part of the world (for further information on agential cuts, see Barad 2007, 2014a; Bozalek and Fullagar 2022). Reality is not already given and preexisting but is a continual relational process of coming into being. Interrogating how processes materialize and what is sedimented in them means that one cannot compare and contrast "this" or "that"—as one cannot take "this" or "that" as given. It is necessary first to establish how "this" and "that" are constituted or framed. "This" and "that" are also in relation to each other rather than separate, so it is not possible to compare them. Analogical and comparative methodologies assume a metaphysics of individualism (Juelskaer, Plauborg, and Adrian 2021).

A relational ontology maintains that humans or entities do not exist before or outside of relationships (Barad 2007), and that agency can be considered only as a performance within a relationship—either between humans or human and nonhuman animals or the material world. Thus, the notion of the intentional individual or of individuality is not considered to be a useful concept and agency is not the attribute of any entity, human or nonhuman, but transcends the Cartesian subject/object distinction; it is an enactment (Barad 2007, 141). Barad distinguishes *interaction* from *intra-action* (a neologism), arguing that intra-action does not assume preexisting, independent entities (or relata). Rather it is through intra-action, or the "mutual constitution of entangled agencies" (Barad 2007, 33), that entities and "subjects and objects come into being" (Haraway 2008, 71). Agency is a form of intra-action—an opening up of possibilities for changes that emanate in the iterative reconfiguring of the world (see also Émilie Dionne's discussion of intra-action and interaction in this volume [chapter 8]).

In summary, then, in relational ontology, individuals and ethical practices do not preexist relationships but come into being through their entanglements and intra-actions—we are ethically entangled and engaged in all that we do. This chapter considers how responsibility, response-ability, and privileged irresponsibility as ethical agencies need to be understood as intra-actions between human and nonhuman entities in reading political ethics of care diffractively through posthuman ethics.

THE POLITICAL ETHICS OF CARE AND POSTHUMAN ETHICS

According to Joan Tronto, care is not merely a disposition but is rather a process and a practice. This is evident in Fisher and Tronto's now famous definition of care: "a species activity that includes everything that we do to maintain, continue and repair our world so that we can live in it as well as possible. This world includes our bodies, ourselves and our environment, all of which we seek to interweave in a complex, life-sustaining web" (Fisher and Tronto 1990, quoted in Tronto 1993, 103).[3] Although this definition of care still tends to center the human, it also brings into focus other-than-human and ecological elements such as the environment, the world, and a web of life. Donna Haraway (2008, 92) writes about an ethics of worlding, which incorporates the richness and responsiveness emanating from species interdependence. This ethics involves a "refusal of innocence and self-satisfaction with one's reasons and the invitation to speculate, imagine, feel, build something better" (Haraway 2008, 92). This is what Haraway (2016) calls a sympoietic (made together with) telling of propositional stories about the origin of ethics—a thinking- and making-with process. Here, ethics is not primarily a rule-based activity, but a propositional, worlding activity; it is "learning to stay with the trouble of living and dying in response-ability on a damaged earth" (Haraway 2016, 2). As well as staying with the trouble, Haraway stresses the importance also of making and stirring up trouble in response to the devastating events happening in the world and of rebuilding "quiet places" (Haraway 2016, 1) in an attempt to enable flourishing, by which she means living and dying well on a damaged planet now and in time to come.

Building on these notions of helping new ways of life to flourish, and new ways of living and composing in an enlarged world, Vinciane Despret has developed what she has called an alter-politics of cosmo-ecology (Despret and Meuret 2016). Despret's philosophy pays attention to other ways of being that involve other beings such as animals, showing how both human and nonhuman are transformed by and transform each other. Humans and other animals are intra-actively modified over time through "the active creation of the possibilities of existence" (Bussolini 2013, 198).

Karen Barad's agential realism views ethics as mattering, which they also see as integrally part of the world's dynamism, which is iteratively remade in each moment. As Barad (2007, 413) puts it, "'This' and 'that,' 'here' and 'now,' don't preexist what happens but come alive with each meeting." We are entangled phenomena of the world, and responding to ethical calls of our attempts to assist flourishing means taking "responsibility for the role that we play in the world's differential becoming" (413).

Reading care ethics through posthuman ethics foregrounds webs or entanglements of relationships and is useful for taking into consideration how we are making and imagining worlds with others, staying with and making trouble, and what might be done to help to bring about better prospects for those who coinhabit our damaged planet. The remainder of the chapter will think-with responsibility, response-ability or responsiveness, and privileged irresponsibility by diffracting the political ethics of care through posthuman ethics deliberations on these concepts.

Responsibility

While Tronto and Fisher provide a broad definition of care, Tronto's (1993) work on a political ethics of care theorizes four phases of care, each with an associated ethical element: caring about (attentiveness), caring for (responsibility), caregiving (competence), care receiving (responsiveness). This section of the chapter focuses on the second phase of care, which relates to taking actions toward meeting the need. Once the need is perceived, understood, and apprehended ("caring about" or attentiveness), there follows the *responsibility* that something should be done about this need. The core moral element associated with this phase is thus responsibility. Tronto differentiates between obligation, which emanates from a sense of duty or formal/legal ties, and responsibility, which is a response after recognizing a need for care. Haraway (2008, 2016) reminds us that responsibility and accountability are never finished and also never solely located in dualistic relationships. Rather, the relationships are multidirectional, include other species (i.e., not only humans), and recognize as well the asymmetry of these relationships. For Haraway (2008, 2015, 2016), taking responsibility means an acknowledgment of non-innocence in our intra-actions with others. Barad (2007) equates responsibility with accountability—and relates this to what matters and what is excluded from mattering. For example, extractivism and colonialism are dependent on a mechanical worldview that regards the land, animals, and plants as resources for human consumption (Ghosh 2021). Barad emphasizes that responsibility is not something one chooses, but precedes intentionality of consciousness, and is not exclusively human either. Responsibility is also not ours alone but is about entanglements with self and other (and not necessarily a human other; we are not the only active beings). Responsibility takes account of the liveliness of what we are a part of at every moment, how we intra-act as part of the world's vitality, and what different reconfigurings might be possible. Barad (2007, 158) asks the pertinent question in relation to responsibility: "What would it mean to acknowledge that the 'able-bodied' depend on the 'disabled' for their very existence? What would it mean to take on that responsibility? What would it mean to deny one's responsibility to the other once there is a recognition that one's very embodiment is integrally entangled with the other?" It is thus important to acknowledge that our privileges are dependent on those of others with whom we are inextricably entangled. Individuality, from this perspective, takes on new valences from a disembodied rational other; rather, the focus is on "having-the-other-in-one's-skin" (Barad 2007, 391) and the responsibility that ensues from that (Barad 2007, 393–394). From this perspective, responsibility is never ours alone. We also need to take responsibility for what is included or excluded from mattering—which lives, for example, are grievable (Butler 2020), and how best to ensure multispecies flourishing.

Responsiveness or Response-ability

Responsiveness is the fourth moral element in Tronto's (1993, 2013) phases of care and is similar to the notion of response-ability and refers to the response from the thing, group, animal, environment, plant, or person being cared for. Responsiveness is the observing of the response and the discernment about whether the care given was adequate or sufficient or should be ongoing. Also new needs may become apparent in the response of the care receiver.

In posthuman ethics response-ability is cultivating the capacity to respond where we render each other capable. Rendering each other capable enlarges the competency of all the players, since we are constituted through each other; for example, in the field of social work, this can be seen when we consider the relations between social workers, clients, theories, geographical places, and so on. Indeed, it is not only human beings rendered or rendering each other capable; Despret (2004) writes about being rendered capable through human-animal relations. The capacity to respond to the other is an important part of rendering each other capable, and this needs to be cultivated for a response-able practice, which is a collective process of potentiality and becoming. Rendering each other capable happens not through duty ethics but through the capacity to respond to what matters—as Haraway expresses it, "a kind of luring, desiring, making-with" (Davis and Turpin 2015, 257). This is a process that involves cultivating ethical (how to flourish together in a complex world of living and dying), ontological (being and becoming, making-with), epistemological (knowing-with, enlarging each other's thinking), political (macro and micro power relations) response-abilities.

Response-ability is always already collective and with others (a making-with or sympoiesis), and attends to what might be but is not yet there (Haraway 2015). Being response-able for Barad (2014b) is about being in touch with the other. As noted earlier, this also extends to nonhuman others. For example, Astrid Schrader shows how response-ability is important in laboratory practices when working with *Pfiesteria piscicida* or dinoflagellate (a supposedly fish-killing microorganism). She shows how response-ability resides not in the social, the researcher themselves, or a particular response but in the "enabling of responsiveness within experimental relatings." So, according to Schrader, response-ability comes about through attentiveness so that responsiveness can be enabled, which brings into view the indeterminacy of the *Pfiesteria*'s beings and doings.

Privileged Irresponsibility

As Tronto (2013) argues, privileged irresponsibility is where some groups of people can afford to ignore the responsibilities they have regarding caring, at the same time as taking it for granted that their needs will be serviced, while others are obligated. I would add that privileged irresponsibility also involves seeing the environment as an unending resource to be exploited by humans for their own needs. For Karen Barad (2019), privileged irresponsibility means ignoring our entangled relationalities of the past that we inherit and the future of which we are a part (as is evident in the section on temporal diffraction and hauntology earlier in the chapter). We are frequently unaware of that in which we have been complicit. We need to remember that the effects of past actions can never be fully amended, so there can never be full redemption for our past, but there must be an accounting for it as we continue to make connections and commit to what matters (Barad 2010). This would require a radical hospitality of openness to all the injustices of the past in the thick now of the present. This is particularly pertinent to those who have a settler history in colonized lands and to those in the Global North who have inadvertently but substantially benefited through colonialism. Barad (2019, 544) issues an invitation to practice radical hospitality, that is "an opening up to all that is possible in the thickness of the Now in rejecting practices of a-voidance, taking responsibility for injustices, activating and aligning with forces of justice, and welcoming the other in an undoing of the colonizing notion of selfhood rather than as a marker of not us, not me."

Plumwood refers to shadow places (also sacrificial and denied places) as unrecognized places that "provide our material and ecological support" but are "likely to elude our knowledge and responsibility" (Plumwood 2008, 139). These include places where there are histories of indiscriminate, increasingly systematic killing and destruction. For example, in Adrienne van Eeden-Wharton's thesis "Salt-Water-Bodies: From an Atlas of Loss," the "harvesting" of whales, seals, seabirds, and guano is intertwined with narratives of settler colonialism, empire, state control, racial segregation, land dispossession, coercive labor practices, militarization, and industrialization (van Eeden-Wharton 2020). Judith Butler's (2004, 2020) question about which lives are grievable and what distinguishes the lives that are not grievable from those that are is a particularly pertinent one here. She asks, "Whose lives count as 'selves' worth defending, that is, eligible for self-defense, the question only makes sense if we recognize pervasive forms of inequality that establish some lives as disproportionately more livable and grievable than others" (Butler 2020, 25).

Responsibility is a kind of doing that does not assume a givenness of anything in advance but takes into account entangled relations with the other. These entanglements lead us to understand how it is never just about the self but rather about how we are implicated in spacetimematterings.[4] We need to take responsibility for what matters and what has been excluded from mattering (Barad 2007) and how this plays out in the past, present, and future.

Addressing privileged irresponsibility thus involves becoming accountable for the past, present, and future by facing the ghosts of the past and our implicatedness in the entangled web of relations that matter. These are the hauntological relations of inheritance. Facing these inheritances and making them visible is not a straightforward process and is a task that takes effort and work. We need to critically sift through the legacies that we have inherited. For example, South Africans and others in the world manage to ignore the ghosts of colonialism and apartheid by continuing with the very practices to which these two regimes have given rise—separating them/ourselves from those who are poor, living with disabilities, or in other ways reminding us of injustice in which we are implicated and thus prefer not to think about. Thom van Dooren (2014, 283) talks about the importance of experiencing grief and loss and says that in order for these to be experienced, "it is not enough for two such beings to have lived alongside each other, in proximity to one another"—they must "have become at stake in each other, bound up with what matters to each other," in some way "have come to inhabit a meaningfully shared world." Entangled empathy would assist in the process of becoming at stake with each other (becoming involved with what matters for the other). "Entangled empathy," which is a "particular form of caring or loving attention, attention that is directed toward another's flourishing" (Gruen 2018, 81), makes it possible to think about whether and how we should respond. Entangled empathy is thus useful for dealing with privileged irresponsibility in that it involves a refinement of perception in order to more accurately become more responsible through an awareness of our entanglements with particular and situated others (Gruen 2018). Entangled empathy "helps us to deepen the disposition to attend in appropriate and meaningful ways to the effects of our actions within complex networks of power and privilege" (Gruen 2015, 94). This, like a justice-to-come, is an ongoing and never-ending process (see also Émilie Dionne's notion of organic empathy in her chapter on corpo-reality in this volume [chapter 8]).

Such radical shifts necessitate new ways of thinking and doing. They require conceptual movements across disciplinary boundaries as well as new formulations of social reproduction, care, recognition, and redistribution. The Anthropocene crisis is manifestly a crisis for life itself and will require an active working together to address privileged irresponsibility, understanding that our entanglements with others in asymmetrical multidirectional relationships not only involve those who are human but have unintentional effects on the entire planet. Collective thinking, knowing, making together (sympoiesis) (Haraway 2016) regarding what really matters and rendering each other capable (Despret 2013), becoming at stake with, intra-acting in ongoing ways, is what is needed.

We continually need to remind ourselves that all are implicated and affected—and responsibility is not ours alone. This, as Alaimo writes, will necessitate new ways of thinking and doing in our precarious world. Alaimo (2016) refers to transcorporeal culpability and responsibility practiced through fraught and tangled materialities of the world.[5] Transcorporeality requires seeking out information about how practices of daily living, such as food and fuel consumption, lead to and result from carbon emissions, extraction, and pollution, all of which affect the ecological system. This is an important consideration and speaks to the need of caring to know about entanglements and connections. We might not know in advance what might happen or be produced, but we need to be vigilant in our responses to encounters.

Addressing privileged irresponsibility necessitates valuing differences, seeing difference within rather than in the other, and understanding differences that matter. It also requires a vigilant stance toward individualism and separability that serves to distance humans and in so doing erase a sense of accountability and responsibility for our entangled relations as part of the damaged planet. Cultivating creativity and curiosity—generative, experimental, and playful responses that are directed toward capacitating all—is important. An openness to our complicit non-innocence is a crucial step in the process in acknowledging our continuing implicatedness in the damaged planet.

CONCLUSION

The relational ontologies of care and posthuman ethics, when diffracted through each other, have the potential to create generative provocations to think otherwise regarding privileged irresponsibility. If the focus is not solely on the human but on the processes of making as well as living and dying on our damaged planet, taking account of and being responsible for our involvement in entangled relations is a first step in addressing privileged irresponsibility. In order to do this, we would have to eschew notions of the autonomous, unencumbered, rational, intentional human subject who has essentialized qualities and is author of their own actions and a view of nature as separate, inert, and passively waiting to be acted upon. From an ethics of care and posthuman ethics perspective, such a subject is fictitious. Both of these approaches to ethics are predicated on a relational ontology that means that there are no preexisting subjects and objects, but that these are continually coming into being through intra-actions. Ethical sensibilities such as responsibility and accountability are thus part of our entangled relations. Rendering each other capable through cultivating response-ability means that ethics affects all parties who affect and are affected by particular practices in the world. As Thom van Dooren and Deborah Bird Rose (2016, 90) have aptly observed, "... there is no singular 'responsible' course of action; there is only the constantly shifting capacity to respond to another. What counts as good, perhaps ethical, response is always context specific and relational. It is always being rearticulated, re-imagined, and made possible in new ways, *inside* ongoing processes of call and response and the worlds that they produce. Here, responsibility is about developing the openness and the sensitivities necessary to be curious, to understand and respond in ways that are never perfect, never innocent, never final, and yet always required."

Diffracting a political ethics of care and critical posthuman ethics in relation to responsibility, response-ability, and privileged irresponsibility and considering this from the practices of everyday life show how a relational ontology matters to ethics in terms of a coextensive entanglement of relations. This chapter has thought-with notions such as "hauntology" (Derrida 1994; Barad 2010), "grievable lives" (Butler 2004, 2020), "shadow places" (Plumwood 2008), "non-innocence" (Haraway 2008, 2016), entangled empathy (Gruen 2015), and "transcorporeal culpability" (Alaimo 2016), to consider ways of becoming more accountable with regard to privileged irresponsibility, where humans will no longer be able to view the world as a resource to be exploited and expropriated, to regard themselves as separate from the damaged planet, or to distance themselves from the past, present, and future.

NOTES

1. Response-ability is used in feminist new materialism and posthumanism to signify the ability to respond, which can be seen as similar to responsiveness in care ethics (Tronto, 1993, 2013).
2. For a fuller discussion of the reflection/diffraction debate, see Bozalek and Zembylas (2017).
3. Thanks to Maggie FitzGerald for pointing out the problematic nature of this "we," which, first, is human-centric and, second, does not accommodate being differently placed as humans. Braidotti (2022) notes that we are in this together but from different positions.
4. Spacetimematterings is the production of space, time, and matter in their iterative reconfigurings—space, time, and matter are subject to diffraction and entanglement. As Barad puts it, "Not only does spacetimemattering mark the inseparability of space, time, ... it is a dynamic ongoing reconfiguring of a field of relationalities among 'moments,' 'places,' and 'things' (in their inseparability), where scale is iteratively (re)made in intra-action" (Barad 2017, G111).
5. Transcorporeal refers to a situated self as part of the material world and problematizes subject/object as the subject is always already part of the world that she/he/they seek to know—drawing on Karen Barad's theory of agential realism. Transcorporeal also refers to human and nonhuman bodies and landscapes that are entangled with each other. As Alaimo (2016, 121) describes it, "Trans-corporeality is a new materialist and posthumanist sense of the human as perpetually interconnected with the flows of substances and the agencies of environments."

REFERENCES

Alaimo, Stacy. 2016. *Exposed: Environmental Politics and Pleasures in Posthuman Times*. Minneapolis: University of Minnesota Press.
Barad, Karen. 2007. *Meeting the Universe Halfway: Quantum Physics and the Entanglement of Matter and Meaning*. Durham, NC: Duke University Press.

———. 2010. "Quantum Entanglements and Hauntological Relations of Inheritance: Dis/continuities, Spacetime Enfoldings, and Justice-to-Come." *Derrida Today* 3:240–268.

———. 2012. Nature's Queer Performativity. *Kvinder, Køn & Forskning* 53: 1–2. https://doi.org/10.7146/kkf.v0i1-2.28067.

———. 2014a. "Diffracting Diffraction: Cutting Together-Apart." *Parallax* 20 (3): 168–187.

———. 2014b. "On Touching—The Inhuman That Therefore I Am (V.1.1)." In *Power of Material / Politics of Materiality*, edited by Susanne Witzgall and Kerstin Stakemeier, 153–164. Berlin: Diaphanes.

———. 2017. "No Small Matter: Mushroom Clouds, Ecologies of Nothingness, and Strange Topologies of Spacetimemattering." In *Arts of Living on a Damaged Planet*, edited by Anna Tsing, Heather Swanson, Elaine Gan, and Nick Bubandt, G103–G120. Minneapolis: University of Minnesota Press.

———. 2018. "Troubling Time/s and Ecologies of Nothingness: Re-turning, Re-membering, and Facing the Incalculable." In *Eco-deconstruction: Derrida and Environmental Philosophy*, edited by Matthias Fritsch, Phillipe Lynes, and David Wood, 206–248. New York: Fordham University Press.

———. 2019. "After the End of the World: Entangled Nuclear Colonialisms, Matters of Force, and the Material Force of Justice." *Theory & Event* 22 (3): 524–550.

Boulet, Jacques. 2021. "Restorative and Regenerative Relational Praxis Must Include the Nonhuman." In *Post-anthropocentric Social Work: Critical Posthuman and New Materialist Perspectives*, edited by Vivienne Bozalek and Bob Pease, 46–57. London: Routledge.

Bozalek, Vivienne, and Simone Fullagar. 2022. In *A Glossary of Doing Postqualitative, New Materialist and Critical Posthumanist Research across Disciplines*, edited by Karin Murris, 30–31. London: Routledge.

Bozalek, Vivienne, and Dorothee Hölscher. 2021. "Higher Education Hauntologies and Spacetimemattering: Response-ability and Non-innocence in Times of Pandemic." In *Higher Education Hauntologies: Living with Ghosts for a Justice-to-Come*, edited by Vivienne Bozalek, Michalinos Zembylas, Siddique Motala, and Dorothee Hölscher, 171–187. London: Routledge.

———. 2022. "From Imperialism to Radical Hospitality: Propositions for Reconfiguring Social Work towards a Justice-to-Come." *Southern African Journal of Social Work and Social Development* 34 (1): 1–20.

Bozalek, Vivienne, and Michalinos Zembylas. 2017. "Diffraction or Reflection? Sketching the Contours of Two Methodologies in Educational Research." *International Journal of Qualitative Studies in Education* 30 (2): 111–127.

Bozalek, Vivienne, Michalinos Zembylas, Siddique Motala, and Dorothee Hölscher. 2021. *Higher Education Hauntologies: Living with Ghosts for a Justice-to-Come*. London: Routledge.

Braidotti, Rosi. 2022. *Posthuman feminism*. Cambridge: Polity.

Bussolini, Jeffery. 2013. "Recent French, Belgian and Italian Work in the Cognitive Science of Animals: Dominique Lestel, Vinciane Despret, Roberto Marchesini and Giorgio Celli." *Social Science Information* 52 (2): 187–209.

Butler, Judith. 2004. *Precarious Life: The Powers of Mourning and Violence*. London: Verso.

———. 2020. *The Force of Non-violence: An Ethico-politico Bind*. London: Verso.

Davis, Heather, and Etienne Turpin, eds. 2015. *Art in the Anthropocene: Encounters among Aesthetics, Politics, Environments and Epistemologies*. London: Open Humanities Press.

Derrida, Jacques. 1994. *Spectres of Marx: The State of the Debt, the Work of Mourning and the New International*. Translated by Peggy Kamuf. London: Routledge.

Despret, Vinciane. 2004. "The Body We Care For: Figures of Anthropo-zoo-genesis." *Body and Society* 10:111–134.

———. 2013. "Responding Bodies and Partial Affinities in Human–Animal Worlds." *Theory, Culture & Society* 30 (7/8): 51–76.

Despret, Vinciane, and Michel Meuret. 2016. "Cosmoecological Sheep and the Arts of Living on a Damaged Planet." *Environmental Humanities* 8 (1): 24–36.

Dionne, Emilie. 2020. "Slowing Down with Non-human Matter: The Contribution of Feminist New Materialism to Slow Scholarship." In *Posthuman and Political Care Ethics for Reconfiguring Higher Education Pedagogies*, edited by Vivienne Bozalek, Michalinos Zembylas, and Joan C. Tronto, 91–106. London: Routledge.

Fisher, Berenice, and Joan C. Tronto. 1990. "Toward a Feminist Theory of Care." In *Circles of Care: Work and Identity in Women's Lives*, edited by Emily K. Abel and Margaret K. Nelson, 35–62. Albany: State University of New York Press.

Fraser, Heather, and Nik Taylor. 2021. "Animals as Domestic Violence Victims: A Challenge to Humanist Social Work." In *Post-anthropocentric Social Work: Critical Posthuman and New Materialist Perspectives*, edited by Vivienne Bozalek and Bob Pease, 161–174. London: Routledge.

Ghosh, Amitav. 2021. *The Nutmeg's Curse: Parables for a Planet in Crisis*. Chicago: University of Chicago Press.

Gruen, Lauren. 2015. *Entangled Empathy: An Alternative Ethic for Our Relationships with Animals*. New York: Lantern Books.

———. 2018. "Just Say No to Lobotomy." In *Animaladies*, edited by Lauren Gruen and Fiona Probyn-Rapsey, 56–94. New York: Bloomsbury.

Haraway, Donna. 1992. "The Promises of Monsters: A Regenerative Politics for Inappropriate/d Others. In *Cultural Studies*, edited by Lawrence Grossberg, Cary Nelson, and Paula Treichler, 295–337. New York: Routledge.

———. 2008. *When Species Meet*. Minneapolis: University of Minnesota Press.

———. 2015. "Anthropocene, Capitalocene, Chthulhucene: Donna Haraway in Conversation with Martha Kenney." In *Art in the Anthropocene: Encounters among Aesthetics, Politics, Environments and Epistemologies*, edited by Heather Davis and Etienne Turpin, 255–270. London: Open Humanities Press.

———. 2016. *Staying with the Trouble: Making Kin in the Chthulucene*. Durham, NC: Duke University Press.

Hoosain, Shanaaz, and Vivienne Bozalek. 2021. "Hauntology, History and Heritage: Intergenerational Trauma in South African Displaced Families." In *Post-Anthropocentric Social Work: Critical Posthuman and New Materialist Perspectives*, edited by Vivienne Bozalek and Bob Pease, 210–222. London: Routledge.

Juelskaer, Malou, Halle Plauborg, and Stine W. Adrian. 2021. *Dialogues on Agential Realism: Engaging in Worldings through Research Practice*. London: Routledge.

Plumwood, Val. 2008. "Shadow Places and the Politics of Dwelling." *Australian Humanities Review* 44 (1): 139–150.

Pugliese, Joseph. 2020. *Biopolitics of the More-Than-Human: Forensic Ecologies of Violence*. Durham, NC: Duke University Press.

Puig de la Bellacasa, María. 2017. *Matters of Care: Speculative Ethics in More Than Human Worlds*. Minneapolis: University of Minnesota Press.

Rogowska-Stangret, Monika. 2020. "Care as a Methodology: Reading Natalie Jereminko and Vinciane Despret Diffractively." In *Posthuman and Political Care Ethics for Reconfiguring Higher Education Pedagogies*, edited by Vivienne Bozalek, Michalinos Zembylas, and Joan C. Tronto, 13–26. London: Routledge.

Schrader, Astrid. 2010. "Responding to *Pfiesteria piscicida* (the Fish Killer): Phantomatic Ontologies, Indeterminacy, and Responsibility in Toxic Microbiology." *Social Studies of Science* 40 (2): 275–306.

———. 2015. "Abyssal Intimacies and Temporalities of Care: How (Not) to Care about Deformed Leaf Bugs in the Aftermath of Chernobyl." *Social Studies of Science* 45 (5): 665–690.

Tronto, Joan C. 1993. *Moral Boundaries: A Political Argument for an Ethic of Care*. New York: Routledge.

———. 2013. *Caring Democracy: Markets, Equality, and Justice*. New York: New York University Press.

van Dooren, Thom. 2014. "Mourning Crows: Grief and Extinction in a Shared World. In *Routledge Handbook of Human-Animal Studies*, edited by Garry Marvin and Susan McHugh, 275–289. London: Routledge.

———. 2019. *The Wake of Crows: Living and Dying in Shared Worlds*. New York: Columbia University Press.

van Dooren, Thom and Deborah Bird Rose. 2016. "Lively Ethography: Storying Animist Worlds." *Environmental Humanities* 8 (1): 77–94.

van Eeden-Wharton, Adrienne. 2020. "Salt-Water-Bodies: From an Atlas of Loss." PhD diss., Stellenbosch University.

10 · "DO YOU REALLY WANT TO KNOW ABOUT THIS?"
Critical Feminist Ethics of Care as a Project of Unsettling

MASAYA LLAVANERAS BLANCO

> It is the responsibility of geographers to find a way both to locate the specific materiality of the scarred, exhausted, raped, and murdered body of the enslaved person and to map that same materiality of pain and suffering still growing on the bodies of human beings on a global scale today.
> —Noxolo, Raghuram, and Madge (2008, 160)

Early in my research about care and human mobilities among Haitian domestic workers in the Dominican Republic (DR), I realized that my interest in how Haitian domestic workers provided care for themselves and for one another took most interlocutors by surprise. One interview stood out. After I explained that, among other themes, I was exploring the selfcare practices of Haitian women, the interviewee, a researcher and public servant, looked at me with disbelief and repeated as if to confirm what she had heard: "Selfcare?," before suggesting that it was unlikely that I would find anything about that (KI1, January 2017).[1] I was also met with disbelief when I started conversations with domestic workers of Haitian descent. Their disbelief often turned into a rhetorical question, "Do you really want to know about this?," as if to confirm that I really was interested in something so private and irrelevant to other people.

Why was it surprising to ask about these women's strategies to provide care to themselves and one another? The precariousness associated with domestic work and their migration and citizenship status may have made talking about care seem trivial. On the one hand, paid domestic work in the DR is subject to profound exploitation and is mostly unprotected by the existing labor code. On the other, the migration and citizenship status of Haitian migrants, or Dominicans of Haitian descent in the DR, compounds their exploitability after decades of violent deportations and denationalization processes (Wooding and Moseley-Williams 2004; Shoaff 2017; Llavaneras Blanco 2018). In this chapter I argue that these structural conditions of exploitability and deportability are not external to the notion of care but are rather the conditions under which care is conceived and put into practice; they determine who provides care, but also who is deserving of what forms of care and under what terms. Such conditionings are the product of historical processes in which gender and racialization have been critical categories of difference that determine belonging, subjectivity, and labor trajectories. I argue that thinking about a critical and feminist ethics of care necessitates that one engages with the structural power relations that shape care practices, in which gender and racialization play a key role.

Robinson (1999, 115) argues that "an ethics of care ... must become aware of the wider structural and institutional causes of human suffering and find ways to integrate an interrogation of these causes into its ethical framework." I engage with Robinson's invitation by investigating the racialized structures that shape the practice and ethics of care among black women of Haitian descent who have worked as domestic workers in the DR. Even though the literature on critical ethics of care refers to the importance of social structures and relations of power, scant attention has been paid to the effects of racialization and colonial legacies in how needs, care labors, and responsibilities are conceived and experienced by subaltern subjects. This chapter elaborates on the effects of racialization, gender, and migratory status in shaping notions of deservingness of care as well as how care is experienced and provided. It builds on Raghuram's call to foster "geographical sensitivities" in how we understand care by focusing on practices of child care, caring for oneself, as well as access to reproductive and sexual health care among women of Haitian ancestry. Existing literature tends to center on care labor provided by domestic workers (often from the Global South) to their employers (often in the Global North). This chapter intentionally shifts the attention toward the care ethics and care practices that women of Haitian descent conduct among themselves in a South-South migration context. It contributes to "unsettling care" (Murphy 2015) by holding it accountable to the racial and gendered violences in which it is emmeshed. On this basis, I argue that for an ethics of care to be feminist, critical, and global, we need to unsettle care by confronting its unevenness and violence.[2]

The chapter is based on fieldwork conducted in the DR and Haiti during different periods in 2016, 2017, and 2018 as well as on historical and theoretical analysis centering the works of Black feminists and feminists from Global South, Indigenous, and anticolonial perspectives. The text builds on interviews and focus groups with 134 women of Haitian ancestry who worked as domestic workers as well as with twenty civil society leaders and public servants. I approached this research from a complex positionality as a light-skinned Latin American woman, not born on the island of Hispaniola.[3]

The first section presents a theoretical framework that centers the deep interrelation between care practices and care ethics. It locates the analysis in the context of postslavery societies in which racialization and gender are historical markers that are (re)produced by an ethics of care. The second section introduces the context of the DR and the situation of women who are Haitian or of Haitian descent and work as domestic workers. It provides necessary context on the intersections of race, gender, and citizenship and migration status. In the third, I discuss care as practiced and experienced among women of Haitian descent who work as domestic workers in their households and communities. I focus on the care practice and ethics of the Movement of Dominican-Haitian Women (MUDHA for its name in Spanish) as an exemplar of a critical feminist ethics of care that is politically situated and cognizant of the racialized, gendered, and legal structures of exclusion in which care exists. In the fourth and final section, I explore the possibilities of care as emancipatory. I conclude by reflecting on the unsettling potential of a critical feminist care ethics that recognizes the oppressive legacies of care and is committed to supporting emancipatory care practices.

CARE IS NON-INNOCENT

Care ethics is deeply implicated in power structures and concrete practices. It is mundane: "located in the actual activities that we carry out for others" (Robinson 2018, 326). The category of gender has been instrumental in unveiling the power dynamics of care and the material process of care practices. The sexual division of labor is at the heart of who cares, who is cared for, and how we embody, distribute, and experience care (Beneria 1979; Picchio 1992; Razavi 2011). Feminists have demonstrated the heavy role played by gender and the sexual division of labor on how care labor is assumed to be a feminine task assigned to women and girls, poorly valued and often unrecognized.[4]

A critical and feminist ethics of care recognizes the importance of gender while also paying attention to other categories of difference such as citizenship, race, and class (Williams 1995; Reddy et al. 2014). Among them, race and racialization are perhaps the least examined despite their centrality in the edifice of care.[5] This neglect speaks of the uneasy implications of race in the ethics and practices of care that Murphy (2015) describes as the "non-innocent genealogies" of care. The absence of race in care ethics is presented under the auspices of an assumed universality of experience among women and, most importantly, an assumed universality of whiteness. The subdued and yet persistent presence is manifest in "the normative white body through which much care is theorized" (Raghuram 2019, 17). Narayan (1995) explains it as follows: "Colonial stereotypes about the hierarchy of races had similarities to existing theories of the hierarchy of gender-where attributes such as physical 'weakness,' smaller craniums, deficient rationality, and moral frailty were ascribed to western women, constructing them as the 'weaker sex' in need of the care, support, and guidance of western men, not unlike the colonized" (134).

The concept of care is necessarily situated: it exists in place. It is inherently relational, it exists in relation to different geohistories whereby care ethics are implicated in relations of coloniality and protection, both of which are often imbricated with each other (Raghuram 2012, 162). Liboiron (Metis/Michif) illustrates this inherent tension when they argue that care is "an uneven relation and can contribute to and/or mitigate unevenness" (Liboiron 2021, 115). The unevenness that is inherent to care exists a priori as well as ex post. This is an important distinction because it underscores the fact that while care can be performed with the stated intention to recognize and even mend this unevenness, the way it is defined and performed may indeed produce deeper inequalities and violence. The implications of this tension are central to the fixing narrative of colonial enterprise. For example, during colonization forced evangelization was framed as salvation, the ultimate form of care. Liboiron illustrates this point powerfully: "From the position of conquest (of people, Land, and souls), genocidal care is an obligation" (115).

Care practices are embodied manifestations of an ethics of care: they are imbued in power relations between carer and cared-for, as much as they are part of social organizations that involve different socioeconomic and political actors.[6] Care ethics are thus not reduced to individual, rule-based relations but are also part of large social processes, all of which are implicated in power. This is relevant to understand that context matters in how care is conceived and experienced. As proposed by Raghuram (2012, 156), "The concept of care does not stand still"; it changes over locations and has diverse genealogies that are contextually and geographically based. In that sense, how care is practiced embodies and manifests the concrete implications of the care ethics prevalent in a given context and enables its reproduction.

Social positionings such as those based on racialization, gender, and class shape the universe of care and the care practices of individuals and communities. This differentiation is significant to one's subjectivity and sense of deservingness, including both relations of care and relations of neglect. As established by Raghuram (2019, 13), "Care-less practices are as productive of subjectivity as careful ones." In other words, one may never seek to access care that one has never received, simply because it might not be part of the universe of what is deemed possible. Similarly, when care has been deeply immersed in violence, it might become indistinguishable from it.

Care is immersed in "pervasive structural relationships of power ... such as those between colonizers and the colonized, [which] tend to foster ideological justifications for the maintenance of such relationships" (Narayan 1995, 136).[7] Care practices are essential to the reproduction of these relationships by virtue of embodying who cares, who is cared for, as well as what care looks like. This was manifest in the context of enslavement, where Black women's care labor was both "coerced and freely given" (Hartman 2016, 171). The exploitation of their labor was inseparable from sexual exploitation and forced reproduction, which were inflicted for the wealth accumulation and reproduction of the conditions of living of slave owners. In that context, care, social reproduction, and subjectivities were packaged together with intimate violence in ways that continue to influence how care labor is conceived and experienced in Black postcolonial spaces. This conflation was made more complex by the care labors that enslaved women conducted with and for their relations: the rearing of their children, the feeding and caring for their families that produced their survival, alongside the normalization of rape and forced reproduction (Scully and Paton 2005).

The continuum of social reproductive labor, sex work, and relational care is condensed in the concept of "Intimate Labour" (Boris and Parreñas 2010). Its coexistence with violence and exploitation is deeply contextualized in the process of postslavery subject making by Sharpe's *Monstrous Intimacies* (2010). During enslavement, Black women's intimate labor was marked by the likelihood of having their children forcefully taken away from them while often being forced to feed and raise other children. Relatedly, Hartman's duality of coerced and freely given care labor plays out in differentiated care practices of affect and violence, volition and coercion. Noxolo, Raghuram, and Madge (2008) engage with this duality by referring to Morrison's novel *Beloved* ([1987] 2004). They focus on a scene in which Sethe, an enslaved woman, is pregnant and breastfeeding an infant. The character describes having her milk running because she is longing for the lactating child that she had sent away in preparation for their escape from the plantation. During this period of longing Sethe is attacked by a group of white boys who take her down and take her milk, eventually whipping her severely for telling on them. The scene exemplifies relations and practices that are deeply emmeshed with colonial exploitation and violence as much as with nurture and nourishment.

Noxolo, Raghuram, and Madge (2008) refer to Sethe's flowing milk as a metaphor for an intrinsic relationality in which the boundaries of the self are irremediably fluid. For oneself, existing responsibly within these fluid boundaries is a constant negotiation with one's relations. In Noxolo, Raghuram, and Madge's terms, "The specific terms of mutuality cannot be directed; they must be negotiated and renegotiated continually, and the politics of these relationalities recognized" (2008, 158). Care is thus inherently part of processes and relations of power, immersed in tensions of violence and affect that need to be recognized and addressed continuously.

Differentiations within care practices are present in the forms of care provision, the subjectivities of carers and care receivers. These distinctions are key manifestations of colonial legacies. Sethe's experience speaks of the same milk that was meant for her child and was forcefully taken by two white boys. In both cases, Sethe's embodied form of care (breastfeeding and nourishment) is provided in very distinct manners, clearly differentiated by degrees of volition. Also on the subject of breastfeeding as part of the exploitation endured by enslaved Black women, Sharpe refers to the "distinction between the wet nurse's (black) breast and the maternal (white) breast" (2010, 163). In that dyad, the wet nurse fulfills a maternal function without the rights and privileges of white motherhood (163). This denial has ethical implications: it keeps the carer at the margins of legality and femininity, shaping her subjectivity and her subjection.

Sheller (2012, 9) argues that "when slavery ended, techniques and practices of sexual domination and biopolitical power remained entrenched." The deep imbrication between subjectivity, subjection, and care in the labor exploitation of Black women continues to exist in the postslavery world. The historical entanglement between race, coloniality, and care emerges into the present through quotidian manifestations of racialization and gendered exploitation. A clear example of that legacy in current-day North America is the case of Shaina Bell, a Black mother of two children who was temporarily detained and brought to court for leaving them unattended in a motel room while she was working a minimum-wage job that she undertook to be able to sustain her family (Good 2021; Ockerman 2021). Bell was criminalized based on the poverty that pushed her to work while leaving the children unattended, which brought into question her ability to care.

In the case of Black women of Haitian descent in the DR, exclusion is manifest by a migration and citizenship regime that discriminates against them based on gender and race. This form of exclusion is at the core of a process that keeps Dominican-Haitians at the margins of citizenship across generations. The next section delves into the complex relationship between gender, race, and care in the DR, from the standpoint of Haitian migrant women and Dominican women of Haitian descent.

BLACKNESS, GENDER, AND CARE IN THE DR

The mainstream Dominican nation-building narrative emphasizes their Hispanic and Catholic heritage and the "Indio," an idealized mix between the Indigenous population and Spanish colonizers (Ricourt 2016; Candelario 2007). This narrative is prevalent in the educational system, the media, and the conventional narrative of the nation's history (Bartlett 2012). In contrast, Blackness, the historical connections to Africa, as well as the legacies of enslavement have been historically excluded from the national project and transposed to Haiti. This narrative of difference is framed as part of a fatal conflict model in which Haitianness was often equated to Blackness and to an irreconcilable "other" (Martínez 2003; Wucker 1999).

The DR instituted a labor migration regime with Haiti that was the product of the U.S. invasion of both countries (Mayes 2019). From the start, this regime had a clear racial component that privileged permanent immigration of people racialized as white from the United States, Europe, and the Hispanic Antilles. In tandem, the regime included individuals of African descent only as part of highly exploitative temporary labor migration schemes linked mostly to sugar production. Any other form of migration for Black newcomers was exorbitantly costly, especially compared to the visa costs applied to white newcomers (Capdevila 2004).[8] Haitian labor was at the heart of this labor migration scheme that produced wealth for the Dominican and Haitian states and elites. Alongside class and race, gender was an essential marker in the labor migration scheme. Women were left out of most of the migration regulations because plantation labor was considered men's work. However, Haitian women were in the DR since the start of the labor migration regime. By 1920 at least 17 percent of the legally recognized Haitian migrant population in DR was female (Hintzen 2017, 39).

Sirana Dolis, longtime Dominican-Haitian activist and founder of MUDHA, explains the authorities' willful ignorance of the presence of Haitian women on sugar plantations as one of economic convenience: "In those times they would buy *braceros* [sugar cane plantation workers] per head as if it was a commodity, so that they would come to work here ... and this implied a cost [to the plantation owners].... But, if women came, the *braceros* would multiply, and those would be the next *braceritos* [small plantation workers]" (interview, August 2016). This account resonates with Hartman's description of enslaved Black women's situation in North America: "Plainly put, subjection was anchored in black women's reproductive capacities" (2016, 168). Women's invisible presence was conveniently based on their labor and their reproductive capacity. They were expected to reproduce (biologically as well as socially) the labor force of the *bateyes*.[9]

Despite their exclusion from formal migration channels, Haitian women were an important part of the political economy of the plantation model. Alongside other forms of labor, intimate labor was at the heart of their arrival to the DR. Family reunification was a key driver, especially in a system that also relied on child labor (a least 7 percent of Haitian migrants in the DR in 1920 were children) (Hitnzen 2017). Women's work in meal preparation was also central. In 1962, a report by a Sugar Company recommended that "one of each ten men [migrant workers], could bring their family with the objective of having one woman in charge of the kitchen for each group of ten men" (my translation, Fondo Presidencia 1960–2001, cited in Hintzen 2017, 47). Sex work was also one of the pull factors that would make private and public plantation authorities recruit women through *buscones* (smugglers) and bring them into the bateyes to provide sexual services either as sex workers or as partners-to-be for workers who already lived there (Martínez 2007; Riveros 2014). As the reign of sugar in Dominican economy receded, women of Haitian ancestry were no longer secluded in rural bateyes but moved to cities, towns, and touristic enclaves. Many of these communities have become urban slums and have grown significantly. Despite this relative urbanization, access to public services is often suboptimal when compared to other rural or urban poor communities.

Up until the 1980s the survival and mobilities of Haitian communities in the DR were shaped by the sugar economy (Lozano and Báez Evertsz 2008). For Haitian women, intimate labor in the form of sex work and the sexual and social reproduction of labor were central to the spatial trajectories. Once sugar production was no longer central, intimate labor continued to be relevant in the form of paid and unpaid domestic work, among others. As of 2018 paid domestic work was the third most representative form of employment among Haitian migrant women (19.1 percent) and the second most among women of Haitian descent

(26.4 percent) (Oficina Nacional de Estadística [ONE] 2018, 344). These are conservative statistics since many women of Haitian ancestry in the DR (migrants or DR-born) are engaged in paid and unpaid care that goes unregistered. They often interweave unpaid care work provided to their families with occasional paid labor: cleaning a home for a day, doing laundry for others while they do their own, watching each other's children, for example. None of these activities are registered in labor statistics, according to which 47.9 percent of Haitian migrants and 76.9 percent of DR-born women of Haitian ancestry are categorized as economically inactive (ONE 2018, 337), and there is scarce representative information about how they sustain their everyday lives and those of their dependents in the DR as well as in Haiti.

Mayes (2019, 155) argues that women of Haitian descent in the DR are at the heart of a citizenship "regime that manages access to nationality and citizenship through the regulation of race and sex." Deeply intertwined with a complex set of intimate labor, their care practices are also enmeshed with their legal exclusion—first, through the absence of a migration category for Haitian women coming to provide their labors in the sugar plantations and, second, more recently, through their exclusion and that of their descendants from the right to nationality. In this way, their legal exclusion is instrumental to the intergenerational reproduction of marginalization. Women's citizenship status is scrutinized in hospitals when they deliver their children, thus leaving it up to hospital staff to determine the right to nationality of newborns depending on "how Dominican" or "how Haitian" the mother appears to be, regardless of her nationality or that of the father (Petrozziello 2019). Furthermore, when fathers are able and willing to follow up with the second step of the birth registration process in a civil registry, they are often required to show the mother's documents in addition to their own (Mayes 2019).[10]

UNEVEN CARE AND VIOLENCE

In this section I engage with the inherent unevenness and potential violence of care (Liboiron 2021) by exploring the question of differentiated care practices in the lives of women of Haitian ancestry in the DR. I explore the ambivalences of care, which includes the racist and gendered violence of care as well as its emancipatory potential. In a context in which intimate labor is deeply linked to survival and exclusion, the question of care for oneself or care for one's dependents is elusive. What care means and who is entitled to it are necessarily mediated by lived experiences crossed by race, gender, and class. The infrastructures of care vary transnationally as well as nationally and locally. They are determined by migratory and citizenship status, racialization, and income level, for example. This is manifest in whether or not someone has access to healthcare and social protection, among other services (Murphy 2015). Furthermore it is manifest in the people's everyday conditions of living such as access to cement floors, running water, and sanitation (Razavi 2011; Raghuram 2012).

Differentiated Care

My exchanges with women of Haitian descent who work as domestic workers were often peppered with references to the differences between the care they provided to their employers, to their own dependents, and to each other. During a visit to research collaborators in a rural community outside Santo Domingo, the youngest grandchild of the household would come running in and out of the house. A much beloved mischievous three-year-old, the child insisted on running barefoot in a courtyard that led to a larger field. My hosts commented humorously on the hassle that it was to get him to wear sandals, and they worried for him because sometimes there was a cow out in the field and the little boy would try to chase it. Our conversation included him lovingly and often pointing out the contrast between how it was to care for this child as compared to the children they had been hired to take care of. Running barefoot and relatively independently in a courtyard was not acceptable for the children they cared for as nannies. Allowing those kids to run without shoes would have been framed as negligence by their employers (anonymized interview DWC21, 2017).

Raghuram (2019, 13) argues that "what may appear careless parenting involves different, perhaps not very easily recognisable forms of caring." This distinction between negligence and difference is a manifestation of the unevenness in which care is practiced and conceived. This is a fine line that is frequently walked by domestic workers, especially among those who are racialized and live with a precarious migration and citizenship status.

Another example of the quotidian instances in which this line is crossed is when domestic workers' paid care labor includes childminding so that their employers, especially mothers, can participate in the labor market. In traditional settings, neighbors and relatives share the same courtyard and watch each other's children in what is referred to as the *lakou* system (Edmond, Randolph, and Richard 2007).[11] In urban and less traditional contexts, it is often the case that domestic workers and other workers in precarious economic and legal circumstances download the responsibility to care to the oldest sibling (especially older sisters). This is another care differentiation that is often brushed over in literatures about transnational care, in which the care demand is framed in terms of middle-class and possibly white or light-skinned women who resort to the market to hire the care labor that they would be socially expected to provide. Even though some works on transnational care chains and care networks include community and subaltern care practices, these are rarely the focus of attention.[12] These scholarly gaps invisibilize care practices among Black, racialized, and poor communities. Such gaps contribute to the criminalization of racialized and poor mothers because there is scarce understanding of how care is conceived and provided in contexts of structural constraint. The care practices of Black and other racialized and poor women are often presented as careless and without context, which contributes to the institutionalization of racialized children because of alleged neglect.[13]

I often visited with women who worked as domestic workers on their days off, on Saturdays and sometimes on Sundays. On Saturdays, those who worked as live-in domestic workers were coming home after one or two weeks in their places of employment. Our conversations took place while they were doing the care work of their households: doing their laundry, mopping the floors. Often this was a time of conversation, not only with me but also with other women, of different generations, keeping each other company while they did their chores or while sharing the load and working together. A washing machine, for example, was made to work without power by two girls moving it manually, while we sat chatting with a larger group.

When my visits did not involve domestic chores, they often included women coiffing each other's hair. Their elaborate hairstyles would often take hours of dedication that would be combined with conversation and childminding. During one of these moments, a research participant confided that she told her employers that she did not know how to embroider hair, even though this was obviously not true. Doing someone's hair is not something that is done as part of one's domestic work, and she implied that there are forms of care and intimate labor that she reserves for herself and her community. It is not that this is a form of care labor that is not monetized. It is possible that one pays a neighbor, for example, to embroider one's hair, or that one does it in exchange for another form of labor. However, there is an important differentiation between who is to receive that labor of care and who is not. This boundary speaks to belonging in a context in which hair is a key racial and ethnic marker between Haitians and Dominicans. Black Haitians are recognized by embroidering their hair in ways that are reminiscent of their African ancestry, whereas Dominicans, including Black Dominicans, have a long history of straightening their hair and relaxing their curls (Candelario 2007).[14]

Sexual and Reproductive Health Care as a Site of Violence and Emancipation

Blackness and Haitian identity and Dominican-Haitian women's claim to Dominican citizenship have been pillars of MUDHA's approach to grassroots organizing. MUDHA's cofounders, Sonia Pierre and Sirana Dolis, drew on their personal trajectories, which informed their understanding of how oppressions based on gender, race, class, and access to nationality were deeply interlinked and had to be addressed as such (Mayes 2019). One of the products of these intersecting oppressions is women's extremely limited access to health care. Faced with the constant possibility of deportation given their precarious citizenship status, most women of Haitian ancestry avoid using public health services unless they are faced with significant emergencies. MUDHA has sought to address this structural exclusion from its early days.

Among its first actions as an independent organization, MUDHA emphasized sexual and reproductive health practices that women in bateyes could carry out to improve their living conditions despite their exclusion from most healthcare services. Among others, this took the form of community workshops teaching women self-cleansing techniques to manage (and when possible, overcome) sexually transmitted infections under conditions of lack of access to running water. Their work also included the provision of some on-site antenatal and maternal health care, through coordination with other national and international organizations, as well as supporting the role of community-based midwives (interviews with Sirana Dolis 2016, and Sirana Dolis and Cristiana Luís Francisca, January 2017).

Historically, MUDHA's approach to working with women has not been limited to facilitating on-site and community based antenatal care, but rather the organization has always centered much of its work on providing legal support for women, especially pregnant women. From the start, the organization initiated its community work by identifying pregnant people and understanding their legal situation. They would make sure to support them in accessing the necessary documentation so that they had a better chance of registering the births of their children and hopefully facilitating their access to nationality, which has been constantly scrutinized for families of Haitian descent. For the most part, accessing this documentation is a cumbersome and costly process that requires several trips to civic registries often in towns far from the communities of residence. Each step of the process often requires multiple visits to different offices, creating transportation costs on top of different fees, missed days of work, and language barriers (Llavaneras Blanco 2018; interview with Dolis, August 2016).

MUDHA has functioned as a broker between women of Haitian ancestry and the Dominican state while keeping a grassroots approach. It developed a care practice that is integrative of the physical, legal, and material realities of the women for whom they work. Its practice demonstrates that care is a fundamental feature of contemporary citizenship (Robinson 2008), which has been built on racialized and gendered forms of exclusion that need to be tackled interconnectedly. MUDHA has managed to remain true to this sophisticated approach as a small community-based organization. It continues to deal with a transnational reality of gendered and racialized violence that exceeds its local capacity within a state that continues to reproduce a racist and gendered structure of exclusion.[15]

According to media sources, directors of the Dominican National Health System estimate that in 2021, 41.7 percent of the maternal mortality registered in Dominican hospitals affected Haitian mothers. They attribute this overrepresentation to Haitian women's arrival to delivery rooms in poor health, which is likely to produce premature births (Pantaleon 2022). In September of the same year, an unofficial government policy further reduced Haitian women's access to antenatal care. The policy requires them to have private insurance by the sixth month of pregnancy in order to access care, which is unlikely due to poverty and precarious migration status (Consejo Nacional de Migración 2023). The National Health System estimates that 56 percent of maternal mortality deaths in the first trimester of 2022 are of Haitian women, showing a spike of fifteen percentage points compared to 2021 (Pantaleon 2022). Given the government policy to reduce access to antenatal care to

Haitian women, it is unsurprising that maternal mortality is rapidly increasing. To make matters worse, in November 2021 the Migration Directorate conducted raids in maternity wards, leading to the deportation of pregnant women attending antenatal appointments and those who had recently gone through labor, in some cases separating mothers and infants (*Listín Diario* 2021a, 2021b; ICHR 2021).

CRITICAL ETHICS OF CARE AS A PROJECT OF UNSETTLING

A feminist ethics of care of global aspirations needs to be held "accountable to the knotted histories of raced and sexed violence, dispossession and privilege" (Murphy 2015, 722). The histories that Murphy speaks of are part of the present and shape the hierarchies and priorities of what is defined as care, who deserves care, and how it is practiced. Reckoning with the violent differentiation between Black Haitian women as a source of care labor and as a group deemed undeserving (or less deserving) of care is an urgent "project of unsettling" (Murphy 2015, 722). It requires the unsettling of the logics that govern access to care and our implications with it. This approach to an ethics of care necessarily calls for coming to terms with and doing the political work of recognizing and acting upon the damage produced by the imperial and colonial legacies in which care practices emerge and continue to exist (Robinson 2018). Such active recognition is necessary to understanding and contextualizing the different genealogies of care ethics. Coming to terms with the non-innocence of care should be a first step toward emancipatory care ethics that is geographically and politically situated.

Raghuram (2019, 13) argues that "care patterns and processes may be unrecognizable across difference" and points out that "the talk of care may be unrecognizable to those for whom care is only a task." How care is defined and made recognizable is situated in multiple intersections that shape its unevenness. In contexts in which health care is equated with political violence, care becomes indeed unrecognizable. Instead, racialized differentiation and the absence of care become normalized as structuring factors not only of the ethics of care but also of what constitutes citizenship. Thus the incredulous comments of my interlocutors at the start of the chapter.

The historical experiences of women in the Black diaspora, past and present, are testament to the centrality of embodiment, care, and reproduction in political subjectivities and political subjection. That was true during times of enslavement and continues to hold true in the present. The body is a site of oppression as much as it is of survival, nurture, and emancipation. Writing about citizenship in post-emancipation Jamaica and Haiti, Sheller (2012, 17) proposes that "understandings of citizenship must encompass not only discursive practices, but also full sexual, sensual and erotic agency of an embodied freedom." Erotic here includes the labor of surviving and sustaining life. It refers to one's freedom of existing, moving, and experiencing joy like the grandchild running in the courtyard.

It is also about the care we provide for each other that is not meant to be shared outside of one's community, implicit in embroidering each other's hair. I do not seek to romanticize exclusion by bringing up these lighter moments of embodied emancipation. In them, I find micropractices of a care ethics that recognize unevenness and create spaces for emancipatory care. MUDHA's approach, in which embodied care and survival are imbricated with political emancipation, is exemplary of the structural implications of a care practice and a care ethics that are politically situated and cognizant of the structures of exclusion in which MUDHA operates.

Anti-Blackness and patriarchal norms constitute structural systems of oppression in which survival and joy become deeply political. Care is at the heart of these systems; it is non-innocent. By recognizing this ambivalence, we are better equipped to identify the unevenness of care and embarking on the work of unsettling care and decentering its universal (white and other racial "majorities") subjects.

ACKNOWLEDGMENTS

This work exists thanks to the generous disposition of the many women that participated in this research, as well as of the three editors of this volume. My deep gratitude to them, especially to Sirana Dolis, Cristiana Luis, and others who remain anonymized because of the constant risk of deportation. I acknowledge the care relations that sustained me and my family through this research. Thanks always to Antulio Rosales, Vera and Ela. All mistakes remain my own.

NOTES

1. I am aware that the term "selfcare" is associated with paid services used by the middle and upper classes (going to a spa, getting a massage). In using it, I am interested in questioning that association and thinking about selfcare as something that is not limited to these class-specific market transactions and that is essential to individuals' sustenance and subjectivity.
2. Relatedly, Harris (this volume, chapter 11) builds on the Movement for Black Lives to speak about the political potential of unsettling care, or what he refers to as an ethical commitment to a world undone; one that requires the capacity to "attend to differences . . . with careful attention and a willingness to be held accountable."
3. I am a Venezuelan woman, parent, migrant, and university professor in Canada. There are cultural proximities between the DR, Haiti, and Venezuela. I am not a speaker of Haitian Creole; most of my conversations with Haitian women were held in Spanish or with the interpretation of Ylemis Jean, a Dominican-Haitian research assistant.
4. See, for example, Lewis (2001), Razavi (2007), and Esquivel (2011).
5. There are, however, significant contributions on the racial implications of care labor, such as Duffy (2011), Glenn (2002), and Raghuram (2019).
6. See Jenson and Saint-Martin's (2003) and Razavi's (2007) approaches to welfare or care diamonds.
7. Koggel (this volume, chapter 1) frames this structural relationship of power in terms of hermeneutical injustice that determines what is legitimate knowledge and what qualifies as valid interpretative resources to understand our place in the world.

8. The link between the temporary labor mobilities of racialized workers and the plantation system was formalized in different pieces of legislation in the DR such as Executive Order No. 372 of 1919 and Law 279 of 1932.
9. *Batey* is the Spanish word used to refer to the barracks provided to sugar cane cutters on plantation properties. Most *bateyes* (plural of *batey*) are no longer producing sugar and exist as Haitian and Dominican-Haitian communities.
10. Birth registrations are a two-tier process in the DR. New parents are given a certification of live birth at the hospital. That certification, provided by hospital staff, identifies newborns as Dominican or foreign; it is paramount to later obtain a birth certification in a registry (the second step of the process). For a step-by-step description of this process, see Llavaneras Blanco (2020, 74).
11. *Lakou* is a Haitian Creole word for courtyard.
12. Fraga and Rodríguez Enríquez's (2022) work on the Argentinean National Care System is a promising example of care research that focuses on community care practices. See also Reddy et al.'s (2014) volume on care in context as well as Vaittinen's (2014) work on care chains as migrants' trajectories
13. This is not exceptional to the DR. According to Indigenous Services Canada, 52 percent of children in foster care are Indigenous, even though Indigenous children account for only 7 percent of all children in Canada (Indigenous Services Canada 2018). Another example is the case of Shania Bell, mentioned in the previous section.
14. Younger generations of Black Dominicans are contesting this pattern by no longer straightening their hair and/or embroidering it.
15. MUDHA also has a transnational presence. It brought the Dominican State to the Inter-American Human Rights System in the case of case of Yean and Bosico in 1998 (Marsteintredt 2016).

REFERENCES

Interviews:
Llavaneras Blanco, Masaya. 2016. Interview with Sirana Dolis, August 31st, MUDHA Office, Santo Domingo, Dominican Republic.
Llavaneras Blanco, Masaya. 2017. Interview with Sirana Dolis and Cristiana Luís Francisca, February 18, MUDHA Office, Santo Domingo, Dominican Republic.
Llavaneras Blanco, Masaya, anonymized interview KI1. 2017. January, Dominican Republic.
Llavaneras Blanco, Masaya, anonymized interview DWC21. 2017. March, Dominican Republic.

Bartlett, Lesley. 2012. "South-South Migration and Education: The Case of People of Haitian Descent Born in the Dominican Republic." *Compare* 42 (3): 393–414. https://doi.org/10.1080/03057925.2011.633738.
Benería, Lourdes. 1979. "Reproduction, Production and the Sexual Division of Labour." *Cambridge Journal of Economics* 3 (3): 203–225.
Boris, Eileen, and Rhacel Salazar Parreñas. 2010. *Intimate Labors Cultures, Technologies, and the Politics of Care*. Stanford, CA: Stanford Social Sciences.
Candelario, Ginetta E. B. 2007. *Black behind the Ears: Dominican Racial Identity from Museums to Beauty Shops*. Durham, NC: Duke University Press.
Capdevila, Lauro. 2004. "Una Discriminación Organizada: Las Leyes de Inmigración. Dominicanas y La Cuestión Haitiana En El Siglo XX." *Tebeto: Anuario Del Archivo Histórico Insular de Fuerteventura*, no. 5: 438–454.
Consejo Nacional de Migración. 2023. "Acta de Reunión del Consejo Nacional de Migración realizada el 28 de septiembre 2021." In OBMICA, *Trato Digno: Nuevos Desafíos para el Debido Proceso en Deportaciones desde la República Dominicana*. Santo Domingo: Editora Búho.

http://tratodigno.obmica.org/wp-content/uploads/2023/03/Nuevos-Desafíos-para-el-Debido-Proceso-en-Deportaciones-desde-la-República-Dominicana.pdf.

Duffy, Mignon. 2011. *Making Care Count: A Century of Gender, Race and Paid Care Work*. New Brunswick, NJ: Rutgers University Press.

Edmond, Yanique M., Suzanne M. Randolph, and Guylaine L. Richard. 2007. "The Lakou System: A Cultural, Ecological Analysis of Mothering in Rural Haiti." *Journal of Pan African Studies* 2 (1): 19–32.

Esquivel, Valeria. 2011. The Care Economy in Latin America: Putting Care at the Centre of the Agenda. United Nations Development Programme.

Fraga, Cecilia, and Corina Rodríguez Enríquez. 2022. "The Pathway towards the National Care System." DAWN. https://dawnnet.org/wp-content/uploads/2022/03/DAWN-DP_36 _The-Pathway-Towards-the-National-Care-System.pdf.

Glenn, Evelyn Nakano. 2002. *Unequal Freedom: How Race and Gender Shaped American Citizenship and Labor*. Cambridge, MA: Harvard University Press.

Good, Brian. 2021. "Charges Officially Dropped Against Black Mother Who Left Her Children in a Motel Room So She Could Go to Work." *DiversityInc*, June 9, 2021. https://www .diversityinc.com/charges-officially-dropped-against-black-mother-who-left-her-children -in-a-motel-room-so-she-could-go-to-work/.

Hartman, Saidiya. 2016. "The Belly of the World: A Note on Black Women's Labors." *Souls* 18 (1): 166–173. https://doi.org/10.1080/10999949.2016.1162596.

Hintzen, Amelia. 2017. "Una Mirada Histórica a Las Mujeres de Los Bateyes de La República Dominicana." In *Género y El Riesgo de Apatridia Para La Población de Ascendencia Haitiana en Los Bateyes de República Dominicana*, 2nd ed., edited by Allison J. Petrozziello, 33–50. Santo Domingo: OBMICA.

InterAmerican Court of Human Rights. 2021. "CIDH expresa preocupación por las mujeres embarazadas expulsadas en República Dominicana y llama al Estado a garantizar el acceso a mecanismos de protección y servicios de salud reproductiva." December 1, 2021. https:// www.oas.org/es/CIDH/jsForm/?File=/es/cidh/prensa/comunicados/2021/320.asp.

Indigenous Services Canada. 2018. "Reducing the Number of Indigenous Children in Care." November 2, 2018. https://www.sacisc.gc.ca/eng/1541187352297/1541187392851.

Jenson, Jane, and Denis Saint-Martin. 2003. "New Routes to Social Cohesion? Citizenship and the Social Investment State." *Canadian Journal of Sociology / Cahiers Canadiens de Sociologie* 28 (1): 77–99. https://doi.org/10.2307/3341876.

Lewis, J. 2001. "The Decline of the Male Breadwinner Model: Implications for Work and Care." *Social Politics: International Studies in Gender, State & Society* 8(2):152–69. doi: 10.1093/sp/8.2.152.

Liboiron, Max. 2021. *Pollution Is Colonialism*. Durham, NC: Duke University Press.

Listín Diario. 2021a. "Deportadas a Haití con un hijo en el vientre." December 1, 2021. https:// listindiario.com/la-republica/2021/12/01/699212/deportadas-a-haiti-con-un-hijo-en-el -vientre.

———. 2021b. "Detienen a 28 haitianas embarazadas en Maternidad de Los Mina." November 12, 2021. https://listindiario.com/la-republica/2021/11/12/696530/detienen-a-28-haitianas -embarazadas-en-maternidad-de-los-mina.

Llavaneras Blanco, Masaya. 2018. "El Convenio 189 de La OIT Desde La Perspectiva de Las Trabajadoras Domésticas Migrantes En República Dominicana: Análisis Cualitativo." Santo Domingo: FES OBMICA.

Llavaneras Blanco, Masaya. 2020. "Fanm Pa Chita: Mobilities, Intimate Labour, and Political Subjectivities among Haitian Women on the Move." PhD diss., Balsillie School of International Affairs, Wilfrid Laurier University, Waterloo, Ontario, Canada.

Lozano, Wilfredo, and Franc Báez Evertsz. 2008. "Políticas Migratorias y Relaciones Domínico-Haitianas: De La Movilidad Insular Del Trabajo a Las Presiones de La Globalización." Retos Del Desarrollo Insular. FLACSO/República Dominicana y CIES-UNIBE.

Martínez, Samuel. 2003. "Not a Cockfight." *Latin American Perspectives* 30 (3): 80–101.

———. 2007. *Decency and Excess: Global Aspirations and Material Deprivation on a Caribbean Sugar Plantation*. Boulder, CO: Paradigm.

Marsteintredet, L. 2016. Mobilisation against International Human Rights: Re- domesticating the Dominican Citizenship Regime. *Iberoamericana: Nordic Journal of Latin American and Caribbean Studies* 44(1), 73–98. https://doi.org/10.16993/ibero.11.

Mayes, April J. 2019. "Black Feminist Formations in the Dominican Republic since La Sentencia." In *Comparative Racial Politics in Latin America*, edited by Kwame Dixon and Ollie A. Johnson, 139–160. New York: Routledge.

Morrison, Toni. (1987) 2004. *Beloved*. New York: Vintage.

Murphy, Michelle. 2015. "Unsettling Care: Troubling Transnational Itineraries of Care in Feminist Health Practices." *Social Studies of Science* 45 (5): 717–737.

Narayan, Uma. 1995. "Colonialism and Its Others: Considerations on Rights and Care Discourses." *Hypatia* 10 (2): 133–140.

Noxolo, Pat, Parvati Raghuram, and Clare Madge. 2008. "'Geography Is Pregnant' and 'Geography's Milk Is Flowing': Metaphors for a Postcolonial Discipline?" *Environment and Planning D: Society and Space* 26:146–168. https://doi.org/10.1068/d81j.

Ockerman, Emma. 2021. "This Mom Was Arrested for Leaving Her Kids to Go to Work at Little Caesars." *Vice*, February 16, 2021. https://www.vice.com/en/article/n7vmyw/this-mom-was-arrested-for-leaving-her-kids-to-go-to-work-at-little-caesars.

Oficina Nacional de Estadística (ONE). 2018. "Segunda Encuesta Nacional de Inmigrantes En La República Dominicana 2017—Informe General." Santo Domingo: ONE.

Pantaleón, Doris. 2022. "El 56% de muertes maternas en el país son de haitianas." *Listín Diario*, April 21, 2022. https://listindiario.com/la-republica/2022/04/21/718160/el-56-de-muertes-maternas-en-el-pais-son-de-haitianas.

Petrozziello, Allison J. 2019. "(Re)Producing Statelessness via Indirect Gender Discrimination: Descendants of Haitian Migrants in the Dominican Republic." *International Migration* 57 (1): 213–228. https://doi.org/10.1111/imig.12527.

Picchio, Antonella. 1992. *Social Reproduction: The Political Economy of the Labour Market*. Cambridge: Cambridge University Press.

Raghuram, Parvati. 2012. "Global Care, Local Configurations—Challenges to Conceptualizations of Care." *Global Networks* 12 (2): 155–174. https://doi.org/10.1111/j.1471-0374.2012.00345.x.

———. 2019. "Race and Feminist Care Ethics: Intersectionality as Method." *Gender, Place & Culture* 26 (5): 1–25. https://doi.org/10.1080/0966369X.2019.1567471.

Razavi, Shahra. 2007. "The Political and Social Economy of Care in a Development Context: Conceptual Issues, Research Questions and Policy Options." UNRISD. https://digitallibrary.un.org/record/603418

———. 2011."Rethinking Care in a Development Context: An Introduction." *Development and Change* 42:873–903.

Reddy, Vasu, Stephen Meyer, Tamara Shefer, and Thenjiwe Meyiwa, eds. 2014. *Care in Context: Transnational Gender Perspectives*. South Africa: Human Sciences Research Council of South Africa Press.

Ricourt, Milagros. 2016. *The Dominican Racial Imaginary: Surveying the Landscape of Race and Nation in Hispaniola*. New Brunswick, NJ: Rutgers University Press.

Riveros, Natalia. 2014. "Estado de La Cuestión de La Población de Los Bateyes Dominicanos En Relación a La Documentación." Santo Domingo: OBMICA.

Robinson, Fiona. 1999. *Globalizing Care: Ethics, Feminist Theory, and International Relations*. Boulder, CO: Westview.

———. 2008. "The Importance of Care in the Theory and Practice of Human Security." *Journal of International Political Theory* 4 (2): 167–188.

———. 2018. "Care Ethics and International Relations: Challenging Rationalism in Global Ethics." *International Journal of Care and Caring* 2 (3): 319–332.

Scully, Pamela, and Diana Paton, eds. 2005. *Gender and Slave Emancipation in the Atlantic World.* Durham, NC: Duke University Press.

Sharpe, Christina Elizabeth. 2010. *Monstrous Intimacies: Making Post-slavery Subjects.* Durham, NC: Duke University Press.

Sheller, Mimi. 2012. *Citizenship from Below: Erotic Agency and Caribbean Freedom.* Durham, NC: Duke University Press.

Shoaff, Jennifer L. 2017. *Borders of Visibility: Haitian Migrant Women and the Dominican Nation-State.* Tuscaloosa: University of Alabama Press.

Vaittinen, Tiina. 2014. "Reading Global Care Chains as Migrant Trajectories: A Theoretical Framework for the Understanding of Structural Change." *Women's Studies International Forum* 47:191–202.

Williams, Fiona. 1995. "Race/Ethnicity, Gender, and Class in Welfare States: A Framework for Comparative Analysis." *Social Politics: International Studies in Gender, State and Society* 2 (2): 127–159. https://doi.org/10.1093/sp/2.2.127.

Wooding, Bridget, and Richard Moseley-Williams. 2004. "Needed but Unwanted: Haitian Immigrants and Their Descendants in the Dominican Republic." London: Catholic Institute for International Relations.

Wucker, Michele. 1999. *Why the Cocks Fight: Dominicans, Haitian, and the Struggle for Hispaniola.* New York: Hill & Wang.

11 · THE OPERATION(S) OF ABOLITIONIST CARE

Healing, Care Ethics, and the Movement for Black Lives

CHRISTOPHER PAUL HARRIS

> We are making the future as well as bonding to survive the enormous pressures of the present, and that is what it means to be a part of history.
> —Audre Lorde

> We are each other's magnitude and bond.
> —Gwendolyn Brooks

November 8, 2016, 11:08 P.M.[1]
D: *ugh*
S: *Y'all this is not f-cking good.*
E: *At all*
E: *He just won FL*
ST: *The most anxious I've been in years. These numbers are weighing heavy on my heart. I'm confused y'all*
J: *This is a nightmare*
E: *Yep. Just violence displayed on a screen.*

November 8, 2016, 11:39 P.M.[2]
C: *I love y'all. We've been through worse and we will get through whatever comes, for real*
S: *Y'all I think I was willfully blind. But I actually did not think that the country hated people like me enough to elect a literal openly racist nationalist.*
S: AND YET HERE WE ARE

November 9, 2016, 1:59 A.M.
R: *I love you all*

November 9, 2016, 1:59 A.M.
RA: *I love you like you was me. And I mean that. Stay safe tonight y'all*
CT: *I love yall.*

November 9, 2016, 2:18 A.M.
F: *Loves, let's go, how we uniting, organizing for change? We have each other.*

Several days later, in a Brooklyn backyard, a group of us assembled around a worn white table and a scattering of chairs for a healing circle. Overtop the comforting seasonal crunch of red, green, and yellow leaves. Through the speakers, rim taps followed the heavy thumps of a kick drum. The hi-hat shutter broke through our silence as the strings' slow swell matched the cadence of our purpose. The swirl of burning bundles of sage cleansed and grounded the invocation,[3] enhanced shortly after when the first verse of Solange's "Cranes in the Sky" began:

> *I tried to drink it away*
> *I tried to put one in the air*
> *I tried to dance it away*
> *I tried to change it with my hair.*[4]

Donald Trump's surprise victory—everything it represented and magnified about the country's commitment to anti-Blackness, white supremacy, and heteropatriarchy—felt like a punch to the face. That there'd be a particularly emotional response to the election of an "openly racist nationalist" by Black folks encountering the results as "violence displayed on a screen" should not be mistaken as a latent belief in the redemptive power of the state or the presidency, dashed by the soon-to-be occupant of the Oval Office. The Obama years made clear, if there were doubts, that the presidency and the state, regardless of who runs them, are instruments of the same structural logic that has oppressed Black people for centuries. Instead, the anguish reads clearest when thought of in the context of Black pain and death. Just months after the murder of Philando Castile and following the steady accumulation of Black bodies since Trayvon Martin's killing, the willful embrace of a man promoting a political agenda driven by white grievance and racial resentment further proved America's continued disregard for Black life and the impossibility of things being otherwise without transformative change.

Given the pernicious and pervasive force of anti-Blackness before and after the election, and no good reason to believe better days might be on the horizon, the healing circle was a moment to remember that, if nothing else, "we have each other." This feeling, the idea that Black people often *have each other*, and that perhaps each other is *all we have*, underscores the centrality of care and care ethics as a liberatory practice in this generation's renewal of the Black Freedom Struggle: the Movement for Black Lives (M4BL). For "Black non/being in the world," to use Christina Sharpe's formulation, care is not a "metaphor" or a moral sentiment but instead an assemblage of methods that "shape, refuse, inform, [and] speak back to material conditions."[5] These conditions are defined by anti-Blackness and its entanglement with racial capitalism, but they are also expressed within the enclosures of CIS heteropatriarchy and the carceral logic of the liberal state. An ethic of care made manifest through a praxis of interdependence that recognizes the self in relation to the collective, and the collective in relation to the self, works to undermine the legitimacy of the sociopolitical past and present—slavery, coloniality, and their afterlives—along with the ideologies that sustain them.

In this context, care must be understood as a form of "repair, maintenance, [and] attention" (Sharpe 2016, 131) that gives way to a concrete analysis of where things stand, a form of study that allows us to sift through the "enormous pressure of our present," to use Audre Lorde's (2007, 144) words, in order to grasp how best to proceed. Such an analysis requires us, in the first instance, to be vigilant about how Black pain and the structural violence(s) of the past come to bear on both the present and the future but have never dominated or defined them in any complete sense (Sharpe 2016, 5, 123). Nevertheless, violence and pain are constitutive of the operations of the capitalist world system, which makes them impossible to redress or eliminate within its purview, what Calvin Warren (2016, 44) describes as our current "cultural space of ethics, relationality, and the sacred." In the face of this cultural space, and its ability to mystify capitalism's extractive and exploitative agenda, "Black care," to borrow Warren's (2016, 44–45) framing, represents a "network of strategies aimed at circulating, communicating, and sharing" slavery's lasting imprint—the oscillation between Black life and Black death—"as a vehicle for endurance" while we sharpen our knives and plot our escape.

If we take escape seriously, if we channel the spirit of insurrection that set fire to the Minneapolis Third Police Precinct during the uprisings in 2020, it should be clear that the goal of this ethic of care is not simply to endure the world as it is or to be content with carving out pockets of reprieve, even as such pockets are, at times, a necessity. It is a world undone, a project that seeks nothing less than mustering the collective will to wrestle away from the precepts of Western modernity, to decenter them such that it becomes possible to see and refuse its internal drive toward destruction and decay, the consequences of which fall disproportionately on Black, Brown, and Indigenous communities, but also distort and undermine freedom for all (Woodly et al. 2021; Collins 1990). None of us have ever truly been free, and so nothing less will do. Consequently, those who advocate for a care ethics that remains committed to a reformed instantiation of our political institutions and modes of governance, as well-intentioned as they may be, miss the mark and fall short of the task (Casalini 2020; Tronto 2013). The demands of the present require an "abolitionist care" and praxis devoted to destroying the capitalist world system altogether (Kaba 2021; Medel 2017).

Without question, the way forward will be littered with land mines, some visible, some buried beneath the surface. But, in the final analysis, we are our own biggest threat. To prepare for the possibility of explosions, especially those unintended eruptions that emerge from unresolved harm, it's necessary to understand that the process and practice of undoing the world and our relationship to it is precisely that, a process, to be learned and experimented with through trial and error, where error often provides valuable lessons about how much of the road we have left to travel, particularly when it comes to how we treat each other.

In what follows, I consider the operation(s) of care in M4BL as I observed them while a member of the New York City chapter of the Black Youth Project 100 (BYP100), one of the movement's most prominent national organizations. Though we did not and could not always care well, the operations I sketch nevertheless gesture to the ways young Black organizers and cultural workers decenter care ethics by centering the Black diasporic experience, drawing inspiration from the teachings of Black feminism.[6] These practices of care, evidence of "a kind of Blackened knowledge" that exceeds Western ethical traditions, include approaches to healing—many reflecting a commitment to African epistemologies—and attempts to create spaces and circulate resources to shoulder pain and promote joy as we prepare for the battles to come (Sharpe 2016, 13). All with the aim of abolishing the institutions, along with the parts of ourselves, that reproduce violence and function according to the paradigms of the world as it is, so that we might more ably move closer to creating the conditions to bring about a liberated future for everyone, one where there's a collective belief that, as Gwendolyn Brooks writes, "we are each other's harvest, we are each other's business, we are each other's magnitude and bond" (Brooks 2005, 129).

WE MUST LOVE AND SUPPORT EACH OTHER: CARE ETHICS AND RELATIONALITY

The election results were not originally the occasion for our gathering. At the time, BYP100 NYC typically held chapter meetings every other Sunday. Chapter meetings bring together both active and prospective members to discuss, provide updates about, and, when necessary, vote on the chapter's work and overall direction. Generally, our meetings opened with a check-in question, such as the query, "What is something that has brought you joy this week?" After this we proceeded with the day's agenda and, more often than not, closed out with the Assata chant, a call-and-response named after its author, the revolutionary freedom fighter Assata Shakur.

> *It is our duty to fight for our freedom.*
> *It is our duty to win.*
> *We must love each other and support each other.*
> *We have nothing to lose but our chains.* (Shakur 2001, 54.)

Unlike other meetings, however, it was decided that the November 13 gathering would be a potluck and kickback.[7] In proposing the idea, chapter leadership wanted a setting that would allow us to eclipse the formalities of a typical meeting. The goal, as I understood it, was to create space for members to get to know each other better: to eat, drink, and chill as a collective even as we maintained our overall desire to map our way toward something like liberation. "Knowing," in this case, was not only about building a stronger rapport but also about establishing trust: trusting that the people you organize with were ready and willing to "throw down" when needed; that they would be willing to take arrest alongside you or help pack the court on your behalf.[8] It was about knowing they were willing to spend long hours talking through and often disagreeing about strategy and that these disagreements would be principled instead of personal.[9] It was about trusting that they were willing to hold you accountable and be held accountable themselves. It was about knowing your comrades were ready to show up for you when the weight of the work proved too heavy.

To "know," in this way, is an essential aspect of successful organizing and organization and institution building in a general sense. But driving the desire to (re)establish trust in this instance were ongoing cycles of interpersonal conflict, political disappointment, and the fallout both produced. Though at the time I'd been a chapter member for only nine months, I'd already witnessed how these cycles of conflict, much of them lingering and unresolved, eroded trust between members, and in the chapter itself. The problems ranged from the immediately actionable to those that were more deeply imbedded in and sourced from a political culture premised on capitalist social relations. Intimate partner violence, abuse between members, and how those abuses were handled by chapter and national leadership were arguably the most damaging. Not far behind, however, was the (largely accurate) perception that trans-identifying members were not being centered and, in fact, were being silenced, despite the organizational rhetoric to the contrary. Then there were all the ways toxic, masculinist behaviors were permeating our spaces in contradiction to our values; notably, these behaviors were carried out not just by male-identifying members, which reveals how the social and cultural logic of masculinity is learned rather than biologically determined. More broadly, we needed to address the justifiable frustration that men were not doing enough to show up for Black women and Black LGBTQ+ folks after their murders. Nor were we doing enough, and I include myself here, to help shoulder the emotional labor of the chapter, particularly in the face of frequent images and reports of Black premature death, labor that generally fell to women and femme-identifying members—what might be usefully labeled the "hidden abode" of Black organizing.[10]

It should come as no surprise that these conflicts mirror or were triggered by the intramural violence and aggression that have long taken place in the Black community along the gradients of class, gender, and sexuality. They were deeply enmeshed in the trauma of secondary marginalization that members experienced—often but not exclusively female-identifying and transgender and gender-nonconforming members—in their everyday lives at the hands of other

Black people, to say nothing of the disregard the rest of the world shows them. The well-warranted anger and hurt members felt, as a result, naturally showed up and reproduced themselves during chapter meetings, dialogues, and functions. Harm had a way of diminishing what many viewed as one of the only spaces they could safely (learn how to) be their full Black selves and, on a practical level, made organizing that much more difficult.

The political frustration was equally vexing, if not less personally charged. Some members felt the chapter's structure and leadership reproduced hierarchies that our political lens was meant to disrupt. For them, core leadership, as it was known, lacked transparency when it came to making decisions on behalf of the chapter in ways that made accountability for those decisions and their subsequent impact on our work difficult to exact. In other words, the deliberative and horizontal foundation of leadership models promoted by organizers like Ella Baker and pursued in the organizational structure of youth led organizations like the Student Nonviolent Coordinating Committee (SNCC) appeared, to some members, as symbolic rather than evidenced in our everyday practices.

Similar concerns about accountability and transparency were leveled at the national organization, especially when it came to decisions about its overall direction and the degree to which the values we claimed aligned with the actions we were taking. On the one hand, these critiques revolved around the organization not being sufficiently "radical," in part because it was too enmeshed in the world of nonprofits and their associated hierarchies to support and promote an abolitionist and anticapitalist agenda guided by Black queer feminist praxis. The relationship between BYP100 and the M4BL organizational ecosystem was also a point of contention, insofar as the latter was seen as taking public positions that did not fully reflect the views of all BYP100 members. At the time, at least, there were no real attempts to garner buy-in or consider objections.

A few of these instances played out publicly through social media, furthering the flames of the issue, the embers of which remain to this day. Since January 2021, for example, several BYP100 chapters have severed their relationship with the organization, citing, among other things, the organization's engagement with electoral politics, lack of transparency around budgeting, interpersonal harm, and an unwillingness to make spaces for, or adequately engage, substantive critique. These issues are by no means exclusive to BYP100. In late November 2020, following the summer of uprisings and, subsequently, a dramatic uptick in donations to movement organizations, ten local chapters of the Black Lives Matter Global Network (BLMGN), known as the BLM 10 (now the BLM10Plus), publicly broke with the organization over a similar lack of transparency and accountability.[11] As they wrote in a subsequent statement released in June 2021, "The issues we raise are bigger than simple complaints about individual leaders, but about the ways liberalism and capitalism have manifested in BLMGN and the current iteration of the Black liberation movement as a whole, co-opting and deradicalizing this critical historic moment of revolutionary possibility."[12] In both instances, the demand for transparency and accountability reflects what had been a growing tension that can be traced back to at least 2016, and, in the case of BYP100 NYC, the decision to have a kickback instead of the usual chapter meeting.

So, beyond a general belief in establishing deeper ties to bolster our organizing work, there was an equally urgent need to create the kind of environment that would make it possible to constructively address and move beyond some of the chapter's internal contradictions. But as the kickback approached and the election results became apparent, there was a general understanding among some of us that the tenor we initially imagined needed to be different—that we would have to ground and reorient ourselves to a new, unexpected political dynamic beyond our control. We carried this need collectively, knowing its traces would be born on our faces, hinted in our laughter, and suggested in our tone. The afternoon of the meeting—before the mac and cheese and soy-soaked brussels sprouts, the veggie lasagna and rotisserie chicken, the chips, dips, and doughnuts, the rum, vodka, champagne, and assorted mixers—we gathered in the backyard. We gathered to summon the strength to heal and find joy in and against a world intent on causing us—and all Black people—harm.

At the outset, the circle's facilitators—both NYC chapter members at the time—asked us to name and "lift up" someone whom we had turned to—in actuality or remembrance—during the difficult week after Election Day. From the table, Jewel picked up a large pitcher of water filled to the brim. The water had two functions: to honor the source of support we identified and invite them, in spirit, to participate in our healing. This part of the circle evoked the ancient libation pouring ritual, which is global in its origins and performance, including West African cultures and religions that then found a place in the cultural practices of the plantation. The latter was BYP100's point of reference. One by one, we held the pitcher close to our bodies, conjured our names (silently or aloud) and poured a splash of water to the ground as the rest recited in unison, "Ashe," before passing the pitcher clockwise to the next person.[13] The still of the moment, the simultaneity of sadness and strength, was a somber ritual of pain, recognition, and care. But the ceremony did not end on that note.

After the pitcher made the rounds, another facilitator—Je Naé Taylor, a member of the D.C. chapter and then a core member of BYP100's Healing and Safety Council—commanded the circle's attention. Her mission was to complete the healing process on an uplifting note. To do this, she began by recounting an anecdote of loss not attached to the present moment. Instead, it was from the past, a Black child in one of her classes killed in 2012. Fighting back tears, Je Naé proceeded to teach us all a chant she had written to help her students, and herself, to get through the pain of her student's premature death—one that, as she explained, still provides her and others uplift: "I Love Being Black." It started slowly as a call-and-response, but gradually picked up energy and volume until everyone was singing as if the song was their own, because for many of us that day, it was:

I love being Black
I said I love being Black
I said I love being Black
I said I love ...
I love the color of my skin
Cuz it's the skin that I'm in
I love the texture of my hair
And I will rock it everywhere
I love being Black
I said I love being Black
I said I love being Black
I said I love ...

The chant turned song seems, in retrospect, a fitting way to conclude the ritual. It permitted us to set aside, even if temporarily, what the election meant—the hurt that it caused—and what President Trump would likely bring about by creating a space for both self and collective care through the affirmation "I love being Black." Like the healing circle itself, the chant was a refusal, a refusal to be weighed down by pain and struggle, to be overcome by contradictions, even though it was necessary to acknowledge them first. It was an active choice to care—for ourselves and each other, drawing on non-Western epistemologies. With and through that care, we were able to find our way to joy and to celebrate our Blackness.

The ceremony marked a turning point in my understanding of the culture of the movement and its relationship to the past. I began to think more deeply about the place of healing, alters, rituals, ancestor veneration, and, more broadly, African cosmology and how this aligned with the dual emphasis on self-care and mental health I'd been observing for some time. They all represent an expression and practice of care. Just as importantly, however, they are tools sourced from African traditions and Black folk culture to acknowledge and move through pain and trauma in a way that not only refuses (white) Western practices and knowledge but does away with them altogether in search of something else. Through their performance, we assert a sense of belonging, a shared membership in, and a spiritual and political devotion to the continuum that is the Black diaspora, and the force of the diaspora's critique. In that sense, communing with the ancestors, returning to and adopting African and Black folk practices, is a process and practice of undoing toward a remade spiritual world in the here and now and a path toward a future yet to come.

HONORING BLACKNESS: CARE ETHICS AND DIFFERENCE

A world undone is an aspiration requiring individual vigilance and collective understanding, especially given how deeply rooted, long-lasting, and all-encompassing violence against Black people and Black communities has been. The effects of pain and trauma extend far beyond one's singular experience, even as its markings appear most pronounced on the individual Black body and how we subsequently interact with others. Black pain and trauma are also collective and generational. They represent the lasting consequences of slavery and colonialism as a shared memory enacted and responded to in the present (Eyerman 2001). The viral visibility of Black death marks the series of violations that has created what Elizabeth Alexander has called the Trayvon generation (Alexander 2022). The ensuing experience of trauma has become a community narrative warranting a community response. Since Trayvon Martin's murder in 2012 and the subsequent emergence of #Blacklivesmatter in 2013, this narrative has helped fortify a sense of being "a people" among younger Black folks, though equipped with new ways of approaching and embodying the full spectrum of Blackness.

Yet as the internal conflicts that roiled BYP100 NYC before (and after) our healing ceremony suggests, pain and trauma are not tied to a sense of "bottom-line Blackness" alone. We cannot reduce them entirely to how anti-Blackness has impacted Black people's lives as if we are all the same. Instead, we cannot shy away from the way pain and trauma are also deeply connected to the violence that has stemmed from—and continues to plague—gender, sexuality, and class-based differences, beyond but especially within the Black intramural. To truly begin healing from these harms and avoid repeating them, as Lorde (2007, 142) instructs, "we must allow each other our differences at the same time as we recognize our sameness." Said somewhat differently, to repair and increase our ability to practice care as a political and ethical commitment to a world undone, we must develop the capacity to attend to differences, along whatever lines they may be drawn, with careful attention and a willingness to be held accountable.

It is here, in this ethic, that the influence of Black feminism shines particularly bright and demonstrates that the arc of Black political thought—in the late twentieth century at least—has in large part advanced through the interventions of Black study and feminist praxis. After all, it was a specified and experientially based analytic within Black radical thought—promoted by Black women and anchored in care for the Black lives lived on the margins of the margins—that most forcefully sought to address the entanglements of identity within the Black community. It was Black radical feminism that demonstrated how those identities, and the conflicts they produce, were intrinsically linked to power. It was Black radical feminism that put forth the argument that if we understand oppression to be interconnected across various nodes of difference, so too is our collective liberation.

Lorde's meditation on difference and remembrance during her 1982 speech, "Learning from the 60s," delivered at Harvard's "Malcolm X Weekend," provides a useful frame and anchor. Lorde reminds us that "in the 1960s, the awakened anger of the Black community was often expressed, not vertically against the corruption of power and true sources of control over our lives, but horizontally toward those closest to us who mirrored our own impotence" (2007, 135–136). In her view, the sixties marked a particularly telling, though by no means unique, moment. The power of Black mobilization, fueled by shifts in Black people's self-understanding, was ultimately undermined by the "scars of oppression that lead us to war against *ourselves in each other* rather than against our enemies" (Lorde 2007, 135–138). Lorde's point here is not to say that these scars led Black people to withhold their fire against anti-Blackness, white supremacy, and other related structures of domination—at least not in totality. Instead, she wants to make clear that pain also tended to sharpen existing differences within the Black community itself. These differences were both ideological and, even more harmfully, rooted in how we inhabit Black flesh—the essence of who we are as Black people in the singular.

Part of what explains these self-defeating practices, Lorde (2007, 136) argues, is that "historically, difference [has] been used so cruelly against us that as a people we [are] reluctant to tolerate any diversion from what was externally defined as Blackness." And this is what makes Black self-fashioning a valuable lens to observe Black political development. From slavery onward, in the division between the free and enslaved, the respectable middle class and the backward Black masses, and the image of the masculinist militant during the Black Power and Black Arts movements, Black people have "policed" each other and, in doing so, (re)produced narrow and or anti-Black notions of Blackness and its possibilities. In Lorde's (2007, 135) reading, this blinded many from fighting "against those oppressive values which we have been forced to take into ourselves," like narrating Blackness as a "problem" or that Black expression was not befitting the proper performance of personhood. Transformation and the pursuit of liberation are equal parts external and internal; it is addressed to an anti-Black world and the anti-Blackness many of us harbor within ourselves.

Lorde's critical reflections on difference, directed in this case toward Black movement in the sixties, outline the parameters that guide current attempts to repair oppression's past and present scars and extract ourselves from their root causes. Acknowledging our differences and the aspects of those differences that make us uncomfortable is just as crucial to healing and undoing the world as recognizing the collective and structural nature of Black pain and trauma. They are, in other words, the key to making scars not only manageable but politically actionable. Regardless of how radical we imagine ourselves or our politic to be, Lorde (2007, 139) urges that we practice watchfulness such that we continually ask, self-reflectively, "In what way do I contribute to the subjugation of any part of those who I define as my people?"

These mediations concerning difference demonstrate the importance of an honest engagement with the past, to honor and care for what it might teach us about becoming something other than what we were and are. In that sense, the past is both a source of pride and a cautionary tale that should inform our present growth and build a better and different future. Lorde (2007, 135–139) puts it this way: "Through examining the combination of [Black] triumphs and errors, we can examine the dangers of an incomplete vision. Not to condemn that vision but to alter it, construct templates for possible futures, and focus our rage for change upon our enemies rather than upon each other.... To learn from their mistakes is not to lessen our debt to them, nor to the hard work of becoming ourselves, and effective." For Lorde, as it was for Frantz Fanon, the past has taught us to understand previous visions of Black liberation as necessarily incomplete. They have been experiments pursued with, and therefore limited to and by "the weapons they possessed at the time," to quote Fanon et al. (2005, 145). Their vision did not have the benefit of what we now know.

What this has meant for M4BL, and what it has meant for the development of Black politics, is clear. Though our positions may be different, this positionality—our difference—is not an excuse to blindly eat our own. Black pain and trauma are insufficient reasons to repeat within the intramural so stridently what has been done to us for centuries. As Lorde poignantly argued in an interview, "I don't have to be you in order to work with you. I don't have to be you to honor your Blackness" (Third World Newsreel 1996). Honoring Blackness does not require a strict view of what Blackness is or how Black people should be; quite the opposite, in fact. However, it does demand we recognize what anti-Blackness has meant for, and the harm it has caused to, all Black life, regardless of what other identity gets affixed to it. A radically inclusive ethics of care toward a world undone also requires a process of undoing the parts of ourselves that remain bound to the principles of the already existing world: anti-Blackness, racial capitalism, CIS heteropatriarchy, and the punitive carceral state. It requires us to understand that, to return once more to Gwendolyn Brooks (2005, 129), "we are each other's magnitude and bond." If we fail to do so, revolution won't just fail, it will never start.

THE TEAR IN THE WORLD: CARE ETHICS AND HEALING

Given the enormity of the challenges we face, the belief that confronting difference and working through generational trauma are essential components of Black struggle has made healing a cornerstone of the movement's political culture. While I encountered this firsthand as a member of BYP100—through ceremonies meant to address harmful events and more quotidian practices of alter making, sage burning, and other grounding exercises—the ethos was never confined to any one organization or to organizations at all. The BLMGN, to take one example, used to have an entire page on its website devoted to healing and "healing justice." While that page has since been replaced with an assortment of related tool kits, the original language provides valuable insight into what makes healing synonymous with radical praxis in the time of #BlackLivesMatter: "In many ways, at its essence BLM is a response to the persistent and historical trauma Black people have endured at the hands of the State. This trauma and pain, unresolved and unhealed lives on in our bodies, in our relationships and in what we create together." From the outset, the statement clarifies that M4BL is a direct response to Black pain as historically perpetuated by the state, the capitalist world system's premier institution, and the extrastate actors the state almost always shields. The residual damage caused by this pain not only "lives on in our bodies" but also infects how we relate to and build with one another. What's being described, then, is slavery, colonialism, and their afterlives, the initial "tear in the world," to use Dionne Brand's (2002) phrasing, and how that tear has subsequently breached Black being and sociality. Calling attention to that breach, to sit with the modes of relating to each other it engenders, facilitates a clarity around the extent to which our social relations are conditioned by the brute force of anti-Blackness and its attendant technologies of domination, a force that demands a response.

In that sense, healing justice also gives way to a more agentic account of living in the wake of slavery and colonialism, not just what has been done to us but, with and through that knowledge, what we must then commit ourselves to do—"wake work," as Christina Sharpe has called it. As Prentis Hemphill (2017), who was formally BLMGN's director of healing justice and likely author of the now deleted page describes, "How we protect and care for each other along the way, how we come through connected and stronger on the other end, are possibly the most critical and meaningful questions we face." The way to counter the persistence of "racial hurt," a cycle passed down and reproduced for generations, is to respond to that hurt with care (King 2008). In the present conjuncture, an ethic of care requires both an "understanding of historical and generational trauma" and the will to create liberatory spaces from which we might begin to seek and adopt practices that run contrary to carceral and otherwise punitive ways of being together; it's how we build collective strength. Regarding Black pain, to give careful attention to it is the terrain through which such imaginaries begin and become possible. The page continued as such: "Cara Page and Kindred Southern Healing Collective, through their work and commitment to our communities, offered and recovered from ancestral knowledge a framework for healing justice that guides and supports BLM's vision. We see healing justice as necessary in a society that criminalizes Blackness, and structurally ensures trauma for Black people while creating no space, time resource for healing. In this context how we treat ourselves, how we treat each other, and how we move through conflict become deeply political explorations in liberation." As was the case with the healing circle I took part in, "ancestral knowledge"—what Black people have used for centuries to create a culture of reinvention beyond the tenets of anti-Blackness—is at the forefront of movement praxis. It "guides and supports" a notion of justice through healing that does not name a juridical or legal term but instead outlines a path toward repair, a road to be with and for each other on the outer bounds of captivity. This kind of care is not secondary to notions of the "political" but is itself a "deeply political act" necessary for and "inseparable from explorations in liberation." In that sense, liberation is a practice, not just a destination; it is something we work toward and develop strategies around, rather than already known or knowable. The page concluded in the following way: "Healing justice requires that we listen beyond the understandings we've been given of spirit and ancestors, and asks us to both recover and create self-determined and effective rituals, processes for the kind of healing we need. Healing justice, then, makes room for the role of healer, for the practice of community care, in our work to get free." Here we are told once more, if any doubt remained, that the movement's points of reference, revision, and innovation are not shaped by structures and institutions that have pathologized Black or other marginalized communities. It is rather grounded in the recovery of practices that have "always sustained us and informed our struggles for liberation." By highlighting the importance of healers, calling on the ancestors, rituals, and other healing processes to guide and sustain our organizing, helping us to build trust and solidarity in service of the battles that lie ahead, they make an argument for and express a commitment to care in ways that prior instances of Black social movement did not or that were otherwise considered of secondary importance to "political" work.

Ultimately, the shift toward healing justice in the movement is premised on the conviction that Black people can no longer afford to let pain got unchecked. Nor can we permit emotional labor, and those who take that labor on, to rest at the margins of political struggle, just as we can no longer allow the historically marginalized to remain on the periphery of our visions for the future or for them to be scapegoats for why those futures are challenging to attain. In M4BL, then, healing makes care operative, often by drawing on tools our ancestors have used for their own survival and sustenance—such as sage, alters, chants, songs, rituals, and ceremonies. It attempts to draw on knowledge and value systems that are not solely or even primarily reliant on Western ideas and values. In that sense, healing is a refusal of the modern world as we know it and represents an opportunity to not only imagine but practice alternative futures, Black futures that are drawn from a past (pain) we have learned to claim.[14] As Prentis Hemphill (2017) poignantly put it, "Healing justice is [an] active intervention in which we transform the lived experience of Blackness in our world."

FUMBLING TOWARD REPAIR: CARE ETHICS AND IMAGINING THE WORLD

In BYP100, the movement's focus on healing justice and its critique of carceral power led to innovations like the Healing and Safety Council (HSC), the organizing core of which has, in recent years, been renamed the Healing and Safety Community Care Circle. Drawing on Christina Sharpe's work (which they directly cite), the change was made to reflect, as written by BYP100 members, a "sincere and thorough ... attempt to move away from carceral, state, and police logics," that are often attached to words like "council" or efforts to offer "advice," a further step afield from the path the capitalist world system presents us (BYP100 2019, 21).

The HSC was originally created in 2014 to adjudicate harm within the organization by using mediation processes grounded in an ethos of community accountability and transformation, to hold space for reimagining justice "from an abolitionist perspective and through diverse practices of Black radical care" (BYP100 2019, 21; Green et al. 2018, 912). When I was involved, each of BYP100's chapters had at least one and ideally two HSC representatives dedicated to supporting this task, and the organization maintained a paid staff member charged with coordinating and advancing this aspect of our work. While the HSC's mandate hinged on intervening when conflict or harm took place, and to do so in ways that do not reproduce the carceral state's desire to exact and profit from Black disposability—a tactic that itself reflects the hold of Black (social) death—this was only one part of a larger goal (Green et al. 2018, 913). The intention was also to *prevent* such harms and conflicts from happening in the first place, to be "a proactive and preventive means for Black queer activists to practice healing in community, collective, and self," in order to help "seed Black liberation organizational work that is radically caring, deeply accountable, and wondrously inclusive" (BYP100 2019, 2).

At our national convenings, for example, the HSC curated dedicated healing rooms where members could access a variety of ways to touch base with and center the self so as to proceed with the sometimes difficult work of being in community. As described by former HSC core members, these included "one-on-one sessions with Reiki practitioners, somatic practitioners, herbalists, tarot-card readers, guided meditations, yoga classes, tables for quiet crafting, and areas simply to rest" (Green et al. 2018, 912). The motivation behind maintaining a healing space was to provide a sanctuary where people who needed to ground themselves, in one way or another, could do so. By offering such an environment, the HSC hoped to help quell any tensions that might arise and cultivate a container for any past trauma people might have brought with them.

One of the most meaningful and potentially enduring ways the HSC has tried to be "proactive and preventive" is by creating a guidebook called *Stay Woke, Stay Whole: A Black Activist Healing Manual*. With editions in 2017 then subsequently updated and expanded in 2019, the manual aimed to be a resource people could hold and take with them, allowing activists in the movement to effectively pursue, as the manual explains, "transformative justice by working through our own hurt and harm so that we are not harming ourselves or others" (BYP100 2017, 2). Both editions include "a compilation of resources, stories, interviews with elders, ancestral healing practices, and other remedies for healing" to concretize the healing process as an integral part of a collective praxis armed with an understanding of Black trauma and pain, and the knowledge that we've inherited a long tradition of Black survival, resistance, and rebellion predicated on community well-being (Green et al. 2018, 916).

Activist- and practitioner-generated tools like *Stay Woke, Stay Whole* are important not only because they offer an invaluable, educative resource for people actively engaged in on the ground organizing work but also because they allow healing practices, and the motivations behind them, to circulate beyond the organizations themselves in ways that aren't reliant on those who already possess such knowledge. It was the first edition of *Stay Woke, Stay Whole*, which has a section devoted to understanding and unpacking examples of how Black people use and have used "spirituality and culture as a mode of resistance," that provided further context for me to think about the different elements at play in the healing circle I participated in after the 2016 election (BYP100 2017, 2). A similar thing can be said about BYP100's *The Black Joy Experience Resource Guide*, which allows for the circulation of chants and other freedom songs prominent in the movement among those not already in the fold.

These and other efforts to outline and implement a healing justice framework beyond and against the punitive and individuating protocols of the capitalist world system demonstrate how and why healing has become a mechanism to decenter care ethics and make care operative in the #time of BlackLivesMatter. They also show that, when it comes to imagining otherwise, a sociality premised on nondomination and horizontal community exchange in league with the plantation politics of the enslaved, the movement is doing more than just toiling in theoretical ideas of what *could* or *should* be. Instead, the aim is to, in Je Naé Taylor's words, "model what a commitment to loving Black lives means" (Green et al. 2018, 922). This commitment is a collective and intramural charge, grounded in a belief that the "weight of care does not belong to one person;" and more broadly that care for all Black people is perhaps the most powerful (and accessible) tool we have to wield in an anti-Black world—a testament to our strength (Green et al. 2018, 922).

Harnessing this power such that it can seed and sustain the revolution we need involves being accountable to each other and ourselves. It consists of acknowledging and learning from differences. It means being vulnerable and open to personal growth. It requires tending to the traumas of the past. The HSC was not impervious to these requirements in reflecting on its own work and trajectory. In a brief letter that opens the second edition of *Stay Woke, Stay Whole*, Christopher Roberts, a scholar of Black memory and one of the HSC's founding members, writes the following: "We would be remiss if we did not say that there have been many times where we failed, where we caused harm when we were asked to help, where we were unable to hold people accountable, where we were unable to be our best selves, where we left people disappointed and hurt. There were many times where we were, as Mariame Kaba and Shira Hassan say, 'fumbling towards repair'" (BYP100 2019, 2; Kaba and Hassan 2019). Roberts's admission is further proof of just how messy this work is, has been, and will be, even when our efforts are aimed in the right direction—against punishment and carcerality. I have witnessed firsthand instances in which the HSC, as an experiment in Black radical care, fell short. But by owning up to past failures, by clearly articulating responsibility for harm and disappointment, Roberts points to how we can fumble toward repair instead of falling back into harmful repetition. This means holding ourselves and each other accountable, yes, but also analyzing and taking steps to address the things that went wrong—care is a form of study.

Taken as a whole, healing as an operation of care in M4BL is deeply connected to Black living precisely because it directly engages Black pain and Black death, which represent the baseline conditions for Black life. We do this with intention and with an understanding of the stakes, stakes that make reform-minded care ethics, a modality of care that remains burdened by Western assumptions about political institutions and governance, inadequate to the task (Casalini 2020; Tronto 2013). Our present demands an abolitionist care and all the messiness that arises when we attempt to live otherwise (Kaba 2021; Medel 2017). As Je Naé Taylor explains, "This is not for the faint. It means meeting people in the darkest and most uncomfortable situations, practicing patience and compassion in trying times.... We are trying, we are daring to imagine the world we want in our lifetime" (Green et al. 2018, 922). A healing justice framework seeks a world that "promote[s] healthy Black people who love themselves," a world that is not yet here but in the making (Green et al. 2018, 922). In other words, it seeks a society that actually cares, which means engaging in a project of "unsettling" Western ethical traditions and replacing them with the knowledges and experiences of those the West has historically plundered, not as an end game, or an answer, or a conclusion, but as a beginning, and a place to start imagining the world from a place of possible futures.

ACKNOWLEDGMENTS

This chapter is a modified version of a chapter that appears in the author's book, *To Build a Black Future*, published with Princeton University Press.

NOTES

1. The following dialogue took place on BYP100 NYC's Group Me, which is a widely used group messaging device, the evening of Donald Trump's election in 2016. Because the names of the people involved in this discussion are not germane to its meaning and play no further role in the narrative, I have chosen to indicate them only by first initial. In instances where the first initial repeats itself, I have elected to include an additional letter from their name.
2. While at this point the election had not been officially called for Trump, things were decidedly pointing in that direction. The AP officially announced Trump as the winner at 2:41 A.M.
3. Sage is often present in movement circles. It is understood to be both cleansing and grounding, and its usage is derived from its historical place in slave medical treatments.
4. Solange Knowles, "Cranes in the Sky," from her 2016 album *A Seat at the Table*.
5. The phrasing and sentiment about care and material conditions are owed to Dr. Ashante M. Reese (@AMReese07) from a Twitter post on January 29, 2021, https://twitter.com/AMReese07/status/1355192387035930628.
6. I'd like to thank Fiona Robinson for offering the language to capture one of this chapter's major themes—that "movements of care cannot always care well."
7. A "kickback" simply refers to a planned social gathering that falls just sort of a full-fledged party.
8. Packing the court refers to galvanizing community support to be present in the courthouse during and after an arraignment. It also often includes care packages for the people who spend time in a holding cell while waiting to see a judge.

9. The idea of "principled struggle," most often attributed to activist and community organizer NTanya Lee, acknowledges that "to learn and to grow, is to struggle," that "struggle is a condition for change and liberation," and that within and beyond the movement we must "work to foster and cultivate spaces... to move through conflict in a way that makes us better" (quoted from BYP100's Freedom Forecast distributed internally in 2018).
10. Hidden abode is a reference to Marx's description of the unseen dimensions of capitalism (Marx and Mandel 1992).
11. For the full statement, see #BLM10, "It Is Time for Accountability," *Statement from the Frontlines of BLM*, November 30, 2020, https://www.blmchapterstatement.com/no1/.
12. For the subsequent statement, see YahNé Ndgo, "Tell No Lies," *Statement from the Frontlines of BLM*, June 10, 2021, https://www.blmchapterstatement.com/no2/.
13. The word "ashe" is frequently used throughout the movement ecosystem. Drawn from the West African Yoruba religion, it is meant in this context to harken back to our collective African roots as well as the power we collectively hold to produce change.
14. For a discussion of another kind of politics of refusal—this time within a Canadian context—see the work by Doucet, Jewell, and Watts in this volume (chapter 7).

REFERENCES

Alexander, Elizabeth. 2022. *The Trayvon Generation*. New York: Grand Central.
Black Youth Project 100. 2017. *Stay Woke, Stay Whole: A Black Activist Healing Manual*, vol. 1.
———. 2019. *Stay Woke, Stay Whole: A Black Activist Healing Manual*, vol. 2.
Brand, Dionne. 2002. *A Map to the Door of No Return: Notes to Belonging*. Toronto: Vintage Canada.
Brooks, Gwendolyn. 2005. *The Essential Gwendolyn Brooks:* Edited by Elizabeth Alexander. New York: Library of America.
Casalini, Brunella. 2020. "Care and Injustice." *International Journal of Care and Caring* 4 (1): 59–73. https://doi.org/10.1332/239788219X15730452949174.
Collins, Patricia Hill. 1990. "The Social Construction of Black Feminist Thought." *Signs: Journal of Women in Culture and Society* 14 (4): 745–773.
Eyerman, Ron. 2001. *Cultural Trauma: Slavery and the Formation of African American Identity*. Cambridge: Cambridge University Press.
Fanon, Frantz, Jean-Paul Sartre, and Homi K. Bhabha. 2005. *The Wretched of the Earth*. Translated by Richard Philcox. Anniversary ed. New York: Grove Press.
Green, Kai M., Je Naé Taylor, Pascale Ifé Williams, and Christopher Roberts. 2018. "#BlackHealingMatters in the Time of #BlackLivesMatter." *Biography* 41 (4): 909–941.
Hall, Joan Wylie, ed. 2004. *Conversations with Audre Lorde*. Jackson: University Press of Mississippi.
Hemphill, Prentis. 2017. "Healing Justice Is How We Can Sustain Black Lives." *HuffPost*, February 7, 2017. https://www.huffpost.com/entry/healing-justice_b_5899e8ade4b0c1284f282ffe.
Kaba, Mariame. 2021. *We Do This 'til We Free Us: Abolitionist Organizing and Transforming Justice*. Chicago: Haymarket Books.
Kaba, Mariame, and Shira Hassan. 2019. *Fumbling towards Repair: A Workbook for Community Accountability Facilitators*. Workbook ed. Chicago: Project NIA.
King, Debra Walker. 2008. *African Americans and the Culture of Pain*. Charlottesville: University of Virginia Press.
Lorde, Audre. 2007. *Sister Outsider: Essays and Speeches*. Repr. ed. Berkeley, Calif: Crossing Press.
Marx, Karl, and Ernest Mandel. 1992. *Capital: Volume 1: A Critique of Political Economy*. Translated by Ben Fowkes. Illustrated ed. London: Penguin.

Medel, China. 2017. "Abolitionist Care in the Militarized Borderlands." *South Atlantic Quarterly* 116 (4): 873–883. https://doi.org/10.1215/00382876-4235084.
Shakur, Assata. 2001. *Assata: An Autobiography*. Chicago: Lawrence Hill Books.
Sharpe, Christina. 2016. *In the Wake: On Blackness and Being*. Illustrated ed. Durham, NC: Duke University Press.
Third World Newsreel. 1996. *A Litany for Survival: The Life and Work of Audre Lorde*. https://video.alexanderstreet.com/watch/litany-for-survival-the-life-and-work-of-audre-lorde-a-90-min.
Tronto, Joan C. 2013. *Caring Democracy: Markets, Equality, and Justice*. 3/13/13 ed. New York: New York University Press.
Warren, Calvin. 2016. "Black Care." *liquid blackness* 3 (6): 36–46.
Woodly, Deva, Rachel H. Brown, Mara Marin, Shatema Threadcraft, Christopher Paul Harris, Jasmine Syedullah, and Miriam Ticktin. 2021. "The Politics of Care." *Contemporary Political Theory* 20 (4): 890–925. https://doi.org/10.1057/s41296-021-00515-8.

12 · WHEN FACTS ONLY GO SO FAR

Decentering What It Means to Know and Understand as a Care-Ethical Researcher in a Polarized, Post-Truth Era

ALISTAIR NIEMEIJER AND MEREL VISSE

> This is a fraud on the American public. This is an embarrassment to our country. We were getting ready to win this election. Frankly, we did win this election.... So our goal now is to ensure the integrity for the good of this nation. This is a very big moment.... We want the law to be used in a proper manner. So we'll be going to the US Supreme Court. We want all voting to stop. We don't want them to find any ballots at four o'clock in the morning and add them to the list. To me this is a very sad moment and we will win this. And as far as I'm concerned, we already have won it.
> —President Trump on election night

On the night of the 2020 presidential election, former president Donald Trump gave a perplexing speech where he talked about his leads in key states and said, "Frankly, we did win this election," appearing to claim victory before many states finished counting votes. According to news organization CNN, it was one of the most factually untrue speeches Trump had delivered up to that point. Ever since, Donald Trump has made the "stolen" 2020 election the centerpiece of his post–White House political life. Virtually every statement he has made has invoked this false claim. What is worrying is that polling has shown it has been effective, not just with the crowd that stormed the Capitol on his behalf on January 6, 2021, but with most members of the Republican Party electorate almost a year and a half later.

This is of course not an isolated incident but a growing trend that appears to be related to an increasing autocratic populism that seems to thrive on polarization and misinformation, also highlighting the rising interest in illiberal and religious conservative views of democracy.[1] In parallel, the uptick in the promulgation of conspiracy theories has already been widely reported and often has more feeding ground in times of crisis and increased polarization—the so-called post-truth era. According to the Institute for Strategic Dialogue, when public figures spread conspiracy theories, the reach of these narratives is expanded exponentially, as they point to research from the Reuters Institute last year that concluded that politicians, celebrities, and public figures generated 69 percent of social media engagement around COVID-19 misinformation, even though they accounted for only 20 percent of the misleading posts. What are sometimes at first marginal ideas confined to the fringes of the web can become a disinformation ecosystem in itself, a manifestation of mass false consciousness in service of a political-economic system that serves specific strategic interests (DiMaggio 2022).

Obviously, this poses problems for liberal democracies, which strongly depend on shared truths and an acceptance of certain facts. How should liberal democracies deal with these post-truth contexts that have as their central aim to destabilize and to make precarious our ways of knowing, where what we know is no longer certain or, conversely, fallacious in its misplaced concreteness? And what does this mean for the care ethical researcher? There is of course no doubt that care ethical researchers might respond that our claims to knowledge—especially moral knowledge of what is good or right—are always "unstable," never fixed, always open to revision, and always plural.[2] But if we indeed assume unstable and plural knowledge, how can we understand, as care ethical researchers, the moral good in particular settings in a time where any claim to knowledge is automatically considered equivocal? How do we as care ethicists balance the polyphony of voices, some backed up by evidence, and some lacking any argument or logic? These questions are especially meaningful if we aim to develop a political care ethics that counters the dominance or opposing power of certain types of knowing, while other types and sources of knowledge are subordinated and obscured (Visse, Abma, and Widdershoven 2015; Visse and Abma 2018). These are the central questions of this chapter.

A NOTE OF COUNSEL TO THE READER

Before you read on, however, we would immediately like to alert the reader. In order for us to practice a so-called decentering of our *own* ways of knowing, reading on will mean embarking on a somewhat capricious journey, at least from a scholarly point of view, because the form that this text takes is perhaps not one of offering up a classical philosophical argument (i.e., introducing a proposition and then giving good reasons, grounds, or evidence for accepting the conclusion). Rather, what we plan to do in the text is to practice a "generative critique" (cf. Jerak-Zuiderent 2015; Verran 2001, 20), whereby one looks for "possibilit[ies] of innovation, a way that things might be done differently to affect futures different from pasts." This may seem ambiguous sometimes, but we favor this form over a more traditional philosophical argument, as we want to show what it means to decenter knowing by generating a shift in experiential perspective. We do so through creating a space for the reader to vicariously live the plural and agonal that may accompany the process of decentering. Aligning with postmodern writers, instead of communicating a clear message, we want to invite readers to generate their own interpretations. Academic scholars have experimented with this approach for quite some time (e.g., Braidotti 1994; Derrida 1967; hooks 1990; Kristeva 1987). So instead of imposing our argument and conclusions, or convincing readers of a (shared) truth, we aim to enable and invite readers to form their own judgments and conclusions through generative critique (Jerak-Zuiderent 2015; Verran 2001, 20). We write evocatively and for openness, demonstrating the possible roles of a care ethical researcher in practice (for a recent excellent guide on how to conduct empirical research "with care," see Brannelly and Barnes 2022). Here, the researcher (or the reader) is not a judge searching for facts steered by an argumentative rationality, evoking a competitive element of either criticizing or defending. Instead, the researcher may become a facilitator of plural narrative perspectives in play, holding them up without losing distinctiveness, interweaving a variety of practical and theoretical voices. With this text, we knit together perspectives as well, but we also hope to maintain the relative independence of the voices and examples, enabling readers to experience the narrated examples from a multiplicity of perspectives.

In what follows, we pay particular attention to how care ethics decenters traditional Euro-Western epistemology, which is characterized by reductionist and positivist views of knowing. We contend that although rational consensus is hard to reach and belief polarization is inevitable, especially during crises such as the COVID-19 pandemic, it might also be seen as a productive possibility, acknowledged as a "dimension of antagonism... to be constitutive of human societies" (Mouffe 2005, 9). A care ethics approach enriched by the notion of plural and *precarious knowing* may provide a further guide to understand and respond to conflictual views. With what we dub "precarious knowing" in our upcoming book (Visse and Niemeijer forthcoming), we join those who decenter dominant Euro-Western, positivist approaches to knowing that imply an absolutist or universal notion of truth, without completely rejecting them. These may lead to deep disagreements in everyday practices and lives. Our approach to precarious knowing is a response to that and acknowledges and actively works with the existence of many truths and many stories and many situations of tension.

CARE ETHICS AS INHERENTLY DECENTERING

Whether it was to argue that women's moral experiences were not reflected in the dominant, masculinist approaches to ethics, which were centered on a rational, atomistic moral agent, or to expand scholarly discussions to the realms of both private and public life, care ethics has always been in the business of decentering traditional approaches to knowing. Indeed, this includes decentering care ethics scholarship itself. For example, second-generation care studies critically analyzed the limitations of first-generation writings and considered the relevance of care beyond the domains of gender and social and healthcare settings (Hankivsky 2005). These authors aimed to disentangle care from care studies' view of care as a set of values or an attitude—and to strive toward an understanding of care and its ethics from a sociopolitical perspective. Politically oriented care ethicists have explored the meaning of a practice-oriented perspective, seeing care as "a collective and political practice that builds up society" (van Nistelrooij 2015, quoted in Leget, van Nistelrooij, and Visse 2019, 18). This implies that care is more than a virtue, bound to persons. Some scholars and researchers perceive care as a paradigm: a way of being that is accompanied by a shift in moral thinking representing something different than a normative theory of moral adjudication (Stake and Visse 2021). These thinkers radically acknowledge the epistemological underpinnings of care as embodied and dialectically connected with our moral, relational selves (Hamington 2012a, 2012b).

Most care ethicists nowadays conceive a caring practice as an inherently collaborative moral practice or a moral ecology formed by normative expectations and negotiated responsibilities (Walker 2007; Visse and Abma 2018). If morality itself consists of practices rather than principles, this also comes with new responsibilities. As Margaret Urban Walker points out, we should "attempt to find out what people are doing in bringing moral evaluation to bear ... on what they and others do and care about, and whether some ways of doing what they are doing are better than others" (Walker 2007, 16). Working from this notion of practice, care becomes an empirically grounded way of being, doing, saying, thinking, and experiencing. Taking seriously the idea that all knowledge is—among other things—contextually and collaboratively mediated and determined, notions of "good care" are bound to moral understandings in specific contexts. Walker (2007) opposes her collaborative-expressive approach to morality to the theoretical-judicial model, the dominant form of ethics in the Western moral theory, expressed in (neo-)Kantian (deontological) and utilitarian ethics. The expressive-collaborative model builds upon the work of Sara Ruddick (1995), whose practicalist notion of truth implies that truth, knowledge, and the evidence required to consider them are socially constructed and embedded practices.

One of the key critical insights of care ethics can thus be formulated as follows: morality and questions about the moral good consist in practices, rather than in principles or essentialist truths, and unfold in sociopolitical contexts. This entails that as care ethical researchers we have to be continually aware that our "modes of understanding" are repeatedly affected and influenced by the time and place we find ourselves in and that our knowledge is continuously "in becoming" and precarious.

EPISTEMICALLY UNSTABLE TIMES

If the COVID-19 pandemic has taught us one thing, it is that crises on such a scale will evidently have destabilizing effects on even the most evidently stable pluralist democracies. For instance, the *Washington Post* alarmingly declared in March 2020 that "coronavirus kills its first democracy" after the Hungarian parliament had voted to give Prime Minister Viktor Orbán the authority to rule by decree in the name of fighting COVID-19 (Tharoor, 2020). Human rights watch organizations have reported that since the coronavirus outbreak began, democracy and human rights have worsened in eighty countries, with particularly sharp deterioration in struggling democracies and highly repressive states (Repucci and Slipowitz 2020).

But even in less repressive more liberal countries, such as the Netherlands, emotions ran high every time (new or additional) restrictive measures were taken, as civilians differed dramatically in their views about what should be done, for whom, when, and why. These views coming up against each other would sometimes lead to violent confrontations between caregivers and (family of) care receivers who disagreed whether safety should always be prioritized over proximity,[3] and even led to riots on the streets in several Dutch cities as a result of an imposed evening curfew (Wikipedia 2023). Most countries were, and are still, vulnerable to this surge in mob mentality and strong antagonism between different factions of society. In the early 1900s, D. H. Lawrence's political novels already warned about "affective contagion" among crowds (Lawtoo 2020), exacerbating contradictions between different groups by (both the lack and the peddling of) (mis)information, all of which ultimately led to an increase in tensions between different factions in society. In the Netherlands, King Willem-Alexander even warned us in his annual speech of 2021 that social debate was increasingly being conducted in a "polarizing" way. The fear of polarization became so great during the pandemic that preventing polarization actually played an important role in the government's consideration of the use of control measures.

Polarization can indeed have undesirable consequences and even be threatening for democracy itself. However, the question is whether polarization can be prevented during a global (health) crisis—such as the COVID-19 pandemic—and what a care ethics approach, characterized by interconnectedness, constructive critique, and gathering for solidarity and support, can offer (Solnit 2017, 18). After all, in such a crisis governments are forced to make difficult choices in short time spans, when it is often unavoidable that one value or practice prevails over the other. While the COVID-19 pandemic crisis has affected people all around the world, it has not affected everyone in the same way. Besides glaring international differences, variations in personal and situational factors resulted in strikingly dissimilar effects even on people within the same country. For instance, in the Netherlands, the values of protection and control were at times so prevalent that the effects were detrimental, especially for those people who are (more) vulnerable to marginalization and precaritization during crises as concerns over safety and public health are likely to trump consideration for inclusion and care. As in most countries, the Netherlands initially adopted a fairly one-sided medicalized conception of risk, primarily aimed at eliminating any possibility of becoming ill, thereby avoiding "catastrophe" (cf. Beck 2006). The result, especially for people receiving residential care, was immediate and grave. The majority of Dutch care providers no longer allowed any visitors at all, afraid of possible health risks for both clients and care staff, and critical questions about banning family visits were not considered relevant, as most care providers had their hands full with all the measures to avoid contamination.

However, since people receiving residential care have few other personal relationship, contact with their families is almost by definition essential. The restrictive measures limited their (already relatively limited) freedom of movement and agency even more. Further, residents often failed to understand the measures and their implications because of their disability. Consequently, the risks faced by people who received residential care in the lockdown were much broader than (somatic) health risks. Their whole lives had been turned upside down, while years had often been spent trying to find a balance in routines and daytime activities wherein they thrive. Psychological, emotional, and relational damage was significant. Unfortunately, there was only limited space for their voices to be heard, if they were even articulated at all. Assuming people receiving (institutionalized) forms of care can always speak for themselves is of course naïve, but the experiences of this particular group had no place in the dominant policy discourse.

It is characteristic of any crisis that situations arise in which values or practices clash and (groups of) citizens do indeed stand up for their values and interests. It is in fact a tenet of any democracy that this is permissible. People are allowed to think radically different about (such) fundamental matters. So the question is not whether polarization (in crisis) can or should be prevented but rather how we can guide the process of polarization, which is so corrosive that it starts to erode the very tenets that allow it in the first place. To postpone resolution in crisis, even to gain understanding from a plural stance can be construed as an avoidance of care. But when it leads to a dominance of certain values and growing polarization, we need to sense the cost of it, the hurt of it, and even the benefit of it. When does polarization diminish to indifference? And should the voice and vote of the presumptuous but fully persuaded not count as much as those of the reasoned and experienced if we are to treat each other with the dignity that should be accorded to all citizens? Who decides which knowledge counts and how much it weighs?

DIFFERENT FORMS OF KNOWING

The current polarized context paradoxically elevates fringe knowledge while also marginalizing and subordinating many forms of knowledge. In the case of the latter, this is however not a recent trend, as many forms of knowing have been either less visible or not considered worthy of attention due to decades of oppression by mainstream, white male, Euro-Western approaches to research. As Vrinda Dalmiya (2016) has so convincingly shown, conventional approaches, specifically in moral theory, projected their knowers as disembedded, abstract, and supposedly neutral reasoners who arrive independently at the same context-free, universal rules. In contrast, the knower of her care-based epistemology uses her experience of concrete situations to reflect on them as well as to tease out ways of behaving appropriately in similar situations in the future (Kirloskar-Steinbach 2018). Dalmiya pushes her knower toward relational humility, being part of messy interpersonal relationships with complex moral and affective demands, practicing perceptiveness to the needs of another. Dalmiya's critique also resonates strongly with a broader discussion within the ethics of care, namely how reflexive we are as care ethical scholars regarding our own position (of privilege), as the feminist tradition that care ethics originates from has been viewed as a form of white feminism (see, for instance, Zakaria 2021; Banarjee 2020). If we want to challenge privilege, diversify, and decenter care ethics and truly build toward (transnational) solidarities, this should always start with a critical reflection on our own identity, positionality, and concomitant theoretical biases.

One example of marginalized knowledge is Indigenous knowledge on health and healing, based on centuries of practices and holistic views of medicine. These forms of medicine, just like other non-Western approaches to medicine (so-called neoteric approaches), are as intricate, sophisticated, and valuable as Euro-Western approaches, and may complement mainstream (allopathic) diagnostic and treatment. Yet these approaches were structurally ignored and oppressed in the United States starting with the closing of Black and female medical schools after the publication of the *Flexner Report*, sponsored by the American Medical Association (Flexner 1910; Gurstelle 2022). Consequentially, Western medical schools became the norm, while Indigenous approaches became estranged from their own cultural forms, which either have been destroyed or are reviled, resulting in severe trauma and public and individual health challenges (Gurstelle 2022). As such, decentering medicine—and science in general—and opening up to learning about Indigenous approaches to knowing may be synonymous with growth and healing. Of course, we can never fully know these approaches having not been socialized in these communities ourselves, but several initiatives to integrate Indigenous viewpoints in medical curricula show an increase of cultural safety and the quality of medicine.

Another example is the continuous oppression of nonverbal, poetic approaches to knowledge development such as arts-based approaches, increasingly reframed as "creative practice-led research" (Vear 2022). Despite a growing interest by qualitative researchers and care ethicists (Thompson 2022; Visse, Hansen, and Leget 2019, 2020; Visse 2017; Hamington and Rosenow 2019; Hamington 2015), many mainstream journals ignore or do not perceive arts-based or creative-practice-led research as viable, rigorous approaches and oppress these by ignoring them, despite successful efforts to develop cohesive frameworks and criteria that foster rigor (Vear 2022). For example, Boydell et al. (2016), who conducted a study around the tensions experienced regarding academic legitimacy and the use of the arts in producing and disseminating research, have argued for the need to transcend "hegemonic conventions" by reconsidering what counts as knowledge in order to support the effective production and dissemination of arts-based approaches.

A third example is related to and deals with the acknowledgment of experiential forms of knowledge in medical research. Scientific medical research has been the exclusive domain of (bio- or para-) medical scientists. Research is often initiated by researchers from a scientific perspective (bottom-up) or by institutes, funding organizations, or patient organizations funding research (top-down). Theme choice, appraisal, and prioritizing are usually made only from the scientific perspective. This is changing with a general trend toward more emancipation and exerting democratic rights by citizens with disabilities or chronic illnesses. "Experiential knowledge" of patients is often seen as essentially different from other more explicit forms of "expert" knowledge such as professional knowledge and scientific knowledge (Baillergeau and Duyvendak 2016). It is a term that has been used widely to account for the experiential and particularistic ways of knowing the world that people draw upon to assess risks, evaluate expert knowledge, and make decisions, particularly in relation to health (Boardman 2014). It is also seen as knowledge that in part can be articulated but in part is also silent or tacit knowledge (Polanyi 1966), which does not originate from applying generalizable rules (knowing how instead of knowing that; cf. Ryle 1945). "Knowledge" here refers not only to experiential data (i.e., bodily awareness of phenomena) but also to insights (viz., connections between the phenomena), memories (of what functioned in the past or not), and expertise (practical savoir faire including an orientation on future action). The contribution of specifically addressing experiential knowledge of patients lies partly in it being the basis for their self-care, as Storni (2015) found that the patient's own knowledge and expertise is critical to integrating clinical knowledge in their everyday chronic self-care. Acknowledging this knowledge as valid also meets a strong need of patients to be understood on their own terms as for "the patient, whether their own knowledge (whatever its source) is acknowledged or accepted by their health-care provider can be crucial" in the patient-caregiver relationship (Papen and Walters 2008, 11). In fact, a growing body of studies assert that experiential knowledge of patients should be an important source of professional learning for practitioners (Gidman 2013; Politi et al. 2013). Experiential knowledge of patients in the health research cycle can lead to legitimacy (as a democratic approach), to an increased likelihood of implementation in practice, and, most importantly, to better decision making and more commitment to the studies' results.

Moving from these three examples on epistemological injustice (cf. Fricker 2017), how does this pertain to the response of the care ethical researcher to polarization and post-truth tendencies? A more generative care ethical research approach liberates us from restrictive, scientifically fixated, singular approaches that neglect parts of our reality. Care ethics research might then be reframed as a decentering approach in a structural, psychological, ethical, but also metaphysical way. Here, decentering relies on a transformed experience and comprehension of plural realities, acknowledging and working with collaborative-expressive human and nonhuman entanglements, in the context of relationality, dependencies, vulnerabilities, materialities, and more. But also with attention to the epistemological power dynamics, *who* or *what* intends, thinks, speaks, acts in a particular context? And, honoring Indigenous views that highlight located, place-based knowing, as Riikka Prattes shows us in her chapter in this volume (chapter 4), *where* is the speaker located, historically and nowadays?

THE "TRUTH" OF MASS PSYCHOLOGY

As corrosive polarization encompasses one of the bigger challenges of the twenty-first century, liberal democracies must look for ways to prevent and/or regulate it, without neglecting the epistemic responsibilities (Sari 2018) that come along with being a sound democracy, falling into the trap of so-called solutions that would in fact preclude any debate. This entails that different social and cultural groups that adhere to different interests and values may and can exist within society and that these groups can and may conflict with each other. This is especially challenging when values collide, when people can't agree on the most basic of facts, and where mass psychology sets in. What we saw during the pandemic (and perhaps preceding that, during the Trump administration) was therefore also an *epistemic* crisis regarding what citizens perceived to be true and false. The pandemic showed not only that different values can clash during a health crisis but also that there are fundamental differences in what knowledge certain groups use to deal with the actual uncertainties of the COVID-19 crisis. This manifested itself, for example, around issues such as the effectiveness of masks (remedial or useless), vaccines, distancing measures, and the risk (and even existence) of the coronavirus. Issues such as fake news and disinformation play(ed) an important role here. For instance, Rerimassie et al. (2021) researched the so-called sensemaking processes of citizens to deal with the uncertainty of the COVID-19 crisis. From this it turned out, among other things, that when dealing with factual uncertainties, citizens often let themselves be informed by people in their social circle and their (and their own) experiences with the coronavirus. But there were also bitter arguments between family member and friends, leading to separation and estrangement. Evidently, mildness or severity of an infection is of great importance. The impact of measures on the living environment of citizens or their friends or family is also a major factor. When the medicine (measures) is worse than the ailment, it can sometime have consequences for how the ailment itself is understood.

We should, however, take heed of Dutch philosopher Sabine Roeser, who argues that (negative) emotions of citizens, strongly reinforcing polarized views, were too easily brushed aside by authorities during the pandemic, which was ultimately a denial of the social impact of the pandemic and the measures to avert it

(Roeser 2022). American sociologist Arlie Hochschild (2016) discovered something similar when she went to the Deep South to study an emerging conservative identity and came away with a more nuanced understanding for the rise of Trumpism. Even though it would seem that many people attracted to Trumpism would actually benefit more from "liberal" policies, she found that it was indeed their precarious circumstances (stagnant wages, a loss of home, an elusive American dream) but also a dominant liberal stream in media and academia that appeared to not only reject but cancel all of their traditional views, which drove them to become attracted to Trumpism as a form of resentment politics. In a sense, a rebuke of Trump and his actions was internalized as a personal attack on his supporters (Thompson 2020).

Clearly, the moral-psychological perspective of affective, contagious, and bodily relations between authorities and the general public has not received the attention it deserves. The sense of overwhelming crisis revealed that the public was not necessarily acting by reason. We turn to D. H. Lawrence (1994, 298) again, who wrote that a "mass is not even formed by reason. The more intense or extended the collective consciousness, the more does the truly reasonable, individual consciousness sink into abeyance."

Nevertheless, Roeser (2022), in addition, argues that important moral knowledge is hidden in the emotions that citizens experience and that they must be taken seriously in order to learn from them. This is noble, but is it within reach? Here too the pluralism of emotions plays an important role in the previous forms of pluralism. The research of Rerimassie et al. (2021) showed, among other things, that the exhausting nature of the pandemic means that citizens like to reason toward an epistemological outcome that brings comfort. Against this background, it is crucial to gain and maintain insight into the different emotions and moral-psychological response of the public as a mass surrounding polarized discussions. We began this chapter by proposing a decentering of "what it means to know" as a response to polarization and with openness to other, less familiar approaches to knowledge development. As Andrea Doucet, Eva Jewell, and Vanessa Watts also point out in this volume, "Care has been taken up mainly as practices and theories and in relation to policies and sociopolitical life, but much less so in relation to our research practices and our ethical, ontological, and epistemological responsibilities as knowers and knowledge makers" (chapter 7).

It is in response to this gap that we have sought to understand how we, as care ethical researchers, can gain insight in the moral good in epistemically unstable times through a polyvocal, collaborative approach to the everyday particularities of life.

GENERATING KNOWLEDGE

But hold on. Are we moving too fast? How can we learn from experiences, objects, and social practices, create openness for other, unfamiliar approaches to knowing without appropriating these, and not take any theory in consideration? Of course, we value concepts and theories. Concepts do matter, and theories do too, especially in our care ethics approach. Conceptual clarification helps us to heuristically make sense of life's concerns. All we are trying to highlight has already been said by Richard Bernstein (1995, 55) when he wrote about the plurality and conflict of metanarratives: "There is not only a conflict of narratives, but a fortiori, a conflict of metanarratives. There are better or worse narratives and metanarratives. And we can give good reasons in support of our claims for what is better." Bernstein invited us long ago rethink our *relationship* with that which we try to understand, including concepts and our own thoughts and experiences. This *relational* approach favors description by means of distinction and clarification instead of explanation by means of reduction. It leaves behind *appropriation* and generalization of knowledge into metanarratives and moves toward understanding particular practices from an experiential stance (Laugier 2018), allowing for naturalistic generalizations (Stake and Trumbull 1982) so that they can speak with their own distinctive voice, part of a dynamic shifting continuum called "practice." Here, naturalistic generalizations are conclusions arrived at through personal engagement in life's affairs or by vicarious experience so well constructed that the person feels as if it happened to them. For instance, consider the Hermann grid illusion, a famous optical illusion that deceives a person's vision. When looking at the grid you will find that your eyes are not able to process all the black dots. This is in part because our peripheral vision is far from optimal. As a result, our vision has to make assumptions based on learning, memory, and expectation. And although it's an adaptation that has served us well in terms of survival (by rapidly processing information we can make speedier decisions without having to take in every single bit of visual data available to us), it says something about the way we process the world. But what it also tells us, according to French phenomenologist Bruce Bégout (2005), is that because any phenomenon we try to understand does not exhaust itself, never fully explains what it is, we should also suppress our tendencies as researchers to "capture" completely experiences by appropriating ("extricating"; cf. Prattes this volume [chapter 4]) knowledge or fixating insights into a conceptual structure while generalizing this through theory as if they work the same for everyone.

Returning to the beginning of our chapter, adopting more epistemic humility as researchers would therefore entail that we should continually try to understand "in motion," "think questioningly" (Løgstrup 2007; Visse, Hansen, and Leget 2020) and acknowledge practices as dynamic and shifting continuums instead of solidified entities that are completely knowable. Concepts, here, are alive, and no longer part of the binary theory/practice divide, or indeed any "fact value dichotomies" (cf. Sayer 2016), but are as much a part of understanding "in motion" as experiential and material data, entangled in precarious and responsive practices.

PRECARIOUS KNOWING

Our approach to care ethics is open, multiperspectival, and generative, less focused on deductive explanation, logical consistency, or conceptual coherence and attentive to narrative, nonverbal, intuitive, and experiential modes of knowing. Therefore, we favor bottom-up, particular, naturalistic, experiential, plural, and polyvocal approaches to understanding the moral good. We try to become familiar with the spectacularly mundane: the everyday effects of programs and policies on everyday lives. In doing so, we become connoisseurs (to use Elliot Eisner's term 2017): by using our sensitivities and experiences, leaving the highlands to enter the complexities and messiness of practices, the swampy lowlands (Schön 1987).

In making these claims, we do not plead for yet another system of knowledge but rather make a small and modest attempt at enriching care ethics by acknowledging the precarity and particularity that is inherent to knowing. "Precarity" as in lacking in predictability, causality, and generalizability. Precarious as in particularistic, situational, bound to places and people, and vulnerable to oppression and reduction.

Rather than endeavoring to present alternative answers to questions in the precise form of a problem and solution that often leads to attempts to convince others and evokes polarized stances, listening with care, listening analytically, without offering "alternatives" or "answers" requires maintaining openness—a move that, as Isabelle Stengers has pointed out, has historically proven to be challenging for modern scholars to master (Stengers 2005). This is, however, what we hope will assist us in preventing polarization by decentering our belief in the righteousness of our own standpoints, so as to minimize the chance of ending up in argumentative debates with winners and losers.This approach has the potential of gaining an analytical sensitivity to consider "what a 'responsible' telling" (Verran 2001, 43; Addelson 1994) of what emergent collective life might be.

Will this give us all the answers as care ethical researchers on what it means to know and understand in our increasingly polarized era? Perhaps not. But our examples, experiences, and thoughts may be the constituents of a political care ethics that paves the way for plural practices of knowing. The challenge is to contribute to dignified communities in our rather fraught democratic and academic landscape while staying true to all those care ethics insights that have already brought us so much.

ACKNOWLEDGMENTS

The authors are hugely indebted to the editors of this volume (in particular Fiona Robinson and Maggie FitzGerald) who have put a great deal of (caring) effort in commenting on previous versions of this chapter, thereby improving it substantially. The authors would also like to thank both Gustaaf Bos and Rodante van der Waal for their helpful comments on an earlier version of the manuscript.

NOTES

1. See, for instance, Serhan (2020) and Sandsmark (2024).
2. As Fiona Robinson pointed out so astutely during the process of writing this.
3. This happened in the United States as well; see, for example, Harper (2021).

REFERENCES

Addelson, Kathryn Pyne. 1994. "Feminist Philosophy and the Women's Movement." *Hypatia* 9 (3): 216–224.

Baillergeau, Evelyne, and Jan Willem Duyvendak. 2016. "Experiential Knowledge as a Resource for Coping with Uncertainty: Evidence and Examples from the Netherlands." *Health, Risk & Society* 18 (7–8): 407–426.

Banarjee, Subrata. 2020. "Identifying Factors of Sexual Violence Against Women and Protection of Their Rights in Bangladesh." *Aggression and Violent Behavior* 52:101384. https://doi.org/10.1016/j.avb.2020.101384.

Brannelly, Tula, and Marian Barnes. 2022. *Researching with Care: Applying Feminist Care Ethics to Research Practice*. Policy Press.

Beck, Ulrich. 2006. "Living in the World Risk Society: A Hobhouse Memorial Public Lecture Given on Wednesday 15 February 2006 at the London School of Economics." *Economy and Society* 35 (3): 329–345.

Bégout, Bruce. 2005. *La découverte du quotidien*. Paris: Allia.

Bernstein, Richard. 1995. "American Pragmatism: The Conflict of Narratives." In *Rorty and Pragmatism: The Philosopher Responds to His Critics*, edited by Herman J. Saatkamp, 54–67. Nashville, TN: Vanderbilt University Press.

Boardman, Felicity K. 2014. "Knowledge Is Power? The Role of Experiential Knowledge in Genetically 'Risky' Reproductive Decisions." *Sociology of Health & Illness* 36 (1): 137–150.

Boydell, Katherine M., Michael Hodgins, Brenda M. Gladstone, Elaine Stasiulis, George Belliveau, Hoi Cheu, Pia Kontos, and Janet Parsons. 2016. "Arts-Based Health Research and Academic Legitimacy: Transcending Hegemonic Conventions." *Qualitative Research* 16 (6): 681–700.

Braidotti, Rosi. 1994. *Nomadic Subjects: Embodiment and Sexual Difference in Contemporary Feminist Theory*. New York: Columbia University Press.

Brannelly, Tula, and Marian Barnes. 2022. *Researching with Care: Applying Feminist Care Ethics to Research Practice*. Bristol: Policy Press.

Dalmiya, Vrinda. 2016. *Caring to Know: Comparative Care Ethics, Feminist Epistemology, and the Mahābhārata*. New Delhi: Oxford University Press.

Derrida, Jacques. 1967. *De la grammatologie*. Paris: Les Éditions de Minuit.

DiMaggio, Anthony R. 2022. "Conspiracy Theories and the Manufacture of Dissent: QAnon, the 'Big Lie,' Covid-19, and the Rise of Rightwing Propaganda." *Critical Sociology* 48 (6): 1025–1048. https://doi.org/10.1177/08969205211073669.

Eisner, Elliot W. 2017. *The Enlightened Eye: Qualitative Inquiry and the Enhancement of Educational Practice*. New York: Teachers College Press.

Flexner, Abraham. 1910. "Medical Education in the United States and Canada." *Science* 32 (810): 41–50.

Fricker, Miranda. 2017. "Evolving Concepts of Epistemic Injustice." In *The Routledge Handbook of Epistemic Injustice*, edited by Ian James Kidd, José Medina, and Gaile Pohlhaus Jr., 53–60. New York: Routledge.

Gidman, Janice. 2013. "Listening to Stories: Valuing Knowledge from Patient Experience." *Nurse Education in Practice* 13 (3): 192–196.

Gurstelle, Krystyna. 2022. "Uneven Paths to Health and Healing: Medicine, Politics and Power in 19th Century America." PhD diss., Drew University. https://digitalcollections.drew.edu/UniversityArchives/ThesesAndDissertations/CSGS/DMH/2022/Gurstelle/openaccess/KGurstelle.pdf.

Hamington, Maurice. 2012a. "Care Ethics and Corporeal Inquiry in Patient Relations." *IJFAB: International Journal of Feminist Approaches to Bioethics* 5 (1): 52–69.

———. 2012b. "A Performative Approach to Teaching Care Ethics: A Case Study." *Feminist Teacher* 23 (1): 31–49.

———. 2015. "Performing Care Ethics: Empathy, Acting, and Embodied Learning." In *Experiential Learning in Philosophy*, edited by Julinna Oxley and Ramona Ilea, 68–80. New York: Routledge.

Hamington, Maurice, and Ce Rosenow. 2019. *Care Ethics and Poetry*. Cham: Springer.

Hankivsky, Olena. 2005. *Social Policy and the Ethic of Care*. Vancouver: University of British Columbia Press.

Harper, Karen Brooks. 2021. "Verbal and Physical Attacks on Health Workers Surge as Emotions Boil during Latest COVID-19 Wave." *Texas Tribune*, September 1, 2021. https://www.texastribune.org/2021/09/01/coronavirus-texas-hospital-attacks-health-workers/.

Hochschild, Arlie Russell. 2016. "The Ecstatic Edge of Politics: Sociology and Donald Trump." *Contemporary Sociology* 45 (6): 683–689.

hooks, bell. 1990. "Marginality as a Site of Resistance." *Out There* 4:341–343.

Jerak-Zuiderent, Sonja. 2015. "Keeping Open by Re-imagining Laughter and Fear." *Sociological Review* 63 (4): 897–921.

Kirloskar-Steinbach, Monika. 2018. "Review of Vrinda Dalmiya's 'Caring to Know.'" *Essays in Philosophy* 19 (2): 1–11.

Kristeva, Julia. 1987. *In the Beginning Was Love: Psychoanalysis and Faith*. New York: Columbia University Press.

Laugier, Sandra. 2018. "What Matters: The Ethics and Aesthetics of Importance." In *Stanley Cavell on Aesthetic Understanding*, edited by Garry L. Hagberg, 167–195. Cham: Palgrave Macmillan.

Lawrence, David Herbert. 1987. *The Plumed Serpent*. Vol. 754. Cambridge: Cambridge University Press.

———. 1994. *Kangaroo*. Cambridge: Cambridge University Press.

Lawtoo, Nidesh. 2020. "Lawrence Contra (New) Fascism." *College Literature* 47 (2): 287–317.

Leget, Carlo, Inge van Nistelrooij, and Merel Visse. 2019. "Beyond Demarcation: Care Ethics as an Interdisciplinary Field of Inquiry." *Nursing Ethics* 26 (1): 17–25.

Løgstrup, K. E. 2007. *Beyond the Ethical Demand*. Notre Dame, IN: University of Notre Dame Press.

Mouffe, Chantal. 2005. *The Return of the Political*. Vol. 8. London: Verso.

Papen, Uta, and Sue Walters. 2008. *Literacy, Learning and Health*. National Research and Development Centre for Adult Literacy and Numeracy, Department for Innovation, Universities and Skills, London. http://www.nrdc.org.uk.

Polanyi, Michael. 1966. *The Tacit Dimension*. Chicago: University of Chicago Press.

Politi, Mary C., Don S. Dizon, Dominick L. Frosch, Marie D. Kuzemchak, and Anne M. Stiggelbout. 2013. "Importance of Clarifying Patients' Desired Role in Shared Decision Making to Match Their Level of Engagement with Their Preferences." *BMJ* 347: 18–19.

Repucci, Sarah, and Amy Slipowitz. 2020. "Democracy under Lockdown." Freedom House. https://freedomhouse.org/report/special-report/2020/democracy-under-lockdown.

Rerimassie, Virgil, T. F. L. Roedema, Lisa Augustijn, Amelie Schirmer, and Frank Kupper. 2021. "Making Sense of the COVID-19 Pandemic: An Analysis of the Dynamics of Citizen Sensemaking Practices across Europe." Technical Report. https://zenodo.org/record/4507041#.YmkmntPMKUm.

Roeser, Sabine. 2022. "Understanding Risks and Moral Emotions in the Context of COVID-19 Policy Making: The Case of the Netherlands." In *Values for a Post-Pandemic Future*, edited by Matthew J. Dennis, Georgy Ishmaev, Steven Umbrello, and Jeroen van den Hoven, 201–214. Cham: Springer.

Ruddick, Sara. 1995. *Maternal Thinking: Toward a Politics of Peace*. Boston: Beacon.

Ryle, Gilbert. 1945. "Knowing How and Knowing That." *Papers from the Aristotelian Society* 46:1–16.

Sandsmark, Evan. 2024. "Hungary's Illiberal Democracy." Religion, Race & Democracy Lab, University of Virginia. https://religionlab.virginia.edu/projects/hungarys-illiberal-democracy/.

Sari, Yasemin. 2018. "Arendt, Truth, and Epistemic Responsibility." *Arendt Studies* 2: 149–170.

Sayer, Andrew. 2016. "Zugwandte Unterstützung und anteilnehmende Sorge als Weltverhältnis." In *Praxis Der Achtsamkeit: Schluüsselbegruffe der Care—Ethik*, edited by Elisabeth Conradi and Frans Vosman, 631–662. Frankfurt am Main: Campus.

Schön, Donald A. 1987. *Educating the Reflective Practitioner: Toward a New Design for Teaching and Learning in the Professions*. San Francisco: Jossey-Bass.

Serhan, Yasmeen. 2020. "The EU Watches as Hungary Kills Democracy." *The Atlantic*, April 2, 2020. https://www.theatlantic.com/international/archive/2020/04/europe-hungary-viktor-orban-coronavirus-covid19-democracy/609313/.

Solnit, Rebecca. 2017. *The Mother of All Questions: Further Feminisms*. London: Granta Book.

Stake, Robert E., and Deborah J. Trumbull. 1982. "Naturalistic Generalizations." *Review Journal of Philosophy and Social Science* 7 (1): 1–12.

Stake, Robert, and Merel Visse. 2021. *A Paradigm of Care*. Information Age Publishing.

Stengers, Isabelle. 2005. "The Cosmopolitical Proposal." In *Making Things Public: Atmospheres of Democracy*, edited by Bruno Latour and Peter Weibel, 994–1003. Cambridge, MA: MIT Press.

Storni, Cristiano. 2015. "Patients' Lay Expertise in Chronic Self-Care: A Case Study in Type 1 Diabetes." *Health Expectations* 18 (5): 1439–1450.

Tharoor, Ishaan. 2020. "Coronavirus Kills Its First Democracy". *Washington Post*, March 31, 2020. https://www.washingtonpost.com/world/2020/03/31/coronavirus-kills-its-first-democracy/.

Thompson, Derek. 2020. "The Deep Story of Trumpism." *The Atlantic*, December 29, 2020. https://www.theatlantic.com/ideas/archive/2020/12/deep-story-trumpism/617498/.

Thompson, James. 2022. *Care Aesthetics: For Artful Care and Careful Art*. New York: Routledge.

Vear, Craig, ed. 2022. *The Routledge International Handbook of Practice-Based Research*. New York: Routledge.

Verran, Helen. 2001. *Science and an African Logic*. Chicago: University of Chicago Press.

Visse, Merel. 2017. "Nested Tensions in Care." *AMA Journal of Ethics* 19 (4): 399–405.

Visse, Merel, and Tineke A. Abma. 2018. *Evaluation for a Caring Society*. Charlotte, NC: Information Age.

Visse, Merel, Tineke A. Abma, and Guy Widdershoven. 2015. "Practicing Political Care Ethics: Can Responsive Evaluation Foster Democratic Care?" *Ethics and Social Welfare* 9 (2): 164–182.

Visse, Merel, Finn Hansen, and Carlo Leget. 2019. "The Unsayable in Arts-Based Research: On the Praxis of Life Itself." *International Journal of Qualitative Methods* 18. https://doi.org/10.1177/1609406919851392.

———. 2020. "Apophatic Inquiry: Living the Questions Themselves." *International Journal of Qualitative Methods* 19. https://doi.org/10.1177/1609406920958975.

Visse, Merel, and Alistair Niemeijer. Forthcoming. *Precarious Knowing: An Aesthetics of Care and Hope*. Cham: Springer.

Walker, Margaret Urban. 2007. *Moral Understandings: A Feminist Study in Ethics*. Oxford: Oxford University Press.

Wikipedia. 2023. "Dutch Curfew Riots." Last modified October 15, 2023. https://en.wikipedia.org/wiki/2021_Dutch_curfew_riots.

Zakaria, Rafia. 2021. *Against White Feminism: Notes on Disruption*. New York: Norton.

ACKNOWLEDGMENTS

First and foremost, we wish to thank our contributors for their solid work and enthusiasm for this project. Many sincere thanks also to our reviewers, to the series editors, to Peter Mickulas at Rutgers University Press, to Breanne Bandur for the beautiful art for the cover, and to the fantastic interlocutors we had at previous Care Ethics Research Consortium (CERC) conferences. Last but not least, we wish to express our gratitude to Salma El Refaei for her editorial help, and to all the support staff in our respective universities for the behind-the-scenes work that makes research and teaching possible.

NOTES ON CONTRIBUTORS

SOPHIE BOURGAULT is associate professor of political theory at the University of Ottawa (Canada). Current research interests gravitate around the ethics of care; gender, temporality, and work; epistemologies of ignorance; and contemporary feminist theory. In addition to having published numerous book chapters and articles on feminist ethics and epistemic injustice, she has coedited several volumes on care (*Les éthiques de l'hospitalité, du don et du care; In Yet a Different Voice; Care and Emotions* [in Italian, *Cura ed emozioni*]; and *Le care: Ethique féministe actuelle*). She was guest coeditor for a special issue on gender, work, and justice (*Politique et Sociétés*) as well as guest coeditor for the *International Journal of Care and Caring* (with F. Robinson).

VIVIENNE BOZALEK is an emerita professor in women's and gender studies at the University of the Western Cape, and honorary professor in the Centre for Higher Education Research, Teaching and Learning at Rhodes University. Her research interests include the political ethics of care and social justice, posthumanism and feminist new materialisms, innovative pedagogical practices in higher education, and post-qualitative and participatory methodologies. Her most recent coedited books include *Nancy Fraser and Participatory Parity: Reframing Social Justice in South African Higher Education* with D. Hölscher and M. Zembylas, *Posthuman and Political Care Ethics for Reconfiguring Higher Education* with M. Zembylas and J. Tronto, *Post-Anthropocentric Social Work: Critical Posthuman and New Materialist Perspectives* with B. Pease, and *Higher Education Hauntologies: Living with Ghosts for a Justice-to-Come* with M. Zembylas, S. Motala, and D. Hölscher. She is also the editor-in-chief of the journal *Critical Studies in Teaching and Learning*.

VRINDA DALMIYA is a professor in the Philosophy Department at the University of Hawai'i at Mānoa. She has been a fellow at the Indian Institute of Advanced Study, Shimla. Her research interests are in analytic feminist theory with a focus on care ethics, epistemology, and environmental philosophy. She also works in comparative or cross-cultural philosophy. She has published in several anthologies and journals and is the author of *Caring to Know: Comparative Care Ethics, Feminist Epistemology and the Mahabharata* and the coeditor of *Exploring Agency in the Mahābhārata: Ethical and Political Dimensions of Dharma*.

ÉMILIE DIONNE is a social scientist, sociologist of health care, feminist thinker, and political theorist in the Department of Sociology (adjunct professor) at Université Laval and at VITAM—Research Center for Sustainable Health. Combining theoretical and applied research on health care, she uses insights from feminist new materialism, care ethics, material ecocriticism, critical disability studies, science and technologies studies (STS), and critical qualitative methodology to design and conduct research projects that account for their political and ontological participation in shaping shared worlds. Using critical insights from the ethics of vulnerability, she studies various topics in healthcare research, including person-centered care approaches in clinical contexts, the use of digital technology to support and promote health and wellness outcomes, relationality in the care context, and various issues relating to aging. She is the co-director and principal investigator of the FRQS Research Grant "VITA-Lab: Transforming the Social Imaginary of Aging and Older Adults through Art-Based Science."

ANDREA DOUCET is a Canada research chair in gender, work, and care; professor of sociology and women's and gender studies at Brock University; and adjunct research professor at Carleton University and the University of Victoria. She is the author of two editions of *Do Men Mother?*, which was awarded the John Porter Tradition of Excellence Book Award from the Canadian Sociology Association, coauthor of two editions of *Gender Relations: Intersectionality and Social Change* (with Janet Siltanen), and coeditor of *Thinking Ecologically, Thinking Responsibly: The Legacies of Lorraine Code* (with Nancy Arden McHugh). She is project director and principal investigator of the Reimagining Care / Work Policies Partnership Grant Project and co-coordinator of the International Network of Leave Policies and Research.

MAGGIE FITZGERALD is assistant professor in the Department of Political Studies at the University of Saskatchewan, Canada. Her research focuses on the ethics of care, global ethics and international political theory, decolonial ethics, normative and critical international relations theory, and feminist political economy. Her work has appeared in journals such as *Ethics and Social Welfare*, *Journal of International Political Theory*, and *International Journal of Care and Caring*, as well as in edited volumes like *Care Ethics in the Age of Precarity* (edited by Maurice Hamington and Michael Flower). She is the author of *Care and the Pluriverse: Rethinking Global Ethics*.

MARIE GARRAU is senior lecturer (maîtresse de conférences) in social and political philosophy at the Université Paris 1 Panthéon-Sorbonne and member of the research center ISJPS (Institut des Sciences Juridique et Philosophique de la Sorbonne). Her work studies contemporary forms and conceptions of vulnerability, focusing on the political questions related to vulnerability—hence her interest in care ethics, feminist theory, recognition theory, and contemporary republicanism. She has published *Politiques de la vulnérabilité*, *Care et attention*, and, with Alice Le Goff, *Care, justice et dépendance: Une introduction aux théories du care*. Her last book, coedited with Mickaelle Provost, is titled *Experiences vécues du genre et de la race: Pour une phénoménologie critique*.

CHRISTOPHER PAUL HARRIS is an assistant professor in the Department of Global and International Studies at the University of California, Irvine. His first book is *To Build a Black Future*. His other writings have appeared in *South Atlantic Quarterly*, *Contemporary Political Theory*, *Social Science Quarterly*, and *Public*

Seminar. His research interests range from Black political thought, culture, aesthetics, and social movements to broader questions concerning the possibility of revolutionary transformation in the twenty-first century.

EVA JEWELL is Anishinaabekwe from Deshkan Ziibiing (Chippewas of the Thames First Nation) in southwestern Ontario, with paternal lineage from Oneida Nation of the Thames. She is research director at Yellowhead Institute, a First Nation–led policy think tank housed in the Faculty of Arts at Toronto Metropolitan University, where she is also assistant professor in the Department of Sociology. Her scholarship supports community-led inquiry on topics of language, governance, and cultural resurgence among Anishinaabeg people, critical Indigenous perspectives of reconciliation and accountability, and Indigenous perspectives on care.

CHRISTINE KOGGEL is professor of philosophy at Carleton University. Her main research and teaching interests are in the areas of moral theory, practical ethics, feminism, and social and political theory. She has edited or coedited fourteen volumes, including *Care Ethics: New Theories and Applications*; *Gender Justice and Development: Local and Global*; *Examining Injustice: Foundational, Structural, and Epistemic Issues*; and *Relational Theory: Feminist Approaches, Implications, and Applications*. She has published more than forty-five journal articles and chapters, the most recent of which explore topics in development ethics, feminist theory, settler-colonialism, Indigenous issues, and their intersections. She is the former president of the Canadian Society for Women in Philosophy (CSWIP) and board member of the International Development Ethics Association (IDEA) and is a lead coeditor for the *Journal of Global Ethics*.

MASAYA LLAVANERAS BLANCO is an assistant professor of development studies at the Centre for Global Studies of Huron University College, University of Western Ontario. Her research focuses on the intersections between human mobilities, care, and social reproduction in the Caribbean and Latin America. She is a member of DAWN, a network of feminist activists and researchers from the Global South, on behalf of whom she coedited *Corporate Capture of Development* and is currently coediting *Pandemic Policies and Resistance: Southern Feminist Critiques in Times of Covid-19*. Her work has been published in *Global Social Policy*, *Political Geography*, and *Environment and Planning C: Politics and Space*, among others.

ALISTAIR NIEMEIJER'S line of research focuses on precarious practices of care and well-being of and for the (chronically) vulnerable. He has (co)authored scientific articles in a diverse range of scientific journals and has also contributed to several Dutch media outlets and policy reports on topics related to medical and care ethics. Having both a chronic illness and a young son with Down syndrome and epilepsy, he is intrinsically and professionally motivated to carry out research that is aimed at understanding better what it means to live with a chronic disease or disability and what the everyday aspirations of caregivers entail. Currently he works as an assistant professor in care ethics at the University of Humanistic Studies in Utrecht.

RIIKKA PRATTES is a research fellow at the School of Education Culture and Society at Monash University. Previously, she was a postdoctoral associate at the Program of Gender, Sexuality, and Feminist Studies at Duke University. She is a founding member of the Revaluing Care in the Global Economy network and serves on the network's advisory board. She holds a PhD in social and political thought (Institute for Social Justice at ACU Sydney) and an MA in social and cultural anthropology (University of Vienna). Her research focuses on care ethics, gender (including masculinities), affect and decolonial theory, embodiment, and epistemologies. Her work has appeared in journals such as *Feminist Theory* and *Men and Masculinities*.

FIONA ROBINSON is professor of political science at Carleton University in Ottawa, Canada; her research and teaching focus on critical, feminist, and ethical theory in global politics. She is the author of *Globalizing Care: Ethics, Feminist Theory and International Relations* and *The Ethics of Care: A Feminist Approach to Human Security* and coeditor, with Rianne Mahon, of *Feminist Ethics and Social Politics: Towards a New Global Political Economy of Care*. Her work has been published in numerous journals, including *Review of International Studies*, *International Feminist Journal of Politics*, and *International Journal of Care and Caring*. In 2014, she was the recipient of the inaugural J. Ann Tickner Book Prize for scholarship on gender and feminist international relations.

MEREL VISSE works as associate professor and director at Drew University in the United States and the University of Humanistic Studies in the Netherlands. Since the early 2000s, she has spearheaded innovative cross-disciplinary projects funded by grants, fostering collaboration between intellectual, artistic, and entrepreneurial communities on issues related to care, ethics, and the arts. Dr. Visse coleads the Art & Care Platform Series and publishes in peer-reviewed journals. She has authored and edited books, including *Evaluation for a Caring Society* and the forthcoming *Art for the Sake of Care*. She serves as the visual art section editor for the *International Journal of Education and the Arts*, is on the editorial board for the series *Landscapes: The Arts, Aesthetics and Education*, and is an editor at *Visual Arts Research*. For more information, please visit her website: www.merelvisse.com.

VANESSA WATTS is Mohawk and Anishinaabe Bear Clan, Six Nations of the Grand River. She is an assistant professor of Indigenous studies and sociology at McMaster University and holds the Paul R. MacPherson Chair in Indigenous Studies. Her research examines Indigenist epistemological and ontological interventions on place-based, material knowledge production. She is particularly interested in Indigenous feminisms, sociology of knowledge, Indigenous governance, and other-than-human relations as forms of Indigenous ways of knowing. Her SSHRC Insight Development Grant for her project "An Indigenist Sociology of Knowledge: Indigenous Social Lives in Indigenous Studies, Sociology and Political Science (1895 and Beyond)" interrogates over a century of representations of Indigenous peoples in sociology and political science.

INDEX

abdication, 101–102
abolitionist care, 178–179, 189, 191
accountability, 64, 150, 153–154, 170, 190
acting, 101
active ignorance, 56–57, 69
Adorno, Theodor, 59
advocacy epistemology, 129, 133
affective methodologies, 139–140
Afrocentric epistemologies, 3, 64, 179
agency, 41, 59, 79–80, 86–90, 148–149
agential cuts, 148
agential realism, 148, 150, 155n5
agent-regret, 88–89
Ahmed, Sara, 6
Aki-wayn-zih, 120
Aki-wayn-zih (Baxter), 119–120
Alaimo, Stacy, 154
Alcoff, Linda Martín, 68, 75n15
Alexander, Elizabeth, 184
algorithms, 39
Anderson, Elizabeth, 40
Anderson, Kim, 119–120
Anishinaabeg doodem system, 120
Anishinaabe worldviews, 113
anonymization, 37–40, 44n2. *See also* veiling of particulars
Anthropocene, 139, 145, 153–154
anti-Blackness, 11–12, 171, 177–178, 184–187, 190
arts/artists, 133–134, 138–140
assimilation policies, 25
attention, 140–141
attentive hearing, 35, 97, 99–100, 106, 205. *See also* listening
attentiveness, 70–73, 140–141, 150
Australia, 66–67, 74n5, 74n8
autonomy, 122–123
autonomy myths, 48

Baker, Ella, 181
Barad, Karen, 132–133, 135, 146–152
bateyes, 172n9
Baxter, Eli, *Aki-wayn-zih*, 119–120
Bégout, Bruce, 204
Belcourt, Billy-Ray, 120, 122
Bell, Shaina, 164, 172n13

Beloved (Morrison), 163
Bennett, Jane, 130, 136
Bernstein, Richard, 204
biases, 25, 31–32, 36–38, 107–108n5
Bilodeau, Antoine, 37
Black feminist thought, 10–11, 184
Black Joy Experience Resource Guide, The, 190
#Blacklivesmatter, 184, 186, 190
Black Lives Matter Global Network (BLMGN), 181, 186–187
Blackness, 162–164, 171, 178, 185–186
Black pain, 187–188, 191
Black Youth Project 100 (BYP100), 10, 179–182, 184, 188–190
BLM10Plus, 181
bodies (human), 83–85, 97–98, 130–131, 136
bodily absence, 43. *See also* veiling of particulars
"Book of the Women, The" (*Mahabharata*), 78–84. See also *Mahabharata*
Borrows, John, 117
Bourdieu, Pierre, 59; *Masculine Domination,* 55
Bourgault, Sophie, 18, 26, 97–98, 104; "Epistemic Injustice, Face-to-Face Encounters, and Caring Institutions," 17
Bovens, Mark, 38
Boydell, Katherine M., 200–201
Bozalek, Vivienne, 147
Braidotti, Rosi, 155n3
Brand, Dionne, 187
Brison, Susan, 83–84
Brooks, Dwayne, 35–36
Brugère, Fabienne, 37
Busch, Peter A., 39
Butler, Judith, 79, 132, 152–153

Canada, 26–29, 172n13; Indian Act (1876), 27; Indian Residential Schools Settlement Agreement (IRSSA), 26–27; Indigenous health care in, 31, 41; missing and murdered Indigenous women in, 41–43; perceptions of Indigenous Peoples in, 121; settler-colonialism in, 25, 66, 112–113, 120; Truth and Reconciliation Conference (2016), 111. *See also* Truth and Reconciliation Commission final report (Canada)

Index

capitalism, 178, 187
care, 1, 94–95, 103–107, 114, 117–118, 197; and citizenship, 169–170; as critical feminist political theory, 19, 29; dark side of, 113, 120, 162, 166; and emotions, 4; human-centric focus of, 119, 123, 129–131, 141; and Indigenous peoples, 74n6, 113–114, 117–118; and Indigenous worldviews, 28, 118–120, 123; Kittay on, 86; non-Eurocentric, 80; and policy making, 16–17; reciprocal nature of, 120; Sharpe on, 178; situatedness of, 4, 161–162; as social death, 122; Tronto and Fisher on, 16, 122, 129, 134, 149; unevenness of, 162
Care and the Pluriverse: Rethinking Global Ethics (FitzGerald), 26
care discourses, 1, 85
care epistemologies, 97, 99–100, 103–104
care ethical agency, 89
care ethical knowing, 100
care ethicists, 197, 200
care ethics, 1–3, 7, 9, 113, 129, 135–141, 149–154, 160–161, 187, 196–197, 200–203; and the body, 85; and the Buddha's First Noble Truth, 80; and care, 94–95, 105; and care epistemologies, 97; as critical political theory, 19–22; criticisms of, 19–20; and decentering, 94–95; Gilligan on, 120–121; and interdependence, 95–96; ontology of, 95–97; and posthuman ethics, 145, 149–150; and projects of unsettling, 170, 171n2; and time requirements, 35; transformative potential of, 21; and Western ontologies, 66
caregiving, 19, 21–22, 32–33, 54, 88–90
care infrastructures, 166
care knowing, 103–105
Carel, Havi, 35
care-less practices, 162
care practices, 129–130
care recipients, 47–48
carers, 96
care studies, 197
care vanishment, 123
care work, 49, 53–54, 57, 68, 111. *See also* domestic work
caring, 129, 167
Caring Democracy: Markets, Equality, and Justice (Tronto), 7, 48
caring institutions, 17, 40, 43
caring societies, 58, 59–60n1, 96

Caring to Know (Dalmiya), 68
Carson, Rachel, 111
Cartesian cuts, 148
Castile, Philando, 177
childcare, 167
class/race inequalities, 10
Code, Lorraine, 133; *Ecological Thinking*, 111, 128–129
Cohen, Stanley, *States of Denial*, 52
collective consciousness, 203
Collins, Patricia Hill, 3, 64
colonial care, 113, 120–123
colonialism, 7, 113, 120, 123, 161, 163
competence, 150
concepts, 204
"concrete" thinking, 99
Confortini, Catia, 103
conspiracy theories, 194–195
Cordova, V. F., *How It Is*, 119
corpo-real configurations, 129–130, 135
corporeal disposition, 137–141
Coulthard, Glen, 26, 28, 66
courage, 107
COVID-19, 17–18, 89, 198–199, 202–203
Craft, Aimée, 111–112
"Creating Caring Institutions: Politics, Plurality, and Purpose" (Tronto), 16
"creative practice-led research," 200–201
creativity, 154
credibility, 35–36
crises, 198–199
critical feminist care ethics, 161. *See also* feminist care ethics
critical feminist political theory, 19, 29
critical studies on men and masculinities (CSMM), 69
"Crow, Owl, Deer et al. versus the Anishinaabe," 117–118
curiosity, 154
Cusicanqui, Silvia Rivera, 63

Dalmiya, Vrinda, 68, 96, 100, 200; *Caring to Know*, 68; "Why Should a Knower Care?," 2
Das, Veena, 83
Davis, Emmalon, 73
decentering, 5, 94–95, 129, 202; care ethics, 179, 190, 196–197; Euro-Western approaches, 196; in medicine, 200; of self, 95–103; of ways of knowing, 195–196
democracies, 198, 202

Index

departments of care, 21, 28
Derrida, Jacques, 147
Despre, Vinciane, 148–151
dharma, 80–81, 87, 90
diffraction, 146–147
"diffractive methodologies," 10, 115–116, 146–147
disavowal, 52
discretion, 33, 38–39
disinformation ecosystems, 195
Dolis, Sirana, 165, 168
domestic work, 62, 69–70, 75n13; and attentiveness, 70–71; Haitians, 159–160, 165–166; payment for, 62–63, 70, 72. *See also* care work; Haitian migrant domestic workers
dominant collective interpretative resources, 28–29
domination relations, 8, 55–56, 58
Dominican Republic, 164–165, 168–170, 172n8, 172n10, 172n14
Doucet, Andrea, 75n12, 203; "Feminist Sociologies: Diffractive Readings of Histories, Contributions, Futures," 115

echo chambers, 106, 107–108n5
Ecological Thinking (Code), 111
embodied freedoms, 170–171
embodiment, 66–69, 83, 97–99, 107n2, 131–134, 140, 151; and care ethics, 162; and knowledge formation, 63
enslavement, 162–165
entangled empathy, 10, 145, 153, 155
environmental care, 4, 52–53
environmental ethics, 137
epistemic appropriation, 72–73
epistemic bubbles, 106
epistemic capacity, 128–129
epistemic claims, 106
epistemic disobedience, 6, 9, 79
epistemic extractivism, 8, 63–64, 72–73, 100
epistemic humility, 100–102, 204
Epistemic Injustice (Fricker), 31–33, 56
"Epistemic Injustice, Face-to-Face Encounters, and Caring Institutions" (Bourgault), 17
epistemic injustices, 8, 23, 31–32, 201. *See also* hermeneutical injustice; testimonial injustice
epistemic irresponsibility, 2, 5. *See also* "privileged irresponsibility"

epistemic justice, 32–34, 41–43
epistemic vices, 56
epistemic virtue, 34, 36
epistemic vulnerability, 9, 79
epistemological, FitzGerald's definition, 20
epistemology, 128
epistemology of domination, 63–64, 71, 74n3
epistemology of mastery, 63, 66
Epistemology of Resistance (Medina), 56–57
epistemology of separation, 63
erotic agency, 170–171
ethics, 149, 196–197
ethics of care. *See* care ethics
ethics of worlding, 149
ethics/politics of refusal, 56, 122–123, 188
exclusion, 164, 166
exploitability, 159–160, 162–164

face-to-face encounters, 35, 37, 42, 44n1
failure, 86–87, 90, 104–105
familiarity, 36–37, 43
Fanon, Frantz, 186
fatherhood, 69, 75n13
feminist care ethics, 8–9, 66, 110, 114, 116, 118, 120–121, 123, 170; and Indigenous epistemologies, 109, 112–113, 123; and power relations, 160; Tronto on, 118. *See also* critical feminist care ethics
feminist care ethics literature, responding to, 112–113
feminist new materialists (FNM), 129–130, 135–136
feminist relational theory, 19, 22, 29
feminist standpoint epistemology, 2–3
feminist theories, and knowledge production, 115
Finau, Glenn, 119
Finding the Mother Tree: Discovering the Wisdom of the Forest (Simard), 112
Fineman, Martha, 48
Fisher, Berenice, 16, 122, 129
FitzGerald, Maggie, 15–16, 28–29, 84, 155n3; *Care and the Pluriverse: Rethinking Global Ethics*, 26; "Reimagining Government with the Ethics of Care," 18–21
Flexner Report, 200
Flowers, Rachel, 124
Foucault, Michel, 128–129
four Ps, 16–18

Fricker, Miranda, 8, 16, 23, 31, 35–38, 41, 44n1, 107–108n5; *Epistemic Injustice*, 31–34, 56
Friedman, Marilyn, 122

gender, 54–55, 81, 86–87, 164–165. *See also* women
"generative critique" methodologies, 11, 195–196
geographical sensitivities, 160
Gilligan, Carol, 8, 10, 19–21, 58–59, 82, 84, 102, 110–111, 120, 128; *In a Different Voice*, 1, 15; "Letter to Readers, 1993," 15; *Why Does Patriarchy Persist*, 55
Gilson, Erinn, 48
Glenn, Evelyn Nakano, 47
goal-orientedness, 62–63
Graham, Hilary, 118
grief, 81–82, 153
grievable lives, 10, 145, 151–153, 155
Grosfoguel, Ramón, 63

hairstyles, 168, 172n14
Haiti, 164, 168, 172n8
Haitian migrant domestic workers, 10, 159–160, 164–168
Hallenbeck, Jessica, 119
Hamington, Maurice, 37, 97
Haraway, Donna, 121, 137–138, 146, 148–150
Harper, Stephen, 27
Hartman, Saidiya, 163, 165
Hartsock, Nancy, 2
Hassan, Shira, 190
hauntology, 10, 145, 147, 152–153, 155
healing justice, 186–191
health care, 31, 35, 41, 168–170, 200–201
health care cuts, 18
Hekman, Susan, 1
Hemphill, Prentis, 187–188
Henriksen, Helle Z., 39
Hermann grid illusion, 204
hermeneutical injustice, 7, 16, 23–24, 26–27, 29
hermeneutic generosity, 32
heteropatriarchy, 79–80. *See also* patriarchy
Hill, Susan, 117
Hochschild, Arlie, 203
Hölscher, Dorothee, 147
Honig, Bonnie, 78
Hoosain, Shanaaz, 147
How It Is (Cordova), 119
human-animal relations, 151
human exceptionalism, 145

humans, 117, 141, 154; bodies, 83–85, 97–98, 130–131, 136; embodied nature of, 50; mental health of, 136. *See also* bodies
humiliation, 39
humility, 9, 100–103, 106
Hunfeld, Katharina, 26
Hungary, 198

"I Love Being Black" song, 183
imagination, 9, 98–100, 107n2
immanent/dynamic ontology, 134–135
imperialism, and care discourses, 1
In a Different Voice (Gilligan), 1, 15
indeterminacy, 148
Indigenous concepts, marginalization of, 9, 28, 110
Indigenous cosmologies, 116–117, 119
Indigenous epistemologies, 66, 109, 112–113
Indigenous knowledges, 99, 114–115, 121, 124, 200
Indigenous peoples, 26–28, 31, 41, 110, 114; academic perceptions of, 121; Canadian, 25–26, 114, 120–121, 172n13; and care, 74n6, 113–114, 118–119, 123; missing and murdered Indigenous women (Canada), 41–43. *See also* Truth and Reconciliation Commission final report (Canada)
individualization, 140–141
individuals, 80, 134–135, 140, 148
inequality, 152–153
information and communication technology (ICT), 38–39, 43
Institute for Strategic Dialogue, 195
institutional settings, 21–22, 32–33, 41, 54
interdependence, 10–11, 64, 73, 95–96, 120, 151, 178
interspecies communication, 117
intimate labor, 163, 165–167
intra-action, 132
intrinsic relationality, 163
invulnerability myths, 48
Iovino, Serenella, 139

Japan, 138–139
Jewell, Eva, 110, 203; "Calls to Action Accountability," 115
just societies, 47–48

Kaba, Mariame, 190
Karma, 84
Keller, Evelyn Fox, 140

Index

kickbacks, 191n7
Kidd, Ian, 35
King, Hayden, 117
Kirksey, Eben, 138–139
Kittay, Eva, 79, 82, 86
knowing, 7, 9, 65, 72, 105, 180, 199–200; analysis of, 4; and being/doing, 15; and epistemic injustices, 32; limits on, 96–97; and our bodies, 131; and place, 66; precarious, 196, 205; procedural, 74n10, 103; and reflection/reflexivity, 146; settler-colonial contexts of, 22, 25–26, 28; "things," 132; and vulnerability, 53
knowing with care, 11, 103
knowledge, 65–66, 95, 100, 129, 197, 199–201; ancestral, 187–188; appropriation of, 72–73, 204; from care work, 68; experiential, 6, 68–69, 71, 201; folk knowledge, 139; propositional knowledge, 68; and time, 103; unstable, 195; Welch on, 69. *See also* Indigenous knowledges
knowledge practices, 132, 204
knowledge production, 63, 115, 203–204
knowledges, 99–100, 139
Krzywoszynska, Anna, 140
Kumagusu, Minakata, 138–139

labor migration schemes, 164–165
lakou system, 167, 172n11
Laplanche, Jean, 52
Latour, Bruno, 130–131, 136
Laugier, Sandra, 83
Lawrence, D. H., 198, 203
Le Guin, Ursula K., "Marrow," 139
L'Énigme de la femme active (Molinier), 54
"Letter to Readers, 1993" (Gilligan), 15
LGBTQ+ people, and health care, 31, 41
libation rituals, 182–183
liberal democracies, 195, 202
liberal individualism, 20
Liboiron, Max, 162
Lipsky, Michael, *Street-Level Bureaucracy*, 33
listening, 97–100, 139. *See also* attentive hearing
Listening Guide, 110–112, 128–129
Lorde, Audre, 6, 58, 178, 181, 184–186

Madge, Clare, 163
Mahabharata, 8–9, 78–79, 83–87, 90. *See also* "Book of the Women, The" (*Mahabharata*)
male privilege, 3–4, 8
marginalized voices, 4–5, 24–25, 39, 72–73, 200

Marlaloo songline project, 67
"Marrow" (Le Guin), 139
Martin, Trayvon, 177, 184
Masculine Domination (Bourdieu), 55
masculinity, 54–55, 70, 180
material-discursive phenomena, 148
material ecocriticism, 137, 139
maternal mortality, 169–170
maternal thinking, 101
"Maternal Thinking" (Ruddick), 1
matter, 129, 132, 135, 139
Mayes, April J., 166
Medina, José, 8, 24, 35, 58–59; *Epistemology of Resistance*, 56–57
men, 62, 69, 75n13
mending, 38
mental health issues, 135–136
Merleau-Ponty, Maurice, 133–134
metanarratives, 204
Mills, Charles, 56
mno-bmaadziwin, 120
modernity, and colonialism, 7
Molinier, Pascale, 8, 53–54, 58; *L'Énigme de la femme active*, 54
Monstrous Intimacies (Sharpe), 163
Moral Boundaries: A Political Argument for an Ethic of Care (Tronto), 16, 48
moral ecologies, 197
moral failures, 84, 87
moral good, 205
moral injuries, 82
moral life, 80, 89
moral luck, 86–88
moral vulnerability, 79, 86
Moreton-Robinson, Aileen, 66
Morrison, Toni, *Beloved*, 163
mothers, 107n4
Movement for Black Lives (M4BL), 11, 171n2, 177, 179, 181, 186–188, 191
Movement of Dominican-Haitian Women (MUDHA), 161, 165, 168–170, 172n15
multicultural policies, 28
Murdoch, Iris, 36
Murphy, Michelle, 161
mutuality, 163
Myers, Natasha, 139–140

nameless virtues, 88–89
Narayan, Uma, 1, 121, 161
narratives, 204
Native dance, 69, 71

naturalistic generalizations, 204
neoliberalism, 35, 80, 134–135, 140
Netherlands, 198–199, 202–203
Nguyen, C. Thi, 106
Noddings, Nel, 96
"non-innocence," 10, 145, 155, 161
nonverbal communication, 98
noticing, 137, 141
Noxolo, Pat, 163

Obama administration, 177
Onkwehonwe, 117
(onto-)ethics, 141
ontology of precarity, 130–131, 134–135
Oppermann, Serpil, 139
oppression, 10, 25
Orbán, Viktor, 198
orchestra auditions, 38–39
organic empathy, 131, 135–137, 153
organic materials, 136

packing the court, 191n8
Pandora's Hope (Latour), 130
parenting, 167
patriarchy, 55, 102, 171. *See also* heteropatriarchy
Patterson, Orlando, 122
Pfiesteria piscicida, 152
pharmaceutical drugs, 136
Pierre, Sonia, 168
place, 4, 63–64, 66–67, 75n14
place-thought, 119
plants, 140
Plumwood, Val, 152
Poelina, Anne, 67
Pohlhaus, Gaile Jr., 24
polarization, 196, 198–199, 202, 205
police, 36, 42
policy making, 16–18
political care ethics, 195
Pontalis, Jean-Bertrand, 52
positionality, 65–66
posthuman ethics, 145, 149–151
posthumanism, 3, 10
posthumanist ethicists (PE), 129, 135
postmodern writers, 196
post-truth era, 11
power hierarchies, 100–102
power/oppression relationships, 22, 160, 162–164, 171, 202
Prattes, Riikka, 202

precarity, 130–131, 134–135, 159, 168–169, 203, 205
principled struggle, 192n9
privilege, 8, 49–50, 60n4, 69
"privileged irresponsibility," 2, 4, 10, 49, 56–57, 145, 147, 152–155. *See also* epistemic irresponsibility; Tronto, Joan
projection, 52
projects of unsettling, 170, 171n2, 191
psychoanalysis, 52
psychotherapy, 137
public servants, 33, 36, 38, 42
public service ethics, 33
Puig de la Bellacasa, María, 3

race, 161, 177, 184. *See also* Blackness
radical hospitality, 152
Raghuram, Parvati, 94, 106, 160, 162–163, 167, 170
Rancière, Jacques, 133–134, 138
Ranson, Gillian, 69
rapport, 180
rationality, 1
reality, 132, 148
reciprocity, 73
recognition, 35
reconciliation, 26, 123–124
reflection, 146
reflexivity, 146, 200
"Reimagining Government with the Ethics of Care" (FitzGerald), 18–21
relational autonomy, 110, 122–123
relational care practices, 119–120
relational humility, 200
relationality, 19, 57, 116, 155, 202, 204
relational ontologies, 111, 116, 129, 148–149, 154
relational political orientations, 22, 29
relational selves, 116
relational subjectivities, 116
relational values, 39
relationships, 149; dependency relationships, 82; and dominance, 55–56, 58; and epistemic justice, 41–42; and epistemologies, 20; with knowledge, 204; knowledge/ignorance, 65; and vulnerability, 50–51; with yourself, 48
Rerimassie, Virgil, 203
resentment, 113–114
resentment politics, 203
residential care, and COVID-19, 199
"Resisting Hierarchies through Relationality in the Ethics of Care" (Robinson), 18–19

Index

response-ability, 145, 151–152, 154
responsibility, 89–90, 145, 150–151, 153–155
"responsible" telling, 205
responsiveness, 150–152
Reuters Institute, 195
Rey, Jo Anne, 73
Reynolds, Joel Michael, 85
Roberts, Christopher, 190
Robinson, Fiona, 15, 160; "Resisting Hierarchies through Relationality in the Ethics of Care," 18–19
Roeser, Sabine, 202–203
Rose, Deborah Bird, 138–139, 154–155
Ruane, Abigail, 103
Ruddick, Sara, 101, 107n4, 111, 197; "Maternal Thinking," 1

"Salt-Water-Bodies: From an Atlas of Loss" (van Eeden-Wharton), 152
Schrader, Astrid, 151
scientific medical research, 201
Scobie, Matthew, 119
Scribe, Megan, 113
self-care, 6, 159, 168, 171n1
self-erasure, 6
selves, recentering on, 102–103
sensibility, 129, 133–134
settler-colonialism, 110, 120, 122–123; in Canada, 25, 112; and ways of knowing, 22, 25–26, 28
Sevenhuijsen, Selma, 111
sexual harassment, and Carmita Wood, 24–25
shadow places, 10, 145, 152, 155
Shakur, Assata, 179
shared realities, 40
Sharpe, Christina Elizabeth, 178, 187–188; *Monstrous Intimacies*, 163
Sheller, Mimi, 164, 170
silence, 36
Simard, Suzanne, *Finding the Mother Tree: Discovering the Wisdom of the Forest*, 112
Simpson, Audra, 26
Simpson, Leanne Betasamosake, 63, 66, 73
Smith, Linda Tuhiwai, 64
Snider, Naomi, 8, 58–59; *Why Does Patriarchy Persist*, 55
social death, 122, 189
social reproduction theory, 119
social transformation, 59

soil, 130, 136
Solange, "Cranes in the Sky," 177
solidarity, 90, 200
songlines, 66–67, 74n8
South Africa, 147, 153
spatial diffraction, 147
Spivak, Gayatri Chakravorty, 5, 41
standpoint theorists, 65–66
States of Denial (Cohen), 52
Stay Woke, Stay Whole: A Black Activist Healing Manual, 189–190
Stengers, Isabelle, 205
stereotypes, 33, 36–37
Storni, Cristiano, 201
storying, 137–139
storytelling, 137–138, 149
Street-Level Bureaucracy (Lipsky), 33
string figures, 138
structural injustices, 41
Student Nonviolent Coordinating Committee (SNCC), 181
success, 103–105
Sullivan, Shannon, 55

Taylor, Je Naé, 182, 190–191
tears in the world, 187
temporal diffraction, 147
Tessman, Lisa, 79, 82
testimonial injustice, 23, 27, 31–32, 107–108n5
theories, 204
thickness, 141
"things," 132, 142n3
time, 35, 103–104
totalizing views, 142n2
"transcorporeal culpability," 10, 145, 155
transparency, and political movements, 181–182
trauma, 83–84, 136, 184, 186–187
Trayvon generation, 184
Tronto, Joan, 1–2, 8, 15, 17, 19, 35, 37, 47–48, 89, 111, 118, 122, 129, 148, 150–152; *Caring Democracy: Markets, Equality, and Justice*, 7, 48; "Creating Caring Institutions: Politics, Plurality, and Purpose," 16; *Moral Boundaries: A Political Argument for an Ethic of Care*, 16, 48. See also "privileged irresponsibility"
Trump, Donald, 176–177, 191n2, 194, 202
Trumpism, 203
trust, erosion of, 180

Truth, 69, 71, 74n10, 128, 196
Truth and Reconciliation Commission final report (Canada), 7, 16, 26–27, 111. *See also* Canada; Indigenous peoples
Tuck, Eve, 5, 110, 122–123
Turgeon, Luc, 37
2020 presidential election, 194
two-eyed seeing, 110

uncare, 135
uncertainty, 84
United States, 162–164, 203
upward compensation, 34
us/them binaries, 79

van Dooren, Thom, 138–139, 153–155
van Eeden-Wharton, Adrienne, "Salt-Water-Bodies: From an Atlas of Loss," 152
vehicle accidents, 88
veiling of particulars, 32, 37–43, 39–40. *See also* anonymization; bodily absence
Vergès, Françoise, 62
Vienna domestic cleaning study, 62–63, 70
violence, 113, 120, 123, 180–181, 184
virtues, in the *Mahabharata*, 87
"virtuous hearing," 32, 34–36, 41
vulnerability, 48–50, 53–56, 58, 89–90, 135; denials of, 48–53, 56–59; and the *Mahabharata*, 79, 83; and noticing, 137

Walker, Margaret Urban, 197
Warren, Calvin, 178
Watts, Vanessa, 112, 119, 203
we, 141, 155n3
Weil, Simone, 36
Welch, Shay, 68–69, 74n10
Western-centric care ethics, 19, 80
Western ontologies, 66, 68, 112
white feminist scholars, 120
white silence, 118
Why Does Patriarchy Persist (Gilligan and Snider), 55
"Why Should a Knower Care?" (Dalmiya), 2
willful hermeneutical ignorance, 25
Williams, Bernard, 79
Wilson, Elizabeth, 131, 135–136
Wolf, Susan, 88
women, 2, 49, 70, 80–81, 102, 165. *See also* gender
Wood, Carmita, 24–25
Woodly, Deva, 64
world dynamism, 150
world undone, 183–184
would-be knowers, 128–129

Yang, Wayne, 110, 122–123
Yethi'nihstenha Onhwentsya, 117

Zaagidowin, 113
Zouridis, Stavros, 38